MYELOMA BONE DISEASE

Edited by

G. DAVID ROODMAN

University of Pittsburgh Medical Center,
Pittsburgh, PA, USA

D1477404

Humana Press

Editor
G. David Roodman
Department of Medicine
University of Pittsburgh Medical Center
Pittsburgh, PA
USA
roodmangd@upmc.edu

ISBN 978-1-60761-553-8   e-ISBN 978-1-60761-554-5
DOI 10.1007/978-1-60761-554-5
Springer New York Dordrecht Heidelberg London

Library of Congress Control Number: 2010921111

Printed on acid-free paper

Humana Press is part of Springer Science+Business Media (www.springer.com)

MYELOMA BONE DISEASE

CURRENT CLINICAL ONCOLOGY

Maurie Markman, MD, SERIES EDITOR

For other titles published in this series, go to
www.springer.com/series/7631

Preface

Multiple myeloma is the second most common hematologic malignancy and currently affects approximately 50,000 people in the United States. Each year about 20,000 people are diagnosed with myeloma. Although new treatments have been developed, which significantly prolong the survival of patients, myeloma bone disease still remains a major cause of severe morbidity and increased mortality in patients with myeloma. Myeloma bone disease is characterized by "punched out" lytic lesions caused by increased osteoclastic bone destruction accompanied by suppressed or even absent osteoblast activity. Advances in our understanding of both the pathophysiology of myeloma bone disease and the development of novel agents that target specific pathways involved in both the increased osteoclast formation and the suppressed osteoblast activity in myeloma provide new hope for these patients. The treatment of myeloma bone disease was revolutionized by clinical trials that demonstrated the significant benefit of intravenous bisphosphonate therapy in patients with myeloma bone disease. With the identification of many of the cytokines and chemokines involved in myeloma bone disease, novel therapies such as denosumab that blocks RANKL activity, anti-DKK1, which targets the inhibition of osteoblast activity by blocking Wnt signaling inhibition, and the potential anabolic effects of agents such as bortezomib and activin have greatly improved our potential to block the progression or reverse myeloma bone disease. These topics as well as new techniques for imaging myeloma bone disease, the use of new bone markers for monitoring myeloma bone disease, and surgical techniques to ameliorate pain and loss of vertebral height in patients with vertebral compression fractures are highlighted in this volume. With the survival of patients with myeloma increasing, treatments that are directed at preventing the progression of bone disease, fractures, and even repairing lytic lesions will have even a more profound impact on patients with myeloma. In this book, outstanding experts from a variety of backgrounds discuss the presentation of patients with myeloma bone disease, the underlying pathophysiology of both the increased osteoclast activity and the suppressed osteoblast activity that occurs in myeloma, murine models of myeloma bone disease, as well as therapeutic and diagnostic procedures for patients with myeloma bone disease.

Pittsburgh, PA   G. David Roodman

Contents

Contributors

Ashraf Badros Greenebaum Cancer Center, University of Maryland, Baltimore, MD, USA

Bart Barlogie Myeloma Institute for Research and Therapy, Little Rock, AR, USA

Twyla Bartel Department of Radiology, University of Arkansas for Medical Sciences, Little Rock, AR, USA

James R. Berenson Institute for Myeloma & Bone Cancer Research, West Hollywood, CA, USA

Tracy Brown Department of Radiology, University of Arkansas for Medical Sciences, Little Rock, AR, USA

Michelle Chaisson-Blake Amgen Inc., Seattle, WA, USA

Peter I. Croucher Department of Human Metabolism, Faculty of Medicine, Dentistry and Health, University of Sheffield, Sheffield, UK

William C. Dougall Amgen Inc., Seattle, WA, USA

Claire M. Edwards Departments of Cancer Biology and Clinical Pharmacology/Medicine, Vanderbilt Center for Bone Biology, Vanderbilt University Medical Center, Nashville, TN, USA

Joshua Epstein Myeloma Institute for Research and Therapy, University of Arkansas for Medical Sciences, Little Rock, AR, USA

Nicola Giuliani Department of Internal Medicine and Biomedical Science, Hematology and BMT Center, University of Parma, Parma, Italy

Joel S. Greenberger Department of Radiation Oncology, University of Pittsburgh Cancer Institute, Pittsburgh, PA, USA

Mohamad A. Hussein Celgene Corporation, Summit, NJ, USA

Laurie Jones-Jackson Department of Radiology & Radiological Sciences, Vanderbilt University Medical Center, Nashville, TN, USA

Susie Jun Amgen Inc., Thousand Oaks, CA, USA

Suzanne Lentzsch Division of Hematology/Oncology, University of Pittsburgh, Pittsburgh, PA, USA

Gregory R. Mundy Departments of Cancer Biology and Clinical Pharmacology/Medicine, Vanderbilt Center for Bone Biology, Vanderbilt University Medical Center, Nashville, TN, USA

Babatunde Oyajobi Departments of Cellular and Structural Biology, and Medicine, University of Texas Health Sciences Center, San Antonio, Texas, USA

Noopur Raje Division of Hematology-Oncology, Harvard Medical School, Massachusetts General Hospital Cancer Center, Boston, MA, USA

G. David Roodman Department of Medicine/Hematology-Oncology, University of Pittsburgh Medical Center, Pittsburgh, PA, USA

Rebecca Silbermann Department of Medicine/Hematology-Oncology, University of Pittsburgh Medical Center, Pittsburgh, PA, USA

Evangelos Terpos Department of Clinical Therapeutics, University of Athens School of Medicine, Alexandra Hospital, Athens, Greece

Sonia Vallet Division of Hematology-Oncology, Harvard Medical School, Massachusetts General Hospital Cancer Center, Boston, MA, USA

Karin Vanderkerken Department of Hematology and Immunology, Myeloma Center Brussels, Vrije Universiteit, Brussels, Belgium

Ronald C. Walker Department of Radiology & Radiological Sciences, Vanderbilt University Medical Center and Tennessee Valley VA Healthcare System, Nashville, TN, USA

Howard Yeh Amgen Inc., Thousand Oaks, CA, USA

Chapter 1
Clinical Presentation of Myeloma Bone Disease

Rebecca Silbermann and G. David Roodman

Abstract Bone disease in multiple myeloma is characterized by lytic lesions that are frequently associated with fracture, hypercalcemia, and severe pain. Bone pain is the most frequent presenting symptom for patients with multiple myeloma. It is estimated that approximately 60% of patients have bone pain at the time of myeloma diagnosis and 90% of patients develop bone lesions during their disease course. In addition to lytic lesions, patients frequently develop diffuse osteopenia, pathologic fractures, and compression fractures of the spine. Bone disease significantly impacts patient morbidity, performance status, and survival. While there is an association between the number of lytic bone lesions in an individual and their disease burden, an individual's degree of bone disease does not appear to have significant utility in predicting outcomes.

Keywords Multiple myeloma · Myeloma bone disease · Pathologic fracture · Hypercalcemia

1.1 Introduction

Multiple myeloma is a lymphoproliferative disease characterized by the clonal proliferation of plasma cells. In the bone marrow, expansion of this plasma cell population can lead to leukopenia, anemia, and thrombocytopenia, while in the soft tissues plasma cell proliferation can manifest as plasmacytomas, soft tissue masses of plasma cells. Bone disease in patients with myeloma is characterized by lytic lesions that can result in pathologic fractures and severe pain (Fig. 1.1). Other frequent presenting symptoms of myeloma are nonspecific and include fatigue and

G.D. Roodman (✉)
Department of Medicine/Hematology-Oncology, VA Pittsburgh Healthcare System, University of Pittsburgh Medical Center, Pittsburgh, PA 15240, USA
e-mail: roodmangd@upmc.edu

G.D. Roodman (ed.), *Myeloma Bone Disease*, Current Clinical Oncology,
DOI 10.1007/978-1-60761-554-5_1, © Springer Science+Business Media, LLC 2010

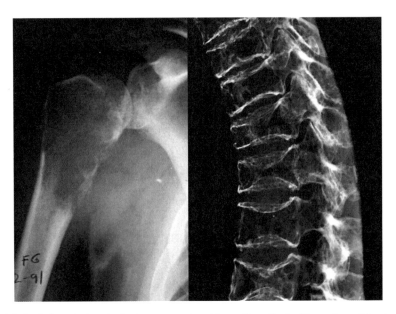

Fig. 1.1 Lytic bone lesions in the humerus and vertebrae of a patient with myeloma (Courtesy of Dr. H. J. Mankin, Massachusetts General Hospital, Boston, MA)

recurrent infections. It is not uncommon for patients to ignore their symptoms or attribute them to other medical problems for months or years before a definitive diagnosis is made as illustrated by the case below.

A 57-year-old male house painter presented to his primary care physician after he was noted to have an abnormality of the left ninth rib on a chest x-ray. The patient had at least 4 months of persistent rib and low back pain which he attributed to an increasingly hectic work schedule and "getting old." Non-steroidal anti-inflammatory drugs (NSAIDs), muscle relaxants, and chiropractic manipulations had been tried on multiple occasions, and the patient felt that his rib pain had improved slightly. However, he did admit to increasing back stiffness and pain, particularly with rapid position changes. Biopsy of the rib lesion demonstrated a plasmacytoma, and skeletal survey revealed multiple lucencies of the frontal bones of the skull and the lumbosacral spine, without definite pathologic fracture. Serum protein electrophoresis demonstrated a monoclonal protein spike in the gamma region measuring 3.7 g/dL, and bone marrow biopsy revealed 80% plasma cell cellularity.

The spectrum of plasma cell neoplasms ranges between the clinically benign monoclonal gammopathy of unknown significance (MGUS) to plasma cell leukemia and includes Waldenstrom's macroglobulinemia, Castleman's disease, and primary amyloidosis, in addition to multiple myeloma. The incidence of myeloma is approximately 4 per 100,000 persons per year in Caucasians (5.3 in men and 3.5 in women) and twice that in African Americans, accounting for approximately 1% of all malignant diseases and approximately 15% of hematologic malignancies. In 2008 it is estimated that 19,920 new cases were diagnosed in the United States and that 10,690 Americans died of the disease. Most patients diagnosed with multiple myeloma are in the seventh decade of life, with 29.2% of cases occurring in patients between the ages of 65 and 74 and 28.2% of cases in patients between the ages of 75 and 84. Diagnosis of patients before the age of 45 is rare (3.9% of cases) [1–3].

1.2 The Incidence of Bone Disease in Myeloma

Myeloma has the highest incidence of bone involvement among malignant diseases, with approximately 60% of patients presenting with bone pain at diagnosis, 90% of patients developing bone lesions during their disease course, and up to 60% of patients developing pathologic fractures [4]. One of the first case descriptions of myeloma was published in 1844 and discussed a 39-year-old woman with fatigue and bone pain due to multiple fractures [5]. At autopsy her bone marrow was described as replaced by a "red grumous matter" [6], and she was found to have significant thinning and destruction of her bones (Fig. 1.2).

While the clinical presentation of myeloma is variable, bone pain, frequently centered on the chest or back and exacerbated by movement, is the most common symptom at presentation. However, approximately 20% of patients are asymptomatic at presentation, with disease identified through routine laboratory studies.

The frequency of bone lesions in myeloma is unique among hematologic malignancies. It is estimated that up to 90% of patients with myeloma have evidence of osteolysis in the form of generalized osteopenia or discrete lytic lesions [7]. In contrast to other tumors that involve bone, myeloma is rarely associated with

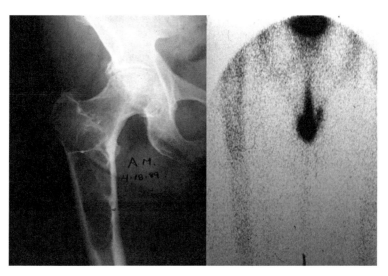

Fig. 1.2 Bone scans in myeloma can underestimate bone involvement. The patient has a large lytic lesion in the right femur and a normal bone scan (Courtesy of Dr. H. J. Mankin, Massachusetts General Hospital, Boston, MA)

osteoblastic lesions except in POEMS syndrome (polyneuropathy, organomegaly, endocrinopathy, monoclonal gammopathy, and skin changes), a multisystem disease occurring rarely in the setting of a plasma cell dyscrasia. Bone lesions from multiple myeloma lead to increased bone resorption and skeletal complications, including hypercalcemia of malignancy, severe bone pain, diffuse osteopenia, pathologic fractures, and cord compression that significantly impact patients' quality of life.

Unlike the bone loss seen in other malignancies, where bone destruction is followed by new bone formation, myeloma bone lesions are purely osteolytic [8]. Any bone can be involved, with lesions most frequently involving the spine (49%), skull (35%), pelvis (34%), ribs (33%), humeri (22%), femora (13%), and mandible (10%) [9]. These lesions do not heal in the majority of patients, and skeletal lesions can progress even when the disease is otherwise controlled with chemotherapy [10].

In a review of 1,027 patients with newly diagnosed multiple myeloma, nearly 80% were noted to have abnormalities on skeletal surveys at the time of diagnosis. Sixty-seven percent of patients had lytic lesions and about 20% had osteopenia, pathologic fractures, or compression fractures of the spine. Twenty-five percent of the remaining patients who did not have radiologic abnormalities at diagnosis developed lytic lesions, pathologic fractures, compression fractures, or osteopenia during subsequent follow-up. Thus, 84% of patients developed skeletal lesions during the course of their disease [11]. In contrast, only two-thirds to three-quarters of patients with solid tumors that can metastasize to bone will develop bone involvement during the course of their disease [12].

In addition to lytic lesions, myeloma patients lose bone more rapidly than age-matched controls. In comparisons of changes in bone mineral density in patients with multiple myeloma receiving glucocorticoid-containing treatments with controls not on steroids, myeloma patients had an approximately 6% reduction in bone mineral density at the lumbar spine with a nearly 10% reduction in bone density at the femoral neck over a 12-month period compared with controls who lost about 1% of bone density at the femoral neck and almost no bone density loss at the lumbar spine (Fig. 1.3) [13].

1.3 Diagnosis of Myeloma Bone Disease

Conventional radiography remains the standard diagnostic procedure for the detection of myeloma-associated skeletal disease and can provide information on disease involvement of both cortical and trabecular bone. The utility of standard radiography to evaluate patients with early disease is limited, however, as lytic lesions can be detected with standard radiography after only 30–50% of trabecular bone is lost and the reproducibility of bone surveys is limited [14,15]. In addition, focal bone loss on radiographs can be obscured by air in the gastrointestinal tract, overlying soft tissues, lungs, and other skeletal structures. Bone scans underestimate myeloma bone disease as they primarily reflect osteoblast activity (Fig. 1.3).

Fig. 1.3 Autopsy specimen demonstrating diffuse myelomatosis of the femur (Courtesy of Dr. H. J. Mankin, Massachusetts General Hospital, Boston, MA)

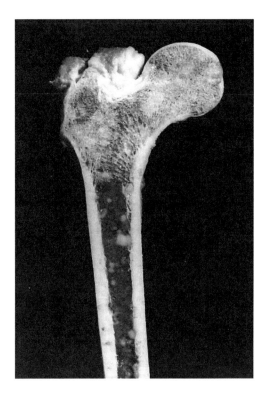

Helical computed tomography (CT) can detect focal bone loss much earlier than conventional x-ray technology and allows the ability to image the marrow space and circumscribed areas of the spine [16]. Multidetector CT (MDCT) of the thoracic and lumbar spine has been used to assess focal vertebral lesions for potential instability. A small study of stage III myeloma patients conducted by Mahnken et al. identified twice the number of potentially unstable vertebral lesions as conventional radiography [17]. Typical findings on CT and conventional radiographs include punched out lytic lesions of the bone, diffuse osteopenia, fractures, and osteosclerosis. PET–CT (positron emission tomography combined with CT using an 18F-labeled deoxyglucose to illustrate quantitative glucose metabolism) can demonstrate focal growth of multiple myeloma before osteolysis occurs and can be used to follow the development of focal osteolytic bone lesions and the effects of treatment.

The role of magnetic resonance imaging (MRI) in evaluation of the bone marrow in patients with plasma cell disorders is growing. Abnormal bone marrow signal intensity on MRI in patients with myeloma is thought to result from increased bone marrow cellularity. Variegated enhancement is thought to represent tumor clusters on a background of normal bone marrow, whereas generalized marrow infiltration is associated with diffuse patterns on MRI images. The presence of bone marrow involvement on MRI correlates with early disease progression, and it is believed that the pattern of marrow involvement may also have prognostic value. In addition, the presence of marrow involvement on MRI in a patient with otherwise normal x-rays appears to be predictive of early disease progression in asymptomatic patients [18, 19]. MRI can also be used to differentiate benign and malignant compression fractures and can provide details of paraspinal and epidural disease involvement.

1.4 Pathogenesis of Myeloma Bone Disease

While bone resorption due to increased osteoclast activation and osteoblast inhibition is a hallmark of multiple myeloma, this process may be intrinsic to plasma cell disorders in general. Normal bone remodeling requires a balanced resorption of damaged bone by osteoclasts and formation of new bone at the site of precursor bone's resorption by osteoblasts, and is mediated by a cytokine network that maintains bone homeostasis. Multiple factors, including hormonal changes, nutrition, genetic factors, and pharmacologic agents, can disrupt the balance between osteoblast and osteoclast activity, leading to abnormalities in bone turnover [20]. In multiple myeloma local cytokines produced by malignant plasma cells increase osteoclast formation and bone resorption systemically and in areas of diffuse tumor infiltration of the marrow. Histologic studies of bone biopsies from patients with myeloma demonstrate that increased osteolytic activity occurs near myeloma cells. This increased bone resorption is thought to release local cytokines that stimulate myeloma cell growth, creating a "vicious cycle" of increased bone resorption leading to an increased tumor burden [21] (Fig. 1.4). Lytic bone lesions result from focal growth of myeloma cells, through mechanisms that remain poorly understood. Increased osteoclast activity also appears to contribute to increased angiogenesis in myeloma as a result of the interaction between myeloma cells and cells of the bone marrow microenvironment and local suppression of osteoblast activity [22].

The RANK/RANKL signaling pathway is central to both normal and malignant bone remodeling. RANK, a transmembrane signaling receptor belonging to the tumor necrosis factor superfamily is expressed on osteoclast precursors. RANK ligand (RANKL) is a membrane-bound NFkB ligand found on osteoblasts and marrow stromal cells and secreted by activated lymphocytes. RANKL binding to the RANK receptor induces osteoclast formation and thus leads to increased osteoclast activity and survival. The RANK/RANKL signaling pathway is normally modulated by marrow stromal cell production of osteoprotegerin (OPG), a soluble decoy receptor for RANKL produced by osteoblasts. RANKL expression is upregulated and OPG expression is decreased in bone marrow biopsies of myeloma patients. In addition it has been demonstrated that circulating levels of OPG and RANKL correlate with myeloma clinical activity, bone disease severity, and prognosis [4, 15, 23] (Fig. 1.5).

Patients with both MGUS and smoldering myeloma have been noted to have increased rates of bone resorption, osteopenia, and osteoporosis with a resultant

The Central Role of the Osteoclast
in Osteolytic Bone Destruction

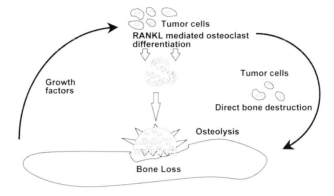

Adapted from Roodman. *N Engl J Med.* 2004;350:1655.

Fig. 1.4 The formation and activity of osteoclasts is induced by both systemic and locally acting factors. Systemic hormones such as parathyroid hormone, 1,25-dihydroxyvitamin D3, and thyroxine stimulate the formation of osteoclasts by inducing the expression of RANKL on marrow stromal cells and osteoblasts. Tumor cells can also stimulate osteoclastogenesis through secretion of factors such as parathyroid hormone-related peptide and factors that increase osteoclast formation (Adapted from Roodman [8])

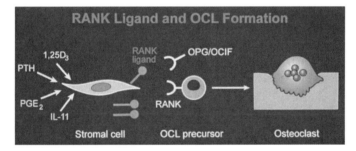

Fig. 1.5 RANKL induces osteoclast formation. 1,25-Dihydroxyvitamin D3, parathyroid hormone (PTH), prostaglandin E-2, and interleukin-11 are osteotropic factors that induce the formation of osteoclasts by up-regulating the expression of RANKL on the surface of marrow stromal cells and osteoclast precursors. RANKL binds to the receptor, RANK, on the surface of osteoclast precursors (Adapted from Roodman [8])

increased risk of fractures [24]. Bataille and colleagues demonstrated that osteoclast number and activity is increased in early myeloma [25]; however, bone resorption in patients with MGUS, a premalignant syndrome without osteolytic lesions that has an annual conversion rate to myeloma of 1%, remained within the normal range. More recent studies of biochemical markers of bone turnover demonstrate that patients with MGUS have reduced levels of the bone formation marker serum bone-specific alkaline phosphatase, compared with patients with benign osteoporosis [26].

Interestingly, osteoblast number and activity is elevated in early myeloma where the tumor burden is low, but reduced in patients with overt disease. Patients with consistently elevated osteoblast activity did not develop lytic bone lesions in spite of elevated osteoclast activity [27]. Progression from MGUS to myeloma appears to be preceded by an increased bone turnover rate, with an uncoupling of bone formation and resorption in the majority of patients. Studies attempting to quantify the degree of bone involvement in individuals with plasma cell dyscrasias based on both biochemical markers of bone formation and bone resorption suggest that there is increased osteoclast activity leading to increased bone resorption even at early stages of plasma cell dyscrasias, as compared with patients with benign osteoporosis. Though it is clear that an alteration in the normal balance of osteoblast and osteoclast activity is common to plasma cell disorders, the severity of any individuals' bone involvement is not predictable at this time.

1.4.1 Bone Disease and Patient Prognosis

While there is an association between a patient's tumor burden and the number of lytic lesions present [28], an individual's degree of bone disease does not appear to have significant utility in predicting outcomes. However, bone disease significantly impacts morbidity, performance status, and survival. The current staging systems for multiple myeloma, the Durie–Salmon system, and the International Staging System (ISS) have attempted to classify a patient's disease state based on markers for tumor burden. The Durie–Salmon system included the presence of lytic bone lesions as assessed by standard radiographs, anemia, hypercalcemia, and the quantification of the monoclonal protein spike and is limited by both the imprecise quantification of the extent of bone lesions afforded by standard radiography and the contribution of factors aside from myeloma that lead to anemia and hypercalcemia. The ISS attempts to simplify risk classification by employing two commonly available blood tests, serum albumin and beta-2 microglobulin, to stratify patients into risk groups with median survival times of 29, 44, and 62 months. Survival data used to develop this staging system was independent of patient age, bone involvement, and treatment protocol [29]. While the ISS is more useful in predicting clinical outcomes in symptomatic patients, characterization of the initial genetic events leading to the development of the disease provides the strongest independent predictor of clinical outcome [30].

The current understanding of the molecular pathogenesis of progression of premalignant MGUS to multiple myeloma can be broadly divided between non-hyperdiploid and hyperdiploid tumors. While the biologic basis for this distinction is not clearly understood, the clinical implications are notable. Approximately 40% of patients have nonhyperdiploid myeloma, (NH-MM), a disease process initiated by the translocation of a variety of oncogenes to the Ig heavy-chain switch region, resulting in ectopic overexpression of a plasma cell oncogene which subsequently immortalizes the plasma cells [31]. The remaining patients are hyper-diploid, (H-MM), with excess chromosome copies present. H-MM is generally a more indolent disease with a better overall prognosis than the nonhyperdiploid form [32]. It presents more frequently in elderly male patients, most of whom have bone lesions. In contrast, patients with the more aggressive NH-MM frequently lack bone lesions.

Specific translocations seen in NH-MM, identified through the use of fluorescence in situ hybridization (FISH) analysis of bone marrow samples, such as $t(4;14)$ are currently used to risk-stratify multiple myeloma patients when planning treatment. This translocation is found in approximately 15% of myeloma cases and linked to a younger patient population, frequent deletion of chromosome 13, and the presence of the IgA isotype [33]. While patients with this genetic subtype are generally very responsive to initial chemotherapy, the population frequently fares poorly due to early relapse. Patients in this subgroup who undergo stem cell transplant frequently relapse within a year and are usually refractory to alkylating agents and steroids. Case series have demonstrated that up to 50% of $t(4;14)$ do not develop bone lesions [34]. It is not clear whether myeloma cells from these patients do not produce cytokines responsible for the development of bone lesions, or if bone lesions do not have time to develop because of the patients' rapid disease progression and increased mortality.

1.5 The Clinical and Economic Burden of Myeloma Bone Disease

The clinical impact of myeloma bone disease on patients is significant. A retrospective analysis conducted by Saad and colleagues [35] of data from patients enrolled on the control arms of randomized trials of zoledronic acid assessed the impact of pathological fractures on survival in patients with malignant bone disease and included 513 myeloma patients in a study group of 3,049 patients. Myeloma patients had a higher incidence of fracture (43%) over the study period compared with patients with breast cancer, lung cancer, and prostate cancer. Myeloma patients with pathologic fractures had a 20% increased risk of death compared to other patients, and those with a skeletal-related event (including pathologic fracture or spinal cord compression syndrome) prior to entry into the study had a much poorer outcome compared to patients without a prior history of skeletal-related events. In addition to patients with prior skeletal events, those who had received radiation therapy to bone or skeletal surgery were more likely to develop new pathologic fractures than patients without prior skeletal events.

The economic burden of metastatic bone disease in general, and myeloma bone disease in particular, is also notable. In a comparison of patients with and without metastatic bone disease, Schulman and Kohles demonstrated that the incremental cost of having bone disease in patients with myeloma was $57,720 per patient. The total cost for patients with myeloma bone disease was estimated at over $950,000,000 [36].

1.6 Other Complications Associated with Skeletal Disease

Neurologic complications associated with bone disease, particularly compression fractures, are significant. Radiculopathy can result from vertebral collapse and resultant nerve compression or tumor expansion in the vertebrae is significant. Two to three percent of patients can develop spinal cord compression, which can be a medical emergency. Vertebroplasty, a technique in which bone cement is injected percutaneously into the vertebral body for pain relief or stabilization, can provide immediate symptomatic relief for patients. Similarly, kyphoplasty, a specialized vertebroplasty technique employing the placement of inflatable bone tamps into the vertebral body to attempt to return the vertebral body to its original height, can improve bone pain and functional activity [37].

Approximately 15–20% of newly diagnosed patients have hypercalcemia, defined as a corrected serum calcium level greater than 11.5 mg/dL due to increased bone resorption, decreased bone formation, impaired renal function, and often exacerbated by immobility. Unlike other malignancies resulting in metastatic disease to the bone, parathyroid-related protein (PTHrP) is rarely overproduced by myeloma cells. The severity of hypercalcemia in patients with myeloma is not correlated with serum PTHrP levels and instead reflects tumor burden [38]. Symptomatic hypercalcemia can result in anorexia, nausea, vomiting, confusion, fatigue, constipation, renal stones, depression, and polyuria and is suggestive of a high tumor burden. Hypercalcemia in myeloma can be exacerbated by renal impairment due to an inability to filter the increased circulating calcium released by bone resorption, as well as increased renal tubular calcium reabsorption.

1.7 Treatment of Myeloma Bone Disease

Treatment of myeloma bone disease requires management of both the underlying malignancy and its effects. Bisphosphonates remain the mainstay of treatment for skeletal-related events in multiple myeloma and can decrease bone pain and slow the progression of lytic lesions to some extent. Bisphosphonates inhibit osteoclast activity by blocking osteoclast formation and the induction of osteoclast apoptosis [38]. Intravenous pamidronate and zoledronate have each been found to reduce the number of skeletal events in patients and to reduce the need for radiation therapy. A study of 392 patients with Durie–Salmon stage II disease randomized to intravenous pamidronate versus placebo demonstrated that skeletal-related events at 9 months were significantly lower in the pamidronate group when compared with placebo [39]. These findings were confirmed in a phase II study of zoledronic acid compared with pamidronate in patients with more than one lytic lesion and at least one prior skeletal event, where the number of skeletal events was comparable between groups [40].

Unfortunately, bisphosphonate therapy does not eliminate skeletal-related events and can be associated with side effects such as osteonecrosis of the jaw and renal toxicity. Approximately 70% of patients with myeloma bone disease receive radiation therapy during the course of their disease [8] for management of painful bone lesions, generally with doses of 30 Gy. Several new agents have recently been developed as a result of improved understanding of the pathophysiology of myeloma bone disease.

As described above, the RANK–RANKL interaction has been implicated in osteoclast-mediated bone resorption in myeloma and other pathologic conditions. Denosumab, a monoclonal antibody that binds RANKL, inhibits RANKL–RANK interaction and leads to sustained suppression of osteoclast-induced bone resorption. A phase II trial of denosumab in myeloma patients with either plateau phase or relapsed disease demonstrated that the drug inhibits skeletal-related events while appearing to have little toxicity [41].

Two classes of new drugs that have proven to be highly effective in the treatment of myeloma may also slow the development of skeletal-related events. Bortezomib, a proteasome antagonist that induces myeloma cell apoptosis, has been shown to increase osteoblast activity and new bone formation. A retrospective analysis of three bortezomib trials in patients with relapsed disease demonstrated that patients who had a partial response to bortezomib therapy also had a transient increase in their serum alkaline phosphatase level, as compared with patients who did not respond to therapy [42]. In addition, the increased alkaline phosphatase levels in patients responding to treatment were associated with an increase in bone-specific alkaline phosphatase and parathyroid hormone, suggesting an association with osteoblastic activation [43]. In comparison, immunomodulatory drugs such as lenalidomide, appear to inhibit osteoclast development, suggesting that they may have both anti-myeloma and bone effects [44].

Thus, bone disease has a major impact on both survival and quality of life of myeloma patients. The succeeding chapters will review in detail emerging imaging techniques, novel agents, and model system that contribute to our understanding of the pathophysiology and treatment of myeloma bone disease.

References

1. Kyle RA. Multiple myeloma and related monoclonal gammopathies. In: Mazza JJ, ed. Manual of Clinical Hematology. 3rd ed. Philadelphia, PA: Lippincott Williams & Wilkins; 2002: 247–273.
2. Jagannath S, Richardson P, Munshi NC. Multiple myeloma and other plasma cell dyscrasias. In: Pazdur R, Wagman LD, Camphausen KA, Hoskins WJ, eds. Cancer Management: A Multidisciplinary Approach. 11th ed. Lawrence, KS: CMPMedica; 2008:775–796.
3. Seymour G, Wang M, Lin P, Weber D. Multiple myeloma and other plasma cell dyscrasias. In: Kantarjian HM, Wolff RA, Koller CA, eds. The MD Anderson Manual of Medical Oncology. New York, NY: McGraw-Hill; 2006:175–197.
4. Roodman GD. Skeletal imaging and management of bone disease. Hematology Am Soc Hematol Educ Program. Washington, DC: The American Society of Hematology. 2008:313–319.
5. Kyle RA, Rajkumar SV. Multiple Myeloma. Blood. 2008;111:2962–2972.
6. Kyle RA. Multiple myeloma: an odyssey of discovery. Br J Haematol. 2000;111:1035–1044.

7. Roodman GD. Pathogenesis of myeloma bone disease. Blood Cells Mol Dis. 2004;32: 290–292.

8. Roodman GD. Mechanisms of Bone Metastasis. N Engl J Med. 2004;350:1655–1664.

9. Kyle RA, Therneau TM, Rajkumar SV, Larson DR, Plevak MF, Melton LJ 3rd. Incidence of multiple myeloma in Olmstead County Minnesota: trend over 6 decades. Cancer. 2004;101:2667–2674.

10. Belch AR, Bergsagel DE, Wilson K, et al. Effect of daily etidronate on the osteolysis of multiple myeloma. J Clin Oncol. 1991;9:1397–1402.

11. Kyle RA, Gertz MA, Witzig TE, et al. Review of 1027 patients with newly diagnosed multiple myeloma. Mayo Clin Proc. 2003;78:21–33.

12. Melton LJ III, Kyle RA, Achenbach SJ, Oberg AL, Rajkumar SV. Fracture risk with multiple myeloma: a population-based study. J Bone Miner Res. 2005;20:487–493.

13. Diamond T, Levy S, Day P, Barbagallo S, Manoharan A, Kwan YK. Biochemical, histomorphometric and densitometric changes in patients with multiple myeloma: effects of glucocorticoid therapy and disease activity. Br J Haematol. 1997;97:641–648.

14. Durie BGM, Salmon SE. A clinical staging system for multiple myeloma. Correlation of measured myeloma cell mass with presenting clinical features, response to treatment, and survival. Cancer. 1975;36:842–854.

15. Sezar O. Myeloma bone disease: recent advances in biology, diagnosis and treatment. Oncologist. 2009;14:276–283.

16. Mahnken AH, Wildberger JE, Gehbauer G, et al. Multidetector CT of the spine in multiple myeloma: comparison with MR imaging and radiography. AJR Am J Roentgenol. 2002;178:1429–1436.

17. Mahnken AH, Wildberger JE, Gehbauer G, et al. Multidetector CT of the spine in multiple myeloma: comparison with MR imaging and radiography. AJR Am J Roentgenol. 2002;178:1429–1436.

18. Moulopoulos LA, Dimopoulos MA, Smith TL, et al. Prognostic significance of magnetic resonance imaging in patients with asymptomatic multiple myeloma. J Clin Oncol. 1995;13:251–256.

19. Moulopoulos LA, Dimopoulos MA. Magnetic resonance imaging of the bone marrow in hematologic malignancies. Blood. 1997;90:2127–2147.

20. O'Brien CA, Jia D, Plotkin LI, et al. Glucocorticoids act directly on osteoblasts and osteocytes to induce their apoptosis and reduce bone formation and strength. Endocrinology. 2004;145:1835–1841.

21. Edwards CM, Zhuang J, Mundy GR. The pathogenesis of the bone disease of multiple myeloma. Bone. 2008;42:1007–1013.

22. Roodman GD. Pathogenesis of myeloma bone disease. Leukemia. 2009;23:435–441.

23. Terpos E, Szydlo R, Apperley JF, et al. Soluble receptor activator of nuclear factor kappaB ligand-osteoprotegerin ratio predicts survival in multiple myeloma: proposal for a novel prognostic index. Blood. 2003;102:1064–1069.

24. Berenson JR, Yellin O, Boccia RV, et al. Zoledronic acid markedly improves bone mineral density for patients with monoclonal gammopathy of undetermined significance and bone loss. Clin Cancer Res. 2008;14:6289–6295.

25. Bataille R, Delmas PD, Chappard D, Sany J. Abnormal serum bone Gla protein levels in multiple myeloma: crucial role of bone formation and prognostic implications. Cancer. 1990;66:167–172.

26. Woitge HW, Horn E, Keck AV, Auler B, Seibel MK, Pecherstorfer M. Biochemical markers of bone formation in patients with plasma cell dyscrasias and benign osteoporosis. Clin Chem. 2001;47:686–693.

27. Epstein J, Walker R. Myeloma and bone disease: "the dangerous tango". Clin Adv Hematol Oncol. April 2006;4(4):300–306.

28. Durie BGM, Salmon SE. A clinical staging system for multiple myeloma. Correlation of measured myeloma cell mass with presenting clinical features, response to treatment, and survival. Cancer. 1975;36:842–854.

29. Greipp PR, San Miguel J, Durie BG, et al. International staging system for multiple myeloma. J Clin Oncol. 2005;23:3412–3420.
30. Bergsagel PL, Kuehl WM. Molecular pathogenesis and a consequent classification of multiple myeloma. J Clin Oncol. 2005;23:6333–6338.
31. Bergsagel PL, Kuehl WM, Zhan F, Sawyer J, Barlogie B, Shaughnessy J Jr. Cyclin D dysregulation: an early and unifying pathogenic event in multiple myeloma. Blood. 2005;106:296–303.
32. Fonseca R, Bergsagel PL. Diagnosis and genetic classification of multiple myeloma. In: Rajkumar SV, Kyle RA, eds. Treatment of Multiple Myeloma and Related Disorders. Cambridge: Cambridge university press; 2009:1–18.
33. Jaksic W, Trudel S, Chang H, et al. Clinical outcomes in t(4:14) multiple myeloma: a chemotherapy-sensitive disease characterized by rapid relapse and alkylating agent resistance. J Clin Oncol. 2005;23:7069–7073.
34. Fonseca R, Blood E, Rue M, et al. Clinical and biological implications of recurrent genomic aberrations in myeloma. Blood. 2003;101:4569–4575.
35. Saad F, Lipton A, Cook R, Chen YM, Smith M, Coleman R. Pathologic fractures correlate with reduced survival in patients with malignant bone disease. Cancer. 2007;110:1860–1867.
36. Schulman KL, Kohles J. Economic burden of metastatic bone disease in the US. Cancer. 2007;110:1860–1867.
37. Roodman GD. Diagnosis and treatment of myeloma bone disease. In: Rajkumar SV, Kyle RA, eds. Treatment of Multiple Myeloma and Related Disorders. New York, NY: Cambridge University Press; 2009:64–76.
38. Kimel DB. Mechanism of action, pharmacokinetic and pharmacodynamic profile, and clinical applications of nitrogen-containing bisphosphonates. J Dent Res. 2007;86:1022–1033.
39. Berenson JR, Lichtenstein A, Parker L, et al. Efficacy of pamidronate in reducing skeletal events in patients with advanced myeloma. N Engl J Med. 1996;334:488–493.
40. Berenson JR. New advances in the biology and treatment of myeloma bone disease. Semin Hematol. 2001;334:488–493.
41. Vij R, Horvath N, Spencer A, Taylor K, Saroj V, Smith J, et al. An open label phase 2 trial of Denosumab in the treatment of relapsed or plateau-phase myeloma. Blood. 2007;118:1054A.
42. Zangari M, Esseltine D, Lee CK, et al. Response to bortezomib is associated to osteoblastic activation in patients with multiple myeloma. Br J Haematol. 2005;131:71–73.
43. Zangari M, Yaccoby S, Cavallo F, Esseltine D, Tricot G. Response to bortezomib and activation of osteoblasts in multiple myeloma. Clin Lymphoma Myeloma. 2006;7:109–114.
44. Breitkreutz I, Raab MS, Vallet S, et al. Lenalidomide inhibits osteoclastogenesis, survival factors and bone-remodeling markers in multiple myeloma. Leukemia. 2008;22:1925–1932.

Chapter 2
Imaging of Multiple Myeloma, Solitary Plasmacytoma, MGUS, and Other Plasma Cell Dyscrasias

Ronald C. Walker, Laurie Jones-Jackson, Twyla Bartel, Tracy Brown, and Bart Barlogie

Abstract The significance of medical imaging in multiple myeloma was established in 1975 with the classic description of the Durie–Salmon staging system which incorporated the presence and number of focal osteolytic lesions in the staging scheme. A third of a century later, this staging system remains in use, though augmented by advances in medical imaging. By the early 1980s, CT imaging demonstrated more focal bone lesions than were seen with standard radiographs as well as extramedullary disease. By the 1980s, MRI imaging revealed skeletal disease that was not apparent by either standard x-rays or CT, focal plasmacytomas in bone that had not yet produced focal osteolysis, and diffuse marrow infiltration. Subsequent work throughout the 1990s developed and established MRI as a very powerful tool to demonstrate the full extent of skeletal disease with resolution approaching a few millimeters. MRI was also used to direct biopsies of focal lesions which increased the detection rate of clinically relevant information compared to random marrow biopsies. However, standard MRI lacked the wide field of view of CT and was both considerably more expensive and less widely available than CT. An additional weakness of standard x-rays, CT, and MRI was their limited utility in the demonstration of response to treatment. By the mid- to late 1990s, the utility of ^{18}F-FDG PET and (after 2000) PET/CT was apparent. PET/CT was particularly powerful since it provided a "whole-body" examination combining the utility of CT ("anatomy") with a "metabolic" image that was linked to the Warburg physiology of tumors, at a fraction of the cost of an extensive MRI. Thus, PET and PET/CT can demonstrate both active disease and, very importantly, response to treatment. The PET image fused to the CT portion of the PET/CT also provides a "free" whole-body metastatic bone survey that can reveal not only focal bone lesions but also additional clinically relevant findings (fractures or impending fractures, additional malignancies, occult infections, unsuspected regions of tumor involvement such as extramedullary tumor). Recent work has established the

R.C. Walker (✉)
Professor, Department of Radiology and Radiological Sciences, Vanderbilt University Medical Center, Nashville, TN, USA
e-mail: ronald.walker@vanderbilt.edu

G.D. Roodman (ed.), *Myeloma Bone Disease*, Current Clinical Oncology,
DOI 10.1007/978-1-60761-554-5_2, © Springer Science+Business Media, LLC 2010

fundamental importance of ^{18}F-FDG PET and PET/CT for the baseline evaluation
of patients with multiple myeloma and related plasma cell dyscrasias, as well as for
subsequent evaluations related to patient management. Future directions for imaging research in multiple myeloma will include PET imaging with isotopes other than
^{18}F-FDG and whole-body MRI.

Keywords Imaging · MRI · PET · PET/CT · Skeletal survey · Focal
lesion · Osteolytic lesion · Occult infection · DKK1 · Extramedullary disease (EMD)

2.1 Introduction

Imaging of multiple myeloma (MM) and related plasma cell dyscrasias includes
anatomic-based imaging (conventional x-rays, CT, and MRI), functional imaging
(PET or ^{99m}Tc-sestamibi), and hybrid imaging combining PET or SPECT with CT
(PET/CT or SPECT/CT), also called fusion imaging [1]. While most imaging of
MM and related diseases with PET or PET/CT has used ^{18}F-labeled fluorodeoxyglucose (^{18}F-FDG), other positron-emitting radiopharmaceuticals have been reported
[2, 3], but these have not yet achieved widespread clinical use. Imaging with ^{99m}Tc-
sestamibi (MIBI) is also useful, especially when imaged with SPECT or SPECT/CT,
with uptake related to the intracellular concentration and activity of mitochondria
[4–6].

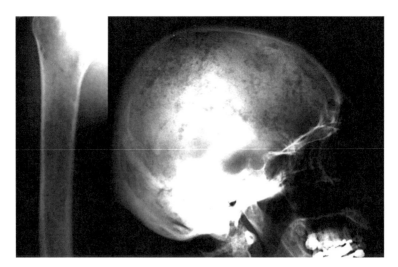

Fig. 2.1 Unchanging focal OL bone lesions of the skull and humerus in a patient with MM in
complete remission for 5 years. Proximal humeral shaft (*left*) and lateral skull (*right*) of a patient
with multiple myeloma demonstrate multiple focal osteolytic lesions that have never healed despite
the patient remaining in complete remission for 5 years. X-ray MBS cannot be used to demonstrate
response to treatment

While the classic hallmark of MM is the focal, destructive, osteolytic (OL) lesion seen on x-ray or CT, there is a systemic, diffuse bone loss that occurs as well, leading to diffuse osteopenia/osteoporosis [7, 8] attributable to both osteoclastic stimulation and osteoblastic anergy resulting from the bone marrow/tumor interaction present in MM. This tumor-induced systemic bone loss is compounded by a treatment-related diffuse loss of bone mass from frequent use of high-dose glucocorticoid medications. Because of the associated destruction of the osteoblast progenitors, the focal OL bone lesions never heal, even if the patient remains in clinical remission for many years, a hallmark of MM bone disease.

2.2 Overview of Imaging – Correlates with Tumor Biology

The underlying biology is reflected in the imaging findings for MM and related plasma cell dyscrasias. There are the obvious changes that result from gross mechanical damage to the skeletal system (insufficiency fractures and lytic bone disease) and soft tissues (extramedullary disease (EMD) and amyloidosis) as well as secondary findings due to immunosuppression resulting from the tumor or its treatment (e.g., infection and avascular necrosis). Most cases of MM are thought to result from progression of monoclonal gammopathy of uncertain significance (MGUS) to smoldering myeloma to symptomatic myeloma. Likewise, the imaging findings also follow a related progression from normal to minimal evidence of disease to gross evidence of widespread, severe disease [9].

A MM-related entity, solitary plasmacytoma, should by definition be limited to one region of involvement, either soft tissue (solitary extramedullary plasmacytoma, SEP) or bone (solitary bone plasmacytoma, SBP). SBP has been considered a frequent harbinger for future MM with a 3% annual conversion rate. However, with more advanced imaging (^{18}F-FDG PET or PET/CT, MIBI, and MRI), it is now apparent that many cases previously thought to be SBP are actually "under-staged" MM or the now recognized variant of MM oxymoronically called "multiple solitary plasmacytomas" [10].

Most plasma cell dyscrasias result from the expansion of a single clone of cells, with resultant monoclonal protein secretion. A small fraction (1–5% at diagnosis) will initially be classified as hyposecretory or nonsecretory [11, 12], either with no or very low levels of secretion of the hallmark M protein. In most of these patients, serum analysis will identify the presence of elevated concentrations of either kappa- or lambda-free light chains with abnormal kappa/lambda ratios. Thus, only about 25% of MM patients initially classified as hypo/nonsecretory are truly nonsecretory [12, 13]. In truly nonsecretory patients, determining the response to treatment is problematic, especially if the nonsecretory status develops during treatment. While true nonsecretory MM at the time of diagnosis is rare, it becomes more common during later clinical stages, reflecting dedifferentiation. In this clinical setting, ^{18}F-FDG PET and MIBI imaging are useful for monitoring disease status and treatment response. MRI can also be useful, though only if progression or relapse is present since the MRI-defined focal lesions respond more slowly than on PET or MIBI imaging [14–17].

2.3 Imaging of Multiple Myeloma

2.3.1 Role of the Metastatic Bone Survey (MBS)

One or more focal OL lesions on x-ray identify specific classic Durie–Salmon stages of MM at baseline and on restaging. The use of x-ray is a mainstay of the classic Durie–Salmon staging (D–S Staging) [18] established in 1975. Since the original D–S staging system was established, medical imaging has made significant advances. Accordingly, Durie has developed the new Durie–Salmon Plus system (Table 2.1), which incorporates newer imaging technology (MRI, PET, or PET/CT and MIBI) [19]. Throughout the development of these newer imaging technologies, hundreds of peer-reviewed reports have described their successful application to the diagnosis and management of MM and related diseases.

The MBS remains in common use and consists of a plain x-ray series of the entire skeleton (skull, vertebral column, ribs, sternum, pelvis, and extremities). While relatively sensitive in the skull and extremities for detection of focal OL lesions, it is less sensitive for detection of focal areas of osteolysis when there are significant overlapping complex structures, such as in the skull base or facial regions,

Table 2.1 Durie–Salmon PLUS staging system (DS+)

Classification	PLUS	New imaging: MRI and/or ^{18}F-FDG PET
MGUS		All negative
Stage IA* (smoldering or indolent)		Can have single plasmacytoma and/or limited disease on imaging
Multiple myeloma stage IB*		<5 focal lesions; mild diffuse disease
Multiple myeloma stage IIA/B*		5–20 focal lesions; moderate diffuse disease
Stage IIIA/B*		>20 focal lesions; severe diffuse disease
	*A Serum creatinine <2.0 mg/dl and no extramedullary disease (EMD)	
	*B Serum creatinine >2.0 mg/dl or extramedullary disease (EMD)	

Adapted from Durie BG, Kyle RA, Belch A, et al. [6]. Used with permission.

vertebral column, pelvis, sternum, and ribs, where mixed densities from complex overlapping skeletal structures, air, solid organs, and GI tract contents can either simulate or obscure focal OL lesions. The MBS is also limited in sensitivity since typically 70% or more loss of bone mass must occur for a focal OL lesion to be visible on x-ray, particularly in the vertebral column [20]. The MBS cannot detect intramedullary tumor that has not produced either focal osteolysis or a secondary feature, such as a pathologic fracture. Severe diffuse osteoporosis/osteopenia can be seen on the MBS, but this is a late finding. The MBS is also virtually useless for the detection of EMD. The MBS is still superior to other imaging modalities for detection of very small (sub-centimeter) focal OL lesions of the distal extremities, such as in the hands, feet, or forearms.

Because the bone lesions from myeloma never heal the MBS is not useful for following response to treatment, though it can reveal relapse if new evidence of disease is identified. The x-ray MBS is especially useful in areas that are problematic for advanced imaging due to imaging artifacts, such as from joint prostheses, spinal fusion hardware, or vertebroplasty cement. Because the x-ray appearance of

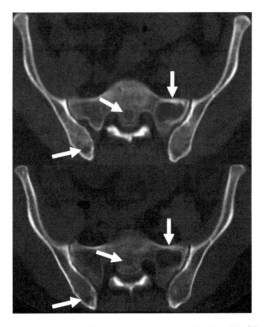

Fig. 2.2 CT MBS cannot demonstrate disease response even after durable CR of 5 years duration. Axial CT images through the upper pelvis in a patient in complete remission for 5 years. Multiple focal osteolytic bone lesions (two indicated by the *upper two arrows* on each image) are present with no evidence of either progression or healing on the *lower image*. At the entry into remission (*upper image*), a biopsy tract is seen on the *right*, traversing a focal osteolytic lesion, with an osteoblastic response induced by the biopsy-related trauma present on either side of the focal osteolytic bone lesion, but not within it, due to permanent destruction of the osteoblast progenitor niche within the focal lesion (*lowest arrow* on each image). On the *lower image*, 5 years later, two new biopsy sites from periodic follow-up examinations are present on the *left* with similar findings (Adapted from Epstein and Walker [9], used with permission)

MM is sometimes distinct from comorbidities, the MBS may serendipitously reveal unsuspected findings, such as evidence of infection and lung cancer.

Accordingly, despite its limitations, the MBS remains a useful tool for the evaluation of the patient with MM and related diseases, especially at baseline. If another x-ray-based imaging modality is used, such as the CT portion of the whole-body PET/CT or a dedicated whole-body musculoskeletal CT, then these latter examinations may largely supplant the classic x-ray-based MBS. Indeed, for patients receiving a whole-body PET/CT as part of staging or restaging, a standard x-ray MBS is probably no longer cost-effective [21, 22].

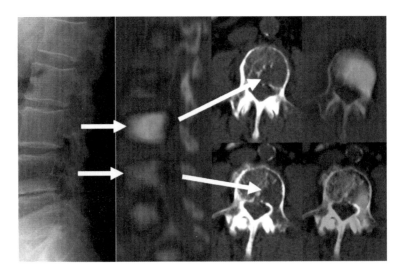

Fig. 2.3 Power of ^{18}F-FDG PET/CT to demonstrate both diffuse and focal lesions of MM as well as the presence of osteolytic bone lesions compared to the MBS. MBS lateral view of the lumbar spine (*left*) fails to demonstrate either the diffuse marrow infiltration or the focal lytic bone lesions (*arrows*) of the L3 and L4 vertebral bodies (axial ^{18}F-FDG PET/CT-fused images, *right*, and corresponding CT-only images, second from *right*). Diffuse increased uptake is also evident on the sagittal fused ^{18}F-FDG PET/CT image (second from *left*), but is not apparent on the lateral MBS x-ray (*left*) (Adapted from Epstein and Walker [9], used with permission)

POEMS syndrome (polyneuropathy, organomegaly, endocrinopathy, presence of abnormal M protein and skin changes) is a poorly understood entity that differs from classic MM in several ways, including superior median survival and the presence of osteosclerotic changes. These osteosclerotic focal lesions are the origin of the name by which POEMS syndrome is also called osteosclerotic myeloma [23–26]. While the diagnosis of POEMS syndrome involves evaluation of several factors, the presence of an osteosclerotic focal bone lesion on x-ray instead of the classic osteolytic lesion of MM should suggest the diagnosis. Occasionally, diffuse osteosclerotic changes occur with MM, though still focal OL lesions can occur. These patterns of either focal osteosclerotic lesions or diffuse osteosclerotic changes with focal OL lesions are rare variants of MM and, thus, are not well understood.

Fig. 2.4 POEMS syndrome
with osteosclerotic focal
skeletal lesions on x-ray.
Axial CT image through the
upper sacrum (*top*) with the
corresponding fused
^{18}F-FDG PET/CT (*bottom*) in
a patient with POEMS
syndrome demonstrate a focal
osteosclerotic lesion of S1 to
the *left* of midline, with no
evidence of increased uptake
above surrounding tissue.
A bone marrow core biopsy
tract is visible in the left
posterior iliac wing

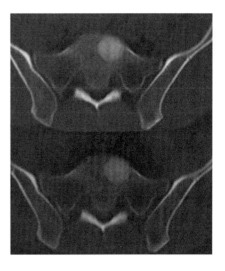

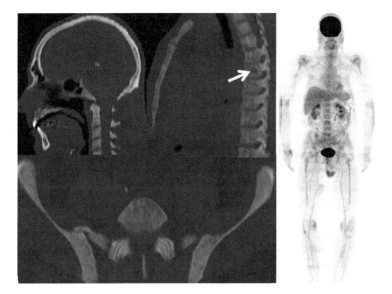

Fig. 2.5 Osteosclerotic MM. Sagittal skull and upper cervical spine (*upper left*), sagittal thoracic
spine and sternum (*upper center*), and axial upper pelvis (*lower left*) demonstrate increased bone
density with loss of the normal marrow space appearance of the adult. There is a focal osteolytic
lesion in an upper thoracic vertebra (*arrow, upper center*). The anterior 3D MIP (maximum intensity projection) ^{18}F-FDG PET image (*right*) demonstrates diffusely increased uptake in the central
hematopoietic marrow space that has also expanded into the mid to distal femora and humeri

2.3.2 Role of MRI

MRI is a well-established and powerful tool for the imaging of MM and related diseases. MRI is also more widely available than PET or PET/CT. MRI has been used for the staging and restaging of MM since the 1980s, with hundreds of peer-reviewed reports in the medical literature and scores of textbook chapters documenting its clinical utility. The basic principles governing the use of MRI in this disease have been established for decades and consist of imaging of the adult distribution of the hematopoietic marrow with a combination of spin-echo T1-weighted (T1-wt, performed typically with "fat suppression" and both with and without gadolinium enhancement) and T2-weighted image sequences, gradient echo, short-tau inversion recovery. The specific protocols will vary between manufacturers and according to the specific model and field strength of the magnetic field, available coils, and other features which are unique to each imaging center. Each imaging center should meet or exceed the image quality standards required for American College of Radiology (ACR) MRI accreditation (www.acr.org) [27–35].

The normal hematopoietic marrow space in adults is comprised of a mixture of tissues, predominately blood and blood-forming elements, fatty tissue, bone and bony support elements, and blood vessels. The appearance of the normal, central, hematopoietic marrow on MRI imaging depends on the patient's age, with younger patients normally having a more "cellular" appearing marrow due to a higher ratio of hematopoietic elements to fat tissue. The normal central marrow appearance of middle-aged to elderly patients, the typical age of the majority of patients with MM and related diseases, has relatively less hematopoietic elements and more fat tissue and will accordingly appear differently on the same MRI sequences. A detailed knowledge of this age-adjusted normal variation in the appearance of the central bone marrow is therefore a prerequisite for proper interpretation of the imaging findings [1, 36]. The overall appearance of the marrow space on MRI is defined as homogenous, heterogeneous, or "variegated" in appearance. Some investigators have also described a "stippled" pattern which seems to be similar to the variegated pattern in appearance and significance. Since tumor infiltration is also associated with an increased blood supply, post-gadolinium T1-wt images in patients with significant MM marrow infiltration demonstrate an increase in T1-wt signal, with the affected marrow space "enhancing" or becoming "bright" in appearance relative to normal skeletal muscle and also relative to the pre-gadolinium T1-wt images. The use of marrow stimulating medications will usually result in a diffuse change in the marrow signal resembling diffuse tumor infiltration, as sometimes will recovery from recent chemotherapy, "chemotherapy rebound." Accordingly, interpretation of the diffuse marrow signal must be made in context to the presence or absence of marrow stimulants or chemotherapy rebound [1].

MRI-defined focal lesions (MRI-FL) are often identified, though the presence of associated focal osteolysis must be established independently by x-ray (preferably CT, especially of the central skeleton, due to its vastly superior accuracy in this location compared to standard x-rays) since MRI does not distinguish between MRI-FL that are associated with focal osteolysis and MRI-FL that are not. Importantly,

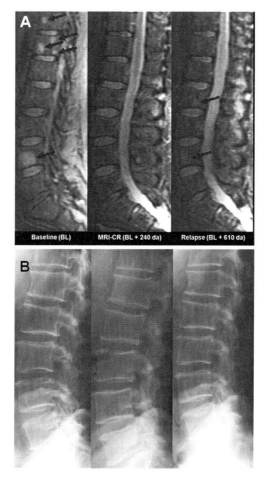

Fig. 2.6 Value of MRI to demonstrate diffuse and focal disease and to demonstrate both treatment response and relapse relative to MBS: Sagittal views of a STIR-weighted MRI series (**a**, *top row*), from *left* to *right*, at time of diagnosis (baseline, BL), complete response (BL + 240 days), and relapse (BL + 610 days). The MRI at DX demonstrates MRI focal lesions (*arrows*, T11, T12, and L4) as well as abnormally increased diffuse marrow signal compatible with diffuse marrow infiltration with MM. Both the diffuse and the focal abnormalities resolve in remission ("MRI-CR") in the central frame. At relapse (*right frame*), the diffuse marrow signal remains within normal range, but there is one recurrent MRI focal lesion (L4, *lower arrow*) and one new MRI focal lesion (*upper arrow*, L2, not present at baseline). The patient's contemporaneous MBS (**b**, *lower row*) remained normal throughout this time period (Adapted from Walker et al. [36], used with permission)

MRI-FL can be obscured by either intense diffuse marrow infiltration by tumor or by marrow stimulation/chemotherapy rebound, since the MRI signal characteristics of a "cellular marrow" are the same as the signal characteristics of MRI-FL due to tumor. Since effective treatment of tumor will rapidly normalize the diffuse

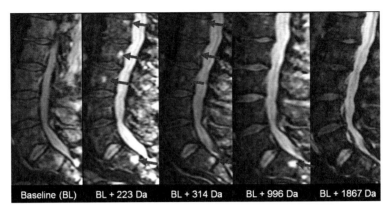

Baseline (BL)   BL + 223 Da   BL + 314 Da   BL + 996 Da   BL + 1867 Da

Fig. 2.7 Unmasking of MRI FL and slow response of MRI FL to treatment: A sagittal STIR-weighted MRI series is shown at baseline (BL), with chronologically ordered follow-up examinations with number of days (Da) relative to the BL examination given below the images. The BL examination demonstrates diffuse, severely increased marrow signal with a "variegated" appearance compatible with diffuse marrow infiltration with tumor. By BL+223 days, most of the diffuse signal had resolved, revealing MRI focal lesions (MRI-FL) at L1, L2, L3, and S1 which had be obscured ("masked") by the diffuse tumor infiltration at baseline. By BL+314 days, the diffuse signal has completely normalized with the MRI-FL continuing to decrease in size and signal intensity, though still apparent. By BL+996 days, only the S1 MRI-FL remained. By BL + 1867 days, all diffuse and focal signal abnormalities had resolved as this patient remained in durable complete remission

marrow signal, whereas the focal lesions resolve much more slowly, these underlying MRI-FL can become visible against the overall marrow background as the diffuse cellular infiltration subsides. This clearing of the diffuse signal that reveals underlying, persistent MRI-FL is termed "unmasking" [36].

Additional findings that are frequently seen with MRI imaging include insufficiency fractures (usually of the vertebral bodies or sacrum), infection (such as discitis), avascular necrosis of the femoral or humeral heads (usually related to dexamethasone therapy), and osteonecrosis of the maxilla or mandible (usually associated with duration of bisphosphonate usage) [1, 36–39].

While MRI is extremely useful for staging and restaging of patients with MM and related diseases, it has limitations. Some patients cannot be scanned if they have implanted devices (pacemakers, defibrillators, neural stimulators, cochlear implants, some prosthetic heart valves, some intracranial aneurysm clips, etc.) that would be unsafe to subject to the magnetic field strength and/or the intense radio frequencies of an MRI scanner. Sometimes a patient can safely be scanned, but portions of the examination are compromised by iatrogenic devices, such as spinal fixation hardware, joint replacements, or vertebroplasty cement. Because MRI imaging requires several minutes to perform, motion artifacts can limit the image quality, sometimes severely, such as in the ribs where the motion of breathing can obscure small lesions. Since MM patients are often in pain, lying still for the duration of a thorough examination of the entire marrow space can be beyond the ability of some patients to withstand without pain medication. Pulsations from the heart and the aorta can cause "phase artifacts" that limit visualization of nearby structures. Additionally, gadolinium must be used with caution in patients who have renal function impairment, a condition commonly encountered in patients with MM, because of the risk of nephrogenic systemic fibrosis. Because of these reasons, the utility of MRI imaging of patients with MM and related diseases is sometimes limited [1, 40–42].

2.3.3 Staging of Multiple Myeloma

MRI is an important staging tool to distinguish truly solitary plasmacytoma of bone from MM and to document the extent and pattern of diffuse marrow involvement. The MRI pattern of MM ranges from a normal appearance to a diffuse, nonfocal tumor infiltration of the marrow space to microfocal ("speckled") appearance and/or to large, macrofocal disease (5 mm or more in size), often occurring in a mixed pattern. MRI imaging can demonstrate "breakout" lesions, focal areas of disease that break through the cortex of bone into the soft tissues (including epidural spread), yet which still occur in the context of and dependence upon the bone marrow microenvironment. MRI can also reveal EMD, though not as well as PET or PET/CT because of the more restricted field of view of MRI and the whole-body field of view of PET or PET/CT [1, 9, 36, 43].

Relative drawbacks of MRI relative to ^{18}F-FDG PET or PET/CT are both the time and the expense for a thorough examination of the skeletal system, requiring separate studies of the calvarium, entire vertebral column, pelvis, shoulder girdles, and sternum. The time required for a thorough MRI examination of these various anatomic regions is longer than for a whole-body PET or PET/CT examination, and the total expense, at least in the USA, is typically much greater for these MRI examinations than for a whole-body PET or PET/CT. The MRI's limited field of view to the specific region being examined and its contraindicated use in some patients (such as in patients with iatrogenic devices that preclude or limit an MRI exam) are significant drawbacks to its use in MM and related diseases, especially compared to the advantages and relative lower cost of whole-body PET/CT, which demonstrates both active skeletal and soft tissue disease and, via the CT portion of the study, includes a "free" CT MBS. MRI's relative advantages compared to ^{18}F-FDG PET and PET/CT are its superior spatial and contrast resolution, typically 2 mm for a high-field system, vs. approximately 5 mm for the PET portion of current PET/CT scanners, and MRI's more widespread availability. As with other malignancies, ^{18}F-FDG PET scanning can be falsely negative in some patients who have recently received treatment, whereas MRI is not as significantly limited in this setting (while the MRI signal abnormalities associated with diffuse tumor infiltration can be rapidly but transiently suppressed by recent chemotherapy, the MRI-defined FL do not respond as quickly). MRI is also superior to other modalities, including PET or PET/CT, for early diagnosis of avascular necrosis [1, 36, 37]. Whole-body MRI is an emerging and exciting technology currently with an undefined role in the staging and restaging of MM and related diseases [44, 45].

Fig. 2.8 Avascular necrosis of the *left* hip. A T1-weighted coronal MRI image through the femoral heads demonstrates a heterogeneous, "speckled," or "variegated" diffuse marrow signal, as well as the characteristic appearance of avascular necrosis of the left femoral head (*arrow*). The MRI appearance of avascular necrosis of the femoral head is typically a small region of sub-cortical "collapse" of the superior, weight-bearing region of the femoral head, as seen in this case. MRI is superior to other imaging modalities for the early diagnosis of avascular necrosis of the femoral or humeral heads (Adapted from Talamo et al. [37], used with permission)

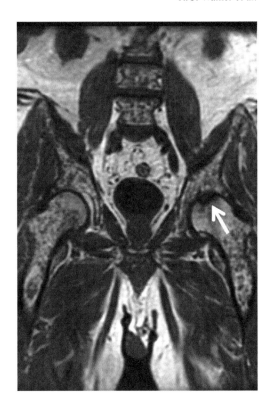

2.3.4 *Role of ^{18}FDG PET or PET/CT*

The ^{18}F-FDG PET imaging protocol for MM and related plasma cell dyscrasias is designed to image the entire marrow space and the soft tissues of the entire body. Imaging begins about 60 min after intravenous injection of the radioisotope, and after the proper dietary and other preparatory measures (described below). It is best to inject the ^{18}F-FDG via direct peripheral venous access rather than to use a central intravenous catheter because the ^{18}F-FDG can be retained to an unknown degree in the catheter tubing, degrading the scan quality overall and possibly obscuring important findings, such as tumor in nearby skeletal or soft tissue structures or an infected thrombus at the tip of the central venous catheter. If direct venous access is not technically feasible, flushing the central catheter with 200 ml of sterile normal saline after ^{18}F-FDG injection is recommended to diminish residual activity in the central catheter [46–49].

In order to image the entire marrow space, ^{18}F-FDG PET and PET/CT imaging of MM and related disorders must span the skull vertex to the feet. Some scanners can accomplish this whole-body examination in one acquisition, but some require two (e.g., mid thighs to the vertex in one examination followed by repositioning the patient for a separate acquisition of the mid thighs to the feet). It is best to begin the PET imaging over the upper thighs and to scan toward the vertex so that the urinary bladder is as empty as possible when imaged (the patient is asked to void immediately before the PET or PET/CT scan). Attenuation correction should be used, either by CT or by ^{68}Ge source rods [50].

As with the use of PET imaging for other malignancies, measuring and documenting the serum glucose level at the time of injection of the radioisotope is essential. Because of frequent use of high-dose glucocorticoid medications in MM and related diseases, high serum glucose levels are common, frequently between 150 and 200 mg/dl or more. This will interfere to some degree with the quality of the PET image through competitive inhibition of the ^{18}F-FDG uptake and will result in reduction of measured SUV values. The use of insulin to lower the blood glucose will have an even greater adverse impact on the scan quality by diverting the ^{18}F-FDG into skeletal muscle and the liver due to insulin-induced increase in glycogen synthesis. Physical exercise, including physical therapy and walking, will have a similar effect, resulting in a poor quality, sometimes even nondiagnostic, examination due to marked muscle uptake induced by glycogen replenishment. Thus, for 24 h prior to a PET or PET/CT scan, the patient should limit physical exertion as much as possible and observe a low-carbohydrate, high-lipid/high-protein diet. Importantly, oral hypoglycemic medications will not adversely affect the quality of the examination and do not need to be withheld from patients who need them. Most patients can take their daily medications with water on the day of the PET or PET/CT examination. However, to avoid stimulation of endogenous insulin, the patients should otherwise remain NPO (including chewing gum or candy mints) for 6 h prior to radioisotope injection [51].

2.3.5 Brown Adipose Tissue

While usually seen in premenopausal females and younger males (e.g., below the age of 30), the activation of brown adipose tissue (BAT) can produce significant, even focal, nodular appearing, intense ^{18}F-FDG uptake that can seriously degrade image quality and, near the areas of BAT, potentially obscure tumor uptake. BAT is usually recognizable by its characteristic distribution (neck, shoulders, mediastinum, upper retroperitoneum, and the paravertebral regions) and by correlation with CT. On PET/CT, especially, the BAT uptake on PET easily correlates to areas of otherwise normal appearing adipose tissue on the accompanying CT. However, correlation between PET and CT on "PET-only" systems is more problematic. If the BAT uptake occurs in areas of abnormal CT density, especially in areas of previously known tumor, then differentiation between BAT uptake and tumor recurrence can be very problematic. If this occurs, or if the patient is known to be likely to have BAT activation (e.g., a premenopausal female), then premedication and other precautionary measures can help minimize BAT uptake. Premedications that have proven useful to block BAT activation include anxiolytic agents (e.g., diazepam or alprazolam) and beta-blockers. Pre-arrangements for safe transportation home (e.g., a driver) must be made for outpatients receiving anxiolytic agents.

Other measures to use to help minimize activation of BAT include avoidance of the cold (BAT is activated by cold, especially the "shivering" response) and the use of nicotine or decongestants (such as ephedrine or pseudoephedrine) for at least 4 h prior to injection of the ^{18}F-FDG. Because many imaging suites are relatively cold because of the environmental demands of the equipment, most centers keep warm blankets available for use by patients [52–57].

PET and PET/CT image acquisition and processing protocols are identical to other "whole-body" protocols used for other malignancies such as melanoma or sarcoma, though specific settings vary between manufacturers and even between units. Accordingly, each imaging center must develop optimized protocols for each system. Each imaging center should meet or exceed the image quality standards required for ACR accreditation (www.acr.org) for PET or PET/CT.

We typically use 555 MBq (15 mCi) of ^{18}F-FDG for PET imaging, injected 60 min prior to initiation of imaging. Like most imaging centers, we will adjust the ^{18}F-FDG dose according to body weight if the patient is unusually small or large

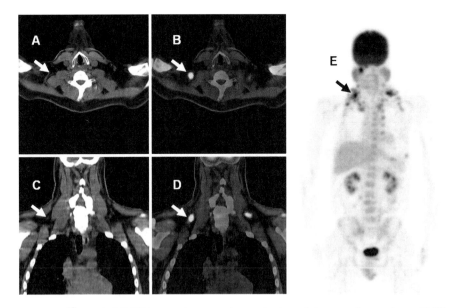

Fig. 2.9 ^{18}F-FDG PET/CT scan demonstrating activation of brown adipose tissue (BAT) (*arrows*). Axial CT (**a**) and fused PET/CT (**b**) images, as well as corresponding coronal images (**c** and **d**, respectively) demonstrate the intense uptake that occurs when BAT is activated. The anterior 3D MIP PET image (**e**) demonstrates the distribution in the neck and chest, though BAT can extend into the upper retroperitoneum to the level of the kidneys. All foci of uptake in this patient were thought to be due to activation of BAT. With CT, the regions of uptake were verified to correspond to areas of normal appearing fatty tissue. However, if the patient had had areas of tumor in these regions, active tumor uptake would not be discernible against the uptake from surrounding BAT. Accordingly, precautions should be taken (as described in the text) to prevent the activation of BAT in patients who are likely to demonstrate this phenomenon, or who have demonstrated activation of BAT on prior PET or PET/CT examinations

(the maximum ^{18}F-FDG amount we inject is 740 MBq, 20 mCi). After radioisotope injection, the patient waits quietly in a semi-recumbent position in a "dosing room" until time for imaging in order to limit muscle uptake.

For PET/CT acquisition, we use "3D" imaging mode to minimize the time needed for acquisition. This is very important for myeloma patients, who are often in significant pain and who will thus have great difficulty remaining completely still for more than the required 20–30 min whole-body (vertex to feet) PET/CT imaging protocol. We perform a CT topogram with helical technique using 120 KV and 30–50 (mA s), the so-called low-dose technique, with the computer automatically adjusting the mA s as needed (the computer increases or decreases the mA s as needed to maintain needed image quality while also minimizing radiation exposure as much as possible).

For the PET acquisition of the PET/CT examination, we will usually image for 3 min per bed position, though if the patient is obese, we will extend this time on an empirically derived "floating scale" to obtain sufficient count statistics for diagnostic image quality. We transfer the image data to dedicated workstations for PET/CT image analysis. We interpret the three data sets (PET, CT) individually and combined ("fused" as PET/CT) since all three provide unique, powerful information [50].

2.3.6 Role of ^{99m}Tc-Sestamibi (MIBI)

MIBI imaging is useful for whole-body imaging of MM and related diseases. The uptake of the radiopharmaceutical is proportional to the concentration of mitochondria within viable cells. Accordingly, areas of greater metabolic activity will, in general, demonstrate increased uptake. Since MIBI uptake is relatively high in normal myocardium, liver, and spleen, and since it is normally excreted in bile, image quality in the region of the heart, liver, spleen, and the bowel (because of rapid biliary excretion) is somewhat impaired. SPECT or SPECT/CT imaging can partially overcome the image quality limitations in these regions, but detection of either bone or EMD in the regions near the heart, liver, spleen, or in the soft tissues of the abdomen or pelvis is to some degree impaired.

MIBI uptake is increased in active disease and normalizes in remission. The uptake of the radioisotope is sometimes blocked in drug-resistant tumor, potentially resulting in a false-negative scan. Despite these limitations, MIBI imaging is proven to be useful in discrimination of MGUS from symptomatic MM and in demonstrating the whole-body extent of disease. Since focal lesions are sometimes visible, MIBI imaging can guide high-yield biopsies. MIBI imaging is complementary to MRI imaging in MM and related diseases, similar to the role of ^{18}F-FDG PET or PET/CT. MIBI imaging may be superior to ^{18}F-FDG PET or PET/CT in demonstrating the full extent of the diffuse component of marrow uptake, and it is certainly less expensive and more widely available. MIBI imaging is particularly helpful if ^{18}F-FDG PET or PET/CT imaging is not available, but probably is not routinely needed in addition to ^{18}F-FDG PET or PET/CT imaging [4, 58–61].

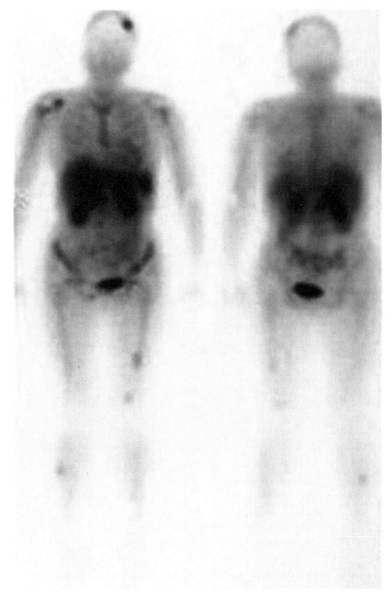

Fig. 2.10 Anterior (*left*) and posterior (*right*) whole-body imaging with ^{99m}Tc-sestamibi (MIBI) in a patient with active MM. Diffuse increased uptake is visible in the axial skeleton with extension into the long bones of the extremities. Focal lesions are also visible in the calvarium, pelvis, right scapula, left femur, right fibula, and proximal humeri. The resolution is inferior to MRI or ^{18}F-FDG PET/CT imaging. Normal uptake in the heart, liver, spleen, and kidneys (and, due to biliary excretion, the GI tract to a variable extent) partially obscures disease in these regions of normal uptake. Some of these limitations can be overcome through the use of SPECT or, especially, SPECT/CT. Despite these limitations, MIBI imaging of MM has proven useful for staging and restaging of MM and for direction of high-yield biopsies as described in multiple reports. MIBI imaging, especially

2.3.7 Clinical Relevance of Imaging in MM and Related Diseases

Imaging is an essential tool in the staging and restaging of MM and related diseases and can also aid in diagnosis by identifying sites for image-guided, high-yield biopsies of focal lesions of the skeletal system and soft tissues. These image-guided biopsies reduce both false-negative and nondiagnostic results by reducing random sampling errors and significantly increase the yield of clinically relevant cytogenetic abnormalities (CGA) over random marrow biopsies, improving identification up-front of patients with high-risk disease [62].

While the various imaging modalities provide overlapping information to some degree, each one also provides both unique and clinically relevant data that are also complementary to the other imaging methods. Imaging of MM and related diseases is divided broadly into baseline staging and subsequent restaging examinations.

In the USA, CMS (Medicare) has approved "broad coverage" reimbursement for imaging of MM for Medicare recipients with ^{18}F-FDG PET and PET/CT imaging at the time of initial staging and for additional PET or PET/CT examinations performed for "subsequent treatment strategy" (the term now used instead of the prior designations of "restaging" and "monitoring response to treatment when a change in treatment is anticipated"). In the USA, the use of PET imaging for diagnosis, such as for monitoring patients with MGUS or with SEP or SBP for progression to MM, is not, as of this writing, reimbursed by CMS except under CED (coverage with evidence development).

A baseline examination should be extremely thorough, ideally comprised of whole-body MBS, whole-body ^{18}F-FDG PET or PET/CT, and an MRI series of the hematopoietic marrow space appropriate to the patient's age. A "CT MBS" that is part of a PET/CT examination is a very cost-effective means of detecting the presence of x-ray focal osteolytic disease since it is provided at no additional cost as part of the whole-body (vertex to feet) PET/CT, frequently revealing focal OL lesions not visible on a standard x-ray-based MBS. Identification of extensive focal osteolytic disease seen on the CT portion of a baseline PET/CT examination of a newly diagnosed MM patient occurs frequently, strongly suggesting that many newly diagnosed patients have had the disease for some time, perhaps years [9, 22, 36].

2.3.7.1 Key Imaging Findings

The findings of great importance in imaging of MM are as follows:

- Identification and quantification of the presence, size, and number of skeletal focal lesions:

Fig. 2.10 (continued)   with SPECT or SPECT/CT, should be strongly considered as a whole-body imaging technique for patients with MM or related diseases when ^{18}F-FDG PET or PET/CT is not available (Adapter from Fonti et al. [61], used with permission)

o Correlation of the location of a focal lesion on MRI with x-ray or CT
  todetermine if focal osteolysis is associated. If not, effective treatment
  can prevent this irreversible end organ damage.
o Identification of areas of high-yield biopsies [36, 62].
  ▪ Focal lesions on MRI
  ▪ Focal lesions on ^{18}F-FDG PET or PET/CT, especially with
    the greatest metabolic activity
  ▪ Suspected areas of EMD
o Identification of areas at high risk for pathologic fractures, allowing possible preemptive action such as vertebroplasty, focal radiation
  therapy, or proper clinical precautions.
o Risk stratification of the patient based on the number of focal lesions
  by MRI or ^{18}F-FDG PET or PET/CT at baseline staging [22, 36].
• Detection of diffuse marrow infiltration (MRI and ^{18}F-FDG PET or PET/CT)
• Detection of the presence of extramedullary tumor, identifying a high-risk subset
  of patients [22]
• Identification of high-risk areas of tumor that may need immediate aggressive
  treatment, such as epidural tumor that could lead to spinal cord compression, a
  destructive lesion of the odontoid process
• Detection of the presence of occult infection [46–49]
• Identification of important but unsuspected comorbid conditions (especially with
  MRI or whole-body PET or PET/CT) such as additional primary malignancies
  (e.g., thyroid, colon, breast, lymphoma, melanoma, or lung) or premalignant
  colon polyps [63]

Focal lesions (FL) are defined as *well-circumscribed areas of increased uptake on
PET or abnormal signal on MRI relative to the marrow background that are thought
to represent areas of tumor involvement, measuring at least 5 mm in diameter.*
This definition specifically excludes focal areas with similar signal characteristics
to MM FL that are not thought to be due to tumor, such as fractures that are not
associated with MM FL, subchondral cysts associated with arthritis, typical benign
bone lesions such as fibrous cortical defects or aneurysmal bone cysts, "Schmorl's
nodes," hemangiomas, suspected sites of infection. Thus, the use of PET/CT is superior to PET-only imaging because of the direct anatomic correlation that PET/CT
provides with an area of focal ^{18}F-FDG uptake [51, 64].

X-ray-based imaging (MBS or CT) is required, by definition, to identify the
anatomic changes associated with end organ damage of focal OL lesions and can
often identify the presence of diffuse osteopenia/osteoporosis. Subtle deformities
are sometimes seen from subacute or chronic insufficiency fractures. Areas at high
risk for fracture, especially of the vertebral column and the lower extremities (such
as the femoral necks), can also sometimes be identified, especially with CT. Since
the skeletal changes associated with MM are irreversible, they cannot be used
to monitor treatment response during restaging, though the identification of new
lesions on x-ray or CT does signify disease progression. Subtle changes in patient

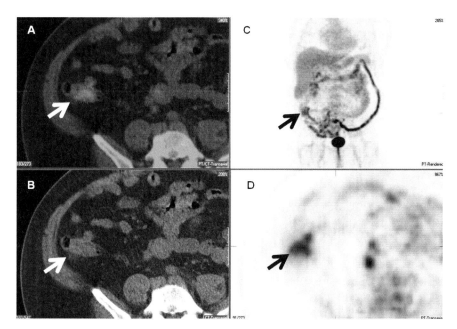

Fig. 2.11 Incidental second malignancy detected on baseline ^{18}F-FDG PET/CT scan for MM. Axial magnified fused (**a**) and CT (**b**) images through the cecum in a patient with newly diagnosed MM demonstrate an area of focal uptake in the cecum (*arrows*) seen on the CT portion to have infiltrating, stranding densities extending into the adjacent fat tissue. On PET-only images (**c**, the anterior 3D MIP image, and **d**, axial image corresponding to **a** and **b**), this area of focal uptake is seen, but the presence of an infiltrative mass is not apparent on the PET-only images and would have been difficult to differentiate from the other GI tract uptake in this patient. Further evaluation with colonoscopy was performed because of the PET/CT appearance, revealing invasive, poor-differentiated adenocarcinoma of the cecum

positioning for standard x-ray MBS can either simulate or obscure focal lesions, especially in the vertebral column where there are overlapping complex soft tissues and bone densities. CT MBS is thus superior to x-ray MBS to verify the presence, absence, or change in size or number of focal OL lesions in most regions [22, 36].

Because x-ray or CT-based MBS rely on anatomic changes, MBS (especially x-ray-based MBS) can under-stage patients compared to imaging by MRI or PET, with these latter two imaging modalities able to detect diffuse and focal lesions before anatomic changes occur. Neither x-ray nor CT-based MBS can assess for diffuse tumor infiltration. X-ray MBS cannot detect EMD, but CT MBS often can [22]. Neither x-ray nor CT-based MBS can determine if a given osteolytic lesion contains active disease or not. Reliance on anatomic imaging can thus be misleading if used to direct treatment or biopsy.

MBS examinations are not useful to demonstrate response to treatment since these focal OL lesions never heal. Accordingly, imaging examinations for restaging should rely on MRI and/or PET or PET/CT. On PET or PET/CT, the diffuse skeletal uptake and the uptake of focal skeletal lesions and of EMD will decrease in "real

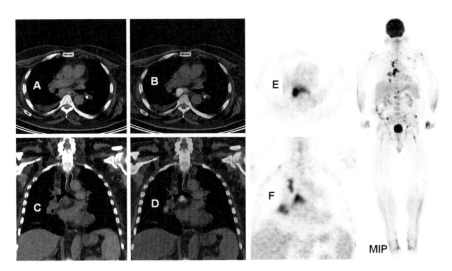

Fig. 2.12 Incidental second malignancy detected on baseline ^{18}F-FDG PET/CT scan for MM. The anterior 3D MIP image (*right*) of this ^{18}F-FDG PET/CT scan demonstrates focal skeletal lesions compatible with this patient's history of newly diagnosed MM. However, the pattern of uptake in the right lung, right hilus, and mediastinum and the presence of a mildly ^{18}F-FDG avid small right pleural effusion were not typical for EMD due to MM (axial CT and fused PET/CT, A and B, as well as coronal CT and fused PET/CT, C and D, with corresponding PET-only axial (**e**) and coronal (**f**) views and (*right*) an anterior 3D MIP view). Further evaluation revealed stage 3A poorly differentiated primary adenocarcinoma of the lung. While most or even all of the skeletal focal lesions may be due to MM, the ^{18}F-FDG PET/CT scan cannot differentiate MM from skeletal metastases from other malignancies

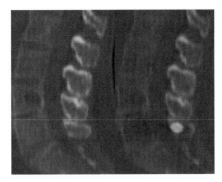

Fig. 2.13 X-ray or CT imaging alone can be very misleading as to disease status. A sagittal CT (*left*) with corresponding fused ^{18}F-FDG PET/CT image in a newly diagnosed MM patient reveals that x-ray, even CT-based x-ray, cannot demonstrate disease activity or the optimum site for biopsy. The sagittal CT image reveals an obvious focal OL lesion at L4 which the fused image reveals to be inactive. While the CT establishes the presence of symptomatic MM, a CT-directed biopsy of the CT focal OL lesion might not yield accurate diagnostic information, especially in regard to clinically relevant cytogenetic abnormalities (CGA) compared to the more metabolically active disease in the vertebral body of L5 or to the most metabolically active lesion in the spinous process of L5, neither of which are apparent on the CT-based imaging modality. Another smaller inactive CT focal OL lesion is present in the posterior aspect of S1

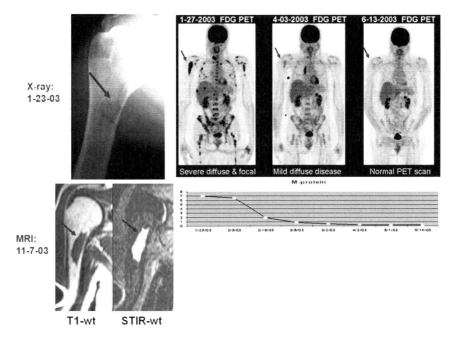

Fig. 2.14 ^{18}F-FDG PET and PET/CT demonstrate response to treatment contemporaneous to tumor response whereas MRI focal lesions (FL) response lags behind. A radiograph of the proximal right humerus (*upper left*) demonstrates a large focal OL lesion (*arrow*) at baseline. The anterior 3D MIP ^{18}F-FDG PET series (*top row, right*) demonstrates normalization of the abnormal diffuse skeletal uptake and the multiple PET-FL contemporaneous to the M protein response (shown by the graph of M protein levels below the PET images). Even though the patient remained in complete remission after the last PET scan, the MRI images of the proximal humerus (*lower left*) continued to demonstrate a large MRI FL for the next several months. In general, the larger the MRI-FL, the longer the patient must remain in remission for the MRI FL to eventually resolve. Since the corresponding MBS or CT OL bone lesion, if present, never resolves, the resolution of an MRI FL represents the replacement of the MRI-FL with fibrous scar tissue which has very low water content (most of the abnormal MRI findings from MM arise from the water in the MM cells) (Adapted from Walker et al. [50], used with permission)

time," contemporaneous to the response of M protein. On MRI, the diffuse marrow infiltration responses contemporaneous to M protein, as well, though focal lesions seen on MRI respond more slowly. In general, the larger the MRI-defined FL, the longer the time required for complete MRI resolution; indeed, despite durable CR lasting many years, some MRI FL never resolve [22, 36].

Both progression of disease and relapse are readily detected on either MRI or PET by an increase in the size and/or number of focal skeletal lesions and/or sites of EMD, or on PET, by an increase in ^{18}F-FDG uptake in the focal skeletal lesions or sites of EMD. Diffuse marrow progression is also readily evident on either MRI or PET as changes compatible with an increase in diffuse marrow infiltration by tumor, but only in the absence of marrow stimulation or chemotherapy rebound. While relapse or progression can occur at sites of previous focal lesions, new focal

Fig. 2.15 Rapid ^{18}F-FDG
PET response. This patient
with newly diagnosed MM
has a baseline PET scan
(anterior 3D MIP image, *left*)
demonstrating severe diffuse
and focal uptake with over
100 PET-FL. As part of an
experimental trial, a repeat
PET scan (anterior 3D MIP
image, *right*) 3 days after
initiation of treatment reveals
that only six PET-FL remain
and that the diffuse marrow
uptake has improved, though
not normalized. While the
diffuse marrow infiltration
seen on MRI would respond
almost as quickly, the MRI
FL would not

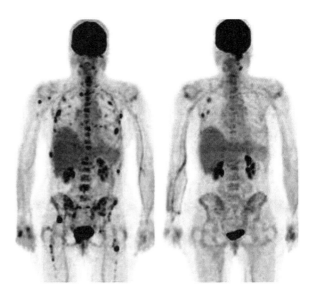

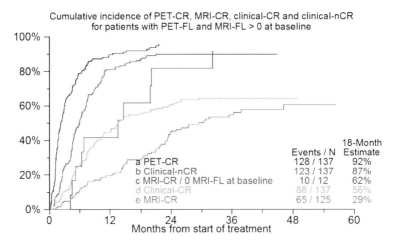

Fig. 2.16 Cumulative incidence of imaging response defined by clinical and imaging data. Cumulative incidence of normalization of the ^{18}F-FDG PET scan (PET-CR), MRI (MRI-CR), clinical response (clinical-CR), and clinical near complete response (clinical-nCR) for patients with PET-FL, 0 MRI-FL at baseline, and baseline MRI-FL >0. PET-CR closely tracks but actually precedes clinical-nCR, with patients with 0 MRI-FL at baseline slightly lagging clinical-nCR. CR and nCR status was determined in accordance with standard criteria [98, 99] (Adapted from Bartel et al. [22], epub ahead of print. Used with permission)

lesions at sites not previously involved with focal disease are also seen at relapse in about half of patients. Patients can relapse with fewer, the same number, or more FL than on prior imaging studies [22, 36].

Although originally intended for solid tumors, standard RECIST guidelines for determining complete response, partial response, stable disease, or relapse/progression are useful [65, 66]. There are shortcomings in WHO and RECIST criteria, leading to recent modification proposals of RECIST (RECIST 1.1) [66–71] and to a proposal for RECIST-like criteria modified for PET (PERCIST) [72]. High numbers of focal lesions on baseline examinations (three or more on PET and eight or more on MRI), confer poor long-term outcome, even in patients

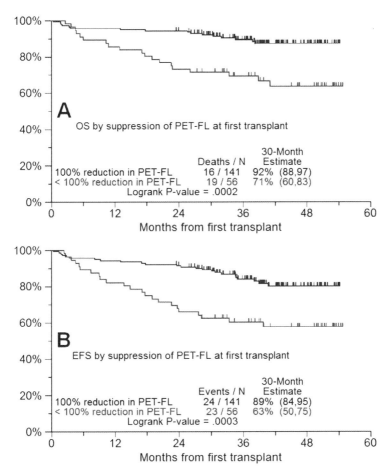

Fig. 2.17 KM analysis demonstrates superior overall survival (**a**, OS) and event-free survival (**b**, EFS) for patients with complete normalization of PET-FL or sites of EMD present at baseline. Normalization of these PET/CT findings confers superior outcome for patients who achieve resolution of the PET-FL and EMD uptake prior to the first of two autologous stem cell transplantations in the clinical trial Total Therapy 3. These results are analogous to results previously reported regarding the importance of achieving a PET-CR prior to stem cell transplantation in patients with malignant lymphoma [85, 100–103] (Adapted from Bartel et al. [22], epub ahead of print. Used with permission)

with gene expression profiling identifying low-risk disease, but does not correlate with short-term response [22]. The presence of EMD confers a very poor prognosis, especially if present at baseline [22]. As with malignant lymphoma, achieving normalization of the ^{18}F-FDG uptake in focal bone lesions and sites of EMD prior to stem cell transplantation is associated with superior durability of remission and improved survival, even in patients who, by gene expression profiling, are at high risk [22].

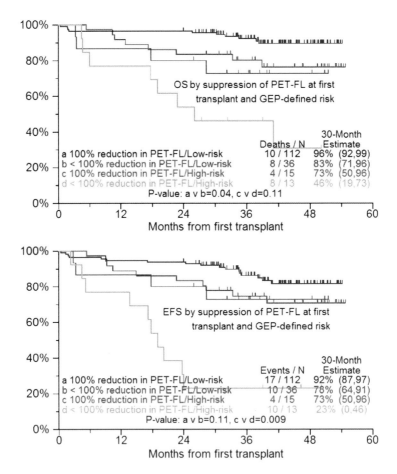

Fig. 2.18 KM analysis of overall survival (OS) and event-free survival (EFS) combining normalization of ^{18}F-FDG PET/CT of skeletal FL and sites of EMD prior to first of two autologous stem cell transplantations as part of the clinical trial Total Therapy 3, with the presence of high-risk disease as defined by gene expression profile [104] (GEP). Significance of normalization of uptake in skeletal focal lesions and sites of EMD had the greatest impact on EFS in high-risk GEP patients ($p = 0.009$) and marginal impact on OS ($p = 0.11$). While normalization of the PET-FL and EMD prior to first autologous stem cell transplantation marginally impacted EFS in the low-risk group ($p = 0.11$), the OS for this group significantly improved ($p = 0.04$). The OS and EFS for GEP high-risk patients who did not achieve PET-CR were particularly poor (Adapted from Bartel et al. [22], epub ahead of print. Used with permission)

2.3.7.2 Clinical Significance of Imaging Findings

Most (85%) MM patients will develop focal lesions during the course of their disease, though a minority of patients at time of diagnosis will have normal imaging examinations without evidence of either diffuse or focal disease of the skeletal system or soft tissues. The presence of more than one focal lesion on MRI, PET, or x-ray (CT or conventional x-ray) establishes the diagnosis of symptomatic MM with the exception of a less common entity known as "multiple solitary plasmacytomas" (an oxymoronic-sounding condition with multiple focal plasmacytoma lesions of bone but without a diffuse infiltration of the bone marrow with plasma cells – a marrow biopsy at a location away from the focal lesions fails to demonstrate tumor). Neither MRI nor PET imaging reliably distinguishes between MM and multiple solitary plasmacytomas since mild diffuse tumor infiltration of the marrow can be indistinguishable from normal marrow appearance. Since biopsy is still required for diagnosis of both MM and multiple solitary plasmacytomas, this is not a significant diagnostic issue [10, 62, 73, 74].

About 5% of patients with a plasma cell dyscrasia have true SEP or SBP. These patients present with only one apparent focal bone or soft tissue lesion (e.g., a solitary vertebral body compression fracture, rib fracture, or swelling). X-ray MBS may not reveal additional lesions. However, most of the patients initially thought to have SEP or SBP are actually under-staged MM patients. Random central marrow biopsy or additional imaging with MRI and/or whole-body ^{18}F-FDG PET or PET/CT will often demonstrate additional sites of tumor, leading to the appropriate diagnosis of symptomatic MM. Proper diagnosis is of obvious importance to patient care since SEP or SBP patients generally do not receive systemic treatment whereas MM patients do, and since the management and prognosis of these distinct entities are very different [10, 75–80].

The number of focal lesions at baseline on MBS, MRI, or ^{18}F-FDG PET is inversely and significantly related to event-free survival. The number of focal lesions at baseline on MBS or ^{18}F-FDG PET, but not MRI, is inversely and significantly related to event-free survival. Accordingly, the number of focal lesions identified at baseline and on follow-up examinations by these various imaging modalities is one of the key imaging findings to document. Indeed, the adverse impact of the number of focal lesions at baseline is second only to the presence of gene expression profile-defined high-risk disease [22, 36].

The physician interpreting an imaging examination for MM should report the number of MRI- or PET-defined focal lesions, and, if PET/CT is used, the presence and approximate number of x-ray focal osteolytic lesions and whether or not a given x-ray focal OL is metabolically active. Similar to reporting the imaging results of other malignancies, standard WHO or RECIST reporting criteria regarding size and location of sites of tumor involvement should be given to allow detailed comparison on subsequent examinations. If there are too many focal lesions (e.g., more than 20) to permit detailed reporting of each one, then the interpreting physician should select a suitable number of "sentinel" lesions (typically 10 or less) for detailed reporting. These sentinel lesions are typically the largest (or, on ^{18}F-FDG PET or PET/CT, the most metabolically active), though lesions of "high interest" (e.g., lesions in

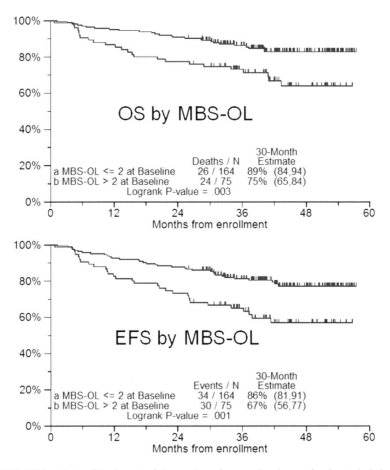

Fig. 2.19 KM analysis of the impact of the number of conventional x-ray focal osteolytic lesions (MBS-OL) at baseline on overall survival (OS) and event-free survival (EFS). More than two MBS-OL seen on baseline MBS significantly impacts both OS ($p < 0.003$) and EFS ($p < 0.001$). These data are derived from the clinical trial Total Therapy 3 (Adapted from Bartel et al. [22], epub ahead of print. Used with permission)

high-risk locations such as near the spinal cord or in an extramedullary location) should be reported regardless of other characteristics. Interestingly, while an increase in size indicates progression of disease, it is the number of focal lesions on MRI or PET, not the maximum size of a specific focal lesion, which inversely correlates with patient outcome [22].

The greatest uptake in focal lesions should be specifically reported, as well as the location of the corresponding focal, so that this area of greatest metabolic activity can be targeted, if possible, for image-guided biopsy. In a large prospective series, Bartel and coworkers [22] found, on univariate analysis, that the maximum uptake of focal lesions (using a cutoff of 4, normalized to lean body mass) on

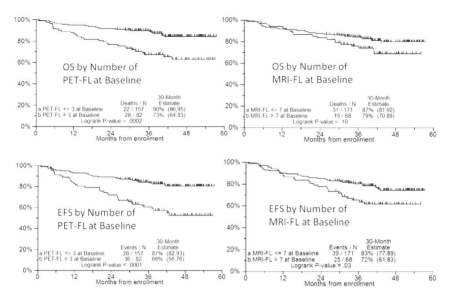

Fig. 2.20 KM analysis of the impact of the number of PET-FL and MRI-FL at baseline on overall survival (OS) and event-free survival (EFS). More than three PET-FL seen on ^{18}F-FDG PET baseline staging significantly impacts OS and EFS. More than seven MRI-FL seen on baseline staging significantly impacts EFS but not OS. These data are derived from the clinical trial Total Therapy 3 (Adapted from Bartel et al. [22], epub ahead of print. Used with permission)

^{18}F-FDG PET/CT imaging at baseline was positively correlated with event-free survival ($p = 0.22$) but not with overall survival, though significance was borderline ($p = 0.52$). Very importantly, failure to completely normalize the PET/CT scan ("PET-CR") prior to the first of two autologous stem cell transplantations significantly and adversely affected both event-free survival and overall survival. Even in gene expression profile-defined high-risk patients, ^{18}F-FDG PET/CT scan normalization prior to the first of two autologous stem cell transplantations had greater positive impact on long-term prognosis than achieving a clinical complete remission. In patients with gene expression profile-defined low-risk, large numbers of PET-FL at baseline significantly and adversely affected outcome [22].

While previous investigators have usually reported maximum SUV values within a defined region of interest (SUVmax) normalized to body weight, modern PET imaging systems allow direct reporting of SUV measurements normalized to lean body mass (LBM). Reporting of SUVmax values from ^{18}F-FDG PET or PET/CT scans normalized to LBM is preferable to body weight for MM patients because body weight can vary widely over the many years that patients with MM must be followed, and because body weight can vary dramatically for patients depending on whether or not they are currently being treated with high-dose dexamethasone. These changes in body weight will change the calculated ^{18}F-FDG SUVmax value normalized to body weight in direct proportion to the difference in body weight between the PET scans, even if there is no change in the actual metabolic rate of the region being measured. Normalization of SUVmax uptake measurements to lean body mass will reduce these artifactual fluctuations in ^{18}F-FDG SUVmax measurements, thereby improving correlation with actual change in tumor metabolic rate. SUVmax normalized to LBM is also reported in other malignancies to correlate better with outcome than SUVmax normalized to body weight. Thus, for both baseline correlation with prognosis and subsequent assessment of response to treatment, SUVmax normalized to LBM should be used for all SUV measurements [22, 81].

Another acceptable method for semi-quantitative reporting of ^{18}F-FDG uptake on PET or PET/CT scans is to report the uptake in a range relative to an internal reference standard, such as uptake in the area of suspected tumor relative to the uptake in an area that is not thought to be involved with tumor, such as a normal appearing region of the liver, or to the mediastinal blood pool. The uptake is then described relative to the reference tissue as being mild (less than the reference tissue), moderate (about the same as the reference tissue), or intense (greater than the reference tissue). Use of a built-in reference tissue helps to compensate for changes in body weight, patient blood sugar at time of radioisotope injection, change in time between radioisotope injection and initiation of the PET or PET/CT scan when comparing examinations, variation in SUV measurements between PET or PET/CT scanners and/or manufacturers, etc. [51, 64].

With low numbers (e.g., 10 or less) of MRI FL, PET-FL, or CT focal OL lesions, it is possible to report the specific number of FLs, the MRI- or CT-defined maximum axial diameter of the larger one(s) as "sentinel" lesions, and single greatest SUVmax (assuming PET or PET/CT is utilized). On follow-up, comparison of these data is helpful to improve objective assessment of response to treatment or to detect relapse or progression. Either MRI or PET can detect relapse or progression, and these two examinations are complementary for this purpose. While the MRI and the PET or PET/CT examinations are often concordant, discordant results must not be dismissed and should be investigated further (e.g., with laboratory or tissue confirmation) [82]. Direct visual comparison of examinations is required since the number of focal lesions can remain the same or even decrease between examinations and yet new focal lesions can appear, strongly suggesting progression or relapse. Likewise, on ^{18}F-FDG PET or PET/CT, the specific lesion with the greatest metabolic activity on a previous scan may remain the same or even decrease in uptake, and yet the uptake in another region of tumor may be increasing, meeting RECIST criteria for progression or relapse.

When progression or relapse on MRI and/or PET or PET/CT is suspected, often standard laboratory evidence is supportive and no further verification is required. However, on short-term follow-up with ^{18}F-FDG PET or PET/CT, sometimes transient increase in ^{18}F-FDG uptake can occur, thought to be due to a treatment-induced inflammatory response that can last for several days to weeks. Accordingly, restaging of patients after treatment with ^{18}F-FDG PET or PET/CT is best done a minimum of 2 weeks, and preferably 4 or more weeks, after completion of a treatment cycle. However, if progression or relapse on treatment is suspected, ^{18}F-FDG PET or PET/CT can often provide verification, and, if indicated, direct biopsy or treatment, such as focal radiation or a change in chemotherapy. Because of this

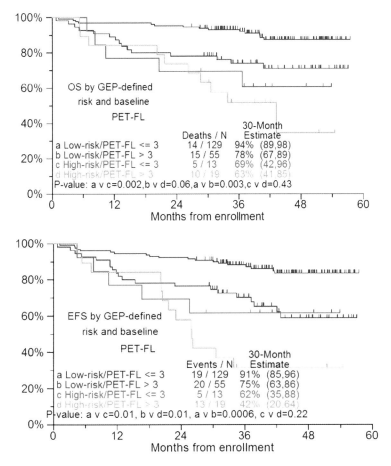

Fig. 2.21 KM analysis of overall survival (OS) and event-free survival (EFS) combining high-risk myeloma as defined by gene expression profiling [104] with the number of ^{18}F-FDG PET/CT-defined focal lesions at baseline examination. The patients are divided into two groups relative to the number of PET-FL, 0–3 and >3. The number of PET-FL at baseline in the low-risk group significantly impacted both OS and EFS but not in the high-risk group. Data were derived from the clinical trial Total Therapy 3 (Adapted from from Bartel et al. [22], epub ahead of print. Used with permission)

treatment-related uptake on ^{18}F-FDG PET and PET/CT, the negative predictive value of PET is superior to the positive predictive value, with treatment-related uptake sometimes persisting for weeks. Radiation therapy-related uptake, in particular, can persist for months, especially in the lungs and pleura. Importantly, the use of PET/CT is superior to PET alone because the CT portion of the PET/CT can demonstrate changes that are not visible on PET-only examinations if there is indolent disease with low ^{18}F-FDG uptake relative to surrounding tissues, such as a CT-visualized increase in tumor size [83–86].

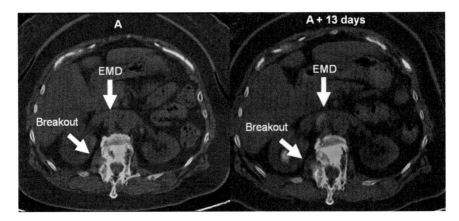

Fig. 2.22 ^{18}F-FDG PET/CT series demonstrating progression of disease on treatment. Axial fused PET/CT image (A) in a patient on treatment prior to progression demonstrates a site of EMD (*vertical arrow*) deep to the left renal vein and a skeletal "breakout" focal lesion to the *right* of the nearby vertebral body (*oblique arrow*). The corresponding axial fused PET/CT image obtained 13 days later during progression on treatment demonstrates increasing size and uptake of both the EMD and the breakout lesion

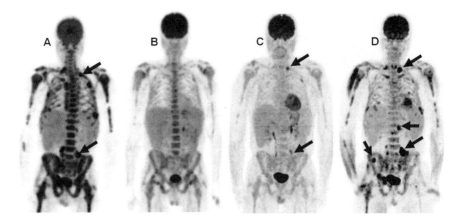

Fig. 2.23 ^{18}F-FDG PET/CT series demonstrating progression of disease on treatment. Anterior 3D MIP at presentation (**a**) demonstrates severe diffuse marrow tumor infiltration as well as EMD of the brachial plexus (*upper arrow*) and lumbar plexus (*lower arrow*). Hepatosplenomegaly is present, perhaps from extramedullary hematopoiesis. (**b**) An anterior 3D MIP image from a PET/CT performed 50 days later on treatment demonstrates resolution of EMD uptake and improving but still present diffuse and focal marrow uptake. Treatment continued with the patient's tumor markers improving, but with a sudden rise in serum lactate dehydrogenase occurring 65 days after presentation; a PET/CT scan obtained at this time (**c**) demonstrates relapsing sites of EMD in the brachial plexus (*upper arrow*) and lumbar plexus (*lower arrow*), even though the diffuse marrow uptake has improved. Despite aggressive and continued treatment, 80 days after presentation a PET/CT (**d**) demonstrates progression of preexistent sites of EMD, new sites of EMD, and marked progression of both diffuse and focal skeletal lesions. This series demonstrates the utility of ^{18}F-FDG PET and PET/CT to demonstrate the presence and site(s) of progression of disease on treatment

2.3.7.3 Extramedullary Disease (EMD)

The identification of EMD is very important because its presence identifies a patient at high risk, with inferior outcome compared to patients of similar stage without EMD. EMD represents a clinical entity that is, relative to medullary tumor, typically less differentiated, often nonsecretory, rapidly progressive, and treatment resistant, by definition capable of growing without dependency on the marrow microenvironment. Median survival for relapsing or refractory patients with EMD is less than 1 year. EMD can be detected with MRI, PET, PET/CT, or MIBI imaging, with PET, PET/CT, and MIBI superior to MRI because of their wider, whole-body fields of view compared to regional MRI examination [22, 61].

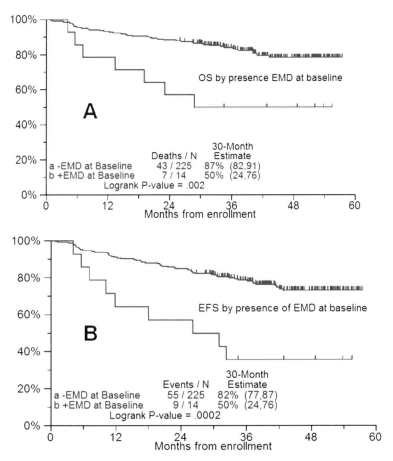

Fig. 2.24 KM analysis of overall survival (**a**), OS, and event-free survival (**b**), EFS, of patients treated in the clinical trial Total Therapy 3 based on the presence or absence of EMD at baseline. The presence of EMD at baseline identifies a high-risk subset of patients in terms of both OS and EFS (Adapted from Bartel et al. [22], epub ahead of print. Used with permission)

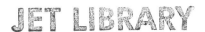

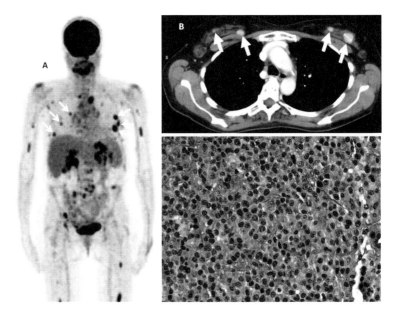

Fig. 2.25 Anterior 3D MIP image (**a**, *left*) from an ^{18}F-FDG PET/CT as part of baseline staging demonstrated extensive diffuse and focal bone disease as well as 21 sites of EMD (eight in the breasts with three in each breast visible on the 3D MIP image, *arrows*). A single axial image from a contrast-enhanced CT (**b**, *upper right*) subsequently performed demonstrated two sites of EMD in each breast. Needle core biopsy of one of the lesions (*lower right*) demonstrates diffuse plasma cell infiltration

2.3.7.4 Detection of Infection

Occult infection is a significant source of morbidity and mortality for patients undergoing treatment for malignancy. The use of chronic pain medication, the frequent use of high-dose glucocorticoid medications, and the frequent presence of tumor-related fever can make detection of infection problematic clinically. Elevation of C-reactive protein can suggest infection but is nonspecific. Chemotherapy frequently produces both significant neutropenia and diminished function of white blood cells, reducing the accuracy of radiolabeled leukocytes to identify the presence or site of infection, especially if the patient has received antibiotics [87]. In this difficult clinical setting, ^{18}F-FDG PET and PET/CT can often detect occult infection as a focal region of uptake. For PET-only scanners, regions of uptake thought to be due to infection rather than tumor are best verified in comparison with both earlier PET scans and contemporaneous additional imaging, such as CT or MRI. With PET/CT, the CT portion of the examination allows immediate correlation of uptake with anatomic appearance and is superior to other imaging methods for detection of occult infection [87]. Fortunately, ^{18}F-FDG PET is effective in detection of infection in clinical settings where other imaging means often fail, such as in patients with significant neutropenia (<1,000 neutrophils/ml)

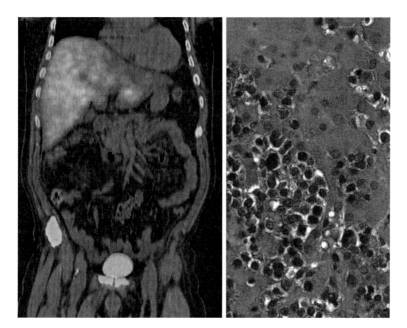

Fig. 2.26 EMD presenting as diffuse liver infiltration as seen on ^{18}F-FDG PET/CT. A coronal PET/CT (*left*) of the abdomen and pelvis in a patient with relapsing MM demonstrates diffuse increased uptake in the liver. A liver biopsy (*right*) demonstrates plasma cell infiltration in the liver parenchyma

or severe immunosuppression (neutrophils, lymphocytes, and/or CD4 counts <100 cells/ml) [49].

^{18}F-FDG PET or PET/CT can also detect, as an "incidental" but clinically relevant finding, clinically silent infections as well as infections not detectable by other methods, such as central venous catheter-associated septic thrombophlebitis, STP, an important source of bacteremia, and, potentially, sepsis. ^{18}F-FDG PET contributes significantly to patient management in this setting by identification of the presence and site of infection, by determination of the extent of infection, and by modification of the diagnostic work-up and/or therapy [46, 49, 87].

^{18}F-FDG PET or PET/CT scans can demonstrate a wide range of infections, including spontaneous STP (without an associated central venous catheter), sinusitis, lung infection, osteomyelitis, discitis, cellulitis, mastoiditis, and infections of the GU or GI tracts. Periodontal abscesses are frequent and must be excluded from tumor involvement of the maxilla or mandible or from osteonecrosis of the mandible or maxilla. While a variety of organisms are responsible for mandibular or maxillary infections, fungal infection in this population ("lumpy jaw" from *Actinomycosis* sp. infection) should be considered, often associated with regions of osteonecrosis [38, 39, 49, 88].

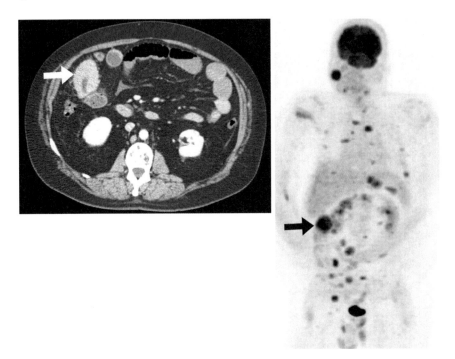

Fig. 2.27 EMD of the small bowel identified with ^{18}F-FDG PET. An anterior 3D MIP image from an ^{18}F-FDG PET scan (*right*) demonstrates extensive focal skeletal disease as well as a metabolically active focal mass in the abdomen (*arrow*). A follow-up diagnostic CT axial image (*left*) demonstrates a site of EMD associated with the hepatic flexure region of the large bowel (*arrow*)

GI tract infections include treatment-associated mucositis/colitis as well as immunosuppression-related entities, such as infectious esophagitis, diverticulitis, and abdominal abscess. While paranasal sinus infection is common, uptake on ^{18}F-FDG PET can be minimal or absent, though air/fluid levels or mucosal thickening with or without uptake can still be seen on the CT portion of the PET/CT. Chronic paranasal sinus retention cysts can be associated with focal uptake on ^{18}F-FDG PET scanning, sometimes quite intense [49].

Patients with hematological malignancies are at high risk for development of lung infections, especially within the first 100 days of stem cell transplantation, occurring in about 7%. Though multiple organisms are responsible (bacterial, viral, and fungal), *Cytomegalovirus* (about 37%) and *Aspergillus* sp. (about 30%) are the two most common pathogens. During the first 30 days after transplant, fungal etiologies caused the majority of pulmonary infections (about 80%). Between days 31 and 100, viral etiologies predominated (about 60%). Interestingly, in one report recipients of allogeneic transplants had a higher probability of developing *Cytomegalovirus* pneumonitis than recipients of autologous or syngeneic transplants ($p < 0.001$). Radiographically, *Cytomegalovirus* pneumonia typically presents with parenchymal

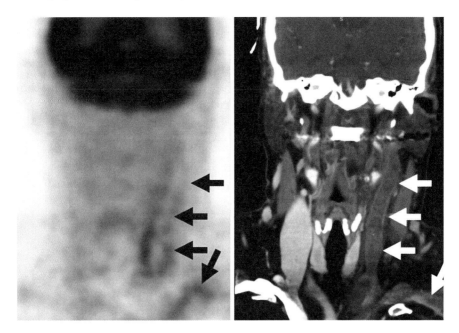

Fig. 2.28 Septic thrombophlebitis (STP) discovered with ^{18}F-FDG PET. A coronal anterior view of the head and neck region (*left*) of a patient with MM and an elevated C-reactive protein demonstrates uptake along the margins of the left common jugular vein (*horizontal arrows*) and the left subclavian vein (*oblique arrow*). A corresponding view from a subsequent contrast-enhanced CT (*right*) demonstrates intraluminal thrombus outlined by the IV contrast in these blood vessels (*corresponding arrows*). The patient had a left subclavian infusion catheter (withdrawn prior to the CT scan) that leads to STP of the left subclavian vein, with propagation into the left innominate vein (not shown) and, in a retrograde fashion, into the left common jugular vein. The patient was on high-dose dexamethasone and narcotic pain medications, with the site of the suspected infection not apparent clinically. Infection was confirmed by culture of the catheter

opacification (90%) and/or with innumerable sub-5 mm nodules (30%), though occasionally x-rays were normal. *Aspergillus* infection commonly presents with nodules, masses, or both [89].

2.4 Imaging of Other Plasma Cell Dyscrasias

2.4.1 Monoclonal Gammopathy of Uncertain Significance (MGUS)

Most authorities consider monoclonal gammopathy of undetermined significance (MGUS) the usual precursor of MM, being indistinguishable from MM based on gene expression profiling and having the same genomic instability. About 1%

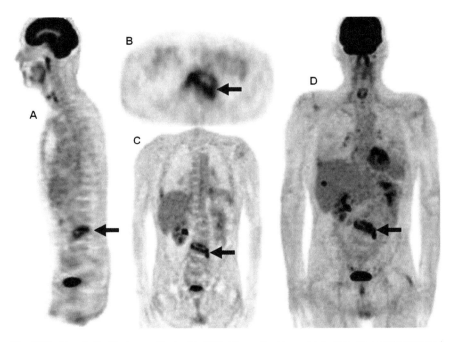

Fig. 2.29 Occult discitis in a patient with MM. The patient is on high-dose dexamethasone and pain medications with chronic back pain. An ^{18}F-FDG PET scan sagittal (**a**), axial (**b**), and coronal (**c**) views through the L2/3 level of the lumbar spine reveals intense uptake in the interspace level (*arrows*) as opposed to the vertebral body, where tumor more commonly occurs. There is extrusion of the region of uptake also seen to the *left* and inferiorly (best seen on the anterior 3D maximum intensity projection, **d**). A CT-guided aspiration verified infection

progress to MM annually. PET scans in MGUS should be normal. Since focal lesions (on x-ray, CT, MRI, PET, or PET/CT) and EMD are not seen in MGUS, the presence of such findings strongly suggests progression to symptomatic MM. ^{18}F-FDG PET or PET/CT, with the wider, "whole-body" field of view compared to MRI, is an excellent means to screen for progression to MM [17, 90].

2.4.2 Solitary Plasmacytoma

Solitary plasmacytoma occurs in two varieties, solitary extramedullary plasmacytoma (SEP), occurring exclusively in the soft tissues, and solitary bone plasmacytoma (SBP), occurring in the skeletal system. SEP has a high cure rate with radiation and is unlikely to progress to MM. On imaging examinations (CT, PET/CT, or MRI) SEP is seen as a nonspecific soft tissue mass (^{18}F-FDG – avid on PET). Biopsy demonstrates a focal plasmacytoma. Patients with SBP progress to MM at about 3% annually. ^{18}F-FDG PET and PET/CT performed for patients with SBP can

Fig. 2.30 Occult infection in a patient with MM. An anterior 3D maximum intensity projection image from a whole-body ^{18}F-FDG PET scan in a patient who is neutropenic from treatment demonstrates increased uptake associated with the pocket of an indwelling infusion catheter (*arrow*). Aspiration and culture revealed infection

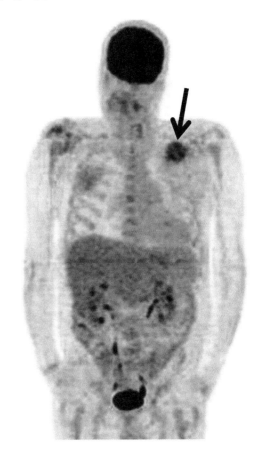

demonstrate additional, unsuspected lesions, upgrading the diagnosis to MM or multiple solitary plasmacytomas. The use of imaging for SBP for staging or restaging is similar to the use of imaging in MM [79, 91, 92].

2.4.3 Castleman's Disease

Benjamin Castleman first described Castleman's disease in 1956, later divided into two subtypes, unicentric and multicentric. Unicentric Castleman's disease has a relatively favorable prognosis and is often diagnosed incidentally. Multicentric Castleman's disease is a polyclonal lymphoproliferative disorder characterized by recurrent fevers, lymphadenopathy, hepatosplenomegaly, and autoimmune phenomena. Multicentric Castleman's disease has a relatively poor prognosis, sometimes progressing to malignant lymphoma. The plasma cell variant of multicentric

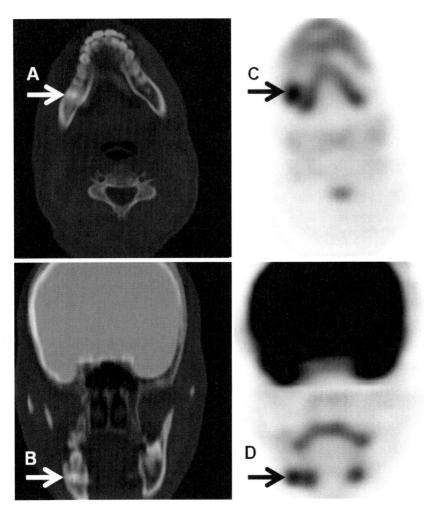

Fig. 2.31 Occult infection in a patient with MM. Axial and coronal fused PET/CT (**a** and **b**) with corresponding PET images (**c** and **d**) demonstrate intense uptake associated with a lytic defect at the base of the posterior right mandibular molar (*arrows*). The ¹⁸F-FDG PET/CT scan was performed as part of the evaluation of this patient with newly diagnosed MM. The patient was to undergo myeloablation in preparation for the first of two autologous stem cell transplantations. The whole-body PET/CT examination allowed detection and subsequent treatment of this patient's occult infection prior to myeloablation

Castleman's disease is frequently associated with HIV infection and sometimes with HHV-8 infection [93–96].

¹⁸F-FDG PET and PET/CT have similar utility in Castleman's disease to their use in lymphoma, demonstrating active regions of disease and response to treatment. ¹⁸F-FDG PET/CT is particularly helpful since the CT images also allow demonstration of adenopathy that may not be ¹⁸F-FDG – avid.

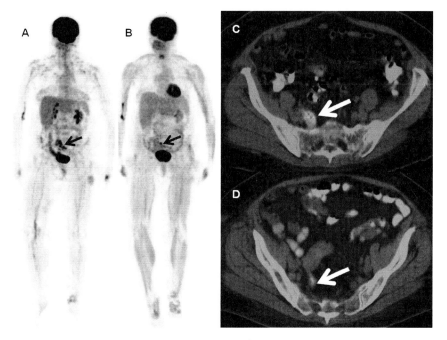

Fig. 2.32 Occult peridiverticular abscess seen with ^{18}F-FDG PET/CT. A patient with MM on high-dose dexamethasone receives a restaging ^{18}F-FDG PET/CT scan (**a**, anterior 3D MIP), revealing an intense focus of activity in the right pelvis corresponding on the axial fused PET/CT image of the pelvis (**c**) to a region of uptake associated with bowel wall thickening and pericolonic stranding characteristic in appearance for a peridiverticular abscess (*arrows*). The patient was asymptomatic due to high-dose dexamethasone and narcotic pain medications, though he did have an elevated C-reactive protein. After treatment, a follow-up ^{18}F-FDG PET/CT scan documents response to treatment in a patient who cannot be followed by clinical examination (**b**, anterior 3D MIP and **d**, axial fused PET/CT). ^{18}F-FDG PET/CT can be used to detect the presence and the site of occult infection, to contribute to the choice of antibiotic selection and treatment regimen, and to document treatment response in this difficult clinical setting, even in patients with severe neutropenia [49]

2.5 Waldenström's Macroglobulinemia

Waldenström's macroglobulinemia (WM) is a variant of non-Hodgkin's lymphoma characterized by a monoclonal lymphoplasmacytic expansion accompanied by secretion of serum monoclonal immunoglobulin M (IgM). Jan G. Waldenström originally described the disease in 1944. WM is uncommon, with about one-tenth the prevalence of MM. WM has an overall better prognosis and median survival than MM. WM is believed to be more common in Caucasians and in men. The median age at diagnosis is 63 years. Analogous to MM, a significant risk factor for development of WM is the presence of IgM-MGUS.The typical findings of WM on ^{18}F-FDG PET and PET/CT are similar to those of lymphoma,

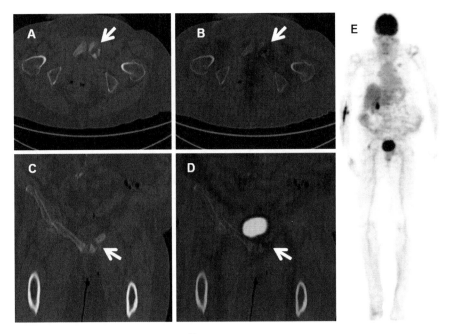

Fig. 2.33 MGUS upgraded to MM by ^{18}F-FDG PET/CT. Axial (**a** and **b**) and coronal (**c** and **d**) CT and fused PET/CT images, respectively, with an anterior 3D MIP (**e**) in a patient with MGUS being evaluated annually for possible conversion to MM demonstrate a focal OL lesion in the left superior pubic ramus on CT and PET/CT (*arrows*) with an associated pathologic fracture. Image-directed biopsy confirmed conversion to symptomatic MM. No other focal lesions were present

with hepatosplenomegaly (especially involving the spleen), lymphadenopathy with increased ^{18}F-FDG nodal uptake, and, rarely, focal lesions of bone similar to MM [97].

2.6 Summary

MRI and ^{18}F-FDG PET or PET/CT scanning in MM and related plasma cell dyscrasias are useful and reliable techniques that assist diagnosis through identification of "high-yield" locations for biopsy and are useful for staging and restaging patients, detecting EMD, and demonstrating response to treatment. Because of the wider field of view of whole-body PET and PET/CT, detection of the sites and number of EMD lesions with PET, PET/CT, or MIBI is superior to MRI, which has a more restricted field of view, though whole-body MRI is a developing technology which may one day allow MRI to be as accurate as PET or PET/CT for the identification of EMD. MRI, PET, and PET/CT are equally effective in secretory or nonsecretory disease, with nonsecretory disease occurring with increasing frequency during the course of the disease, leading to difficulty in the monitoring of disease status.

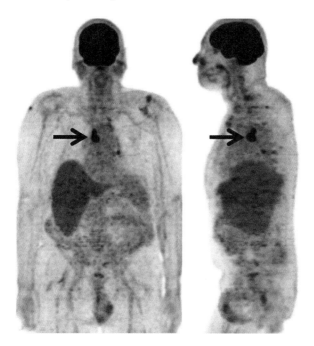

Fig. 2.34 Solitary extramedullary plasmacytoma as seen on ^{18}F-FDG PET/CT. Anterior (*left*) and lateral (*right*) 3D MIP images from a whole-body PET scan demonstrate intensely increased uptake in a mediastinal mass (*arrows*) which was initially discovered by CT (not shown) in a patient with incidental laboratory findings suggesting possible MM. The patient's CT of the chest, abdomen, and pelvis, standard x-ray MBS, and extensive MRI series were otherwise normal. A random marrow biopsy was within normal limits. Biopsy of the mass demonstrated a soft tissue plasmacytoma

^{18}F-FDG PET and PET/CT are especially useful techniques in patients with hematological malignancies for detection of the presence and location of occult infection and for documenting response to treatment of the infection, even in the setting of severe immunosuppression. The information gained by ^{18}F-FDG PET or PET/CT in infectious disease management often contribute to changes in patient management and, by identification of the location of the infection, in the choice of antibiotics.

The presence of a high number of focal lesions, especially gene expression profile-defined high-risk MM and/or the presence of EMD, identifies patients at high risk with poor long-term prognosis who may benefit aggressive monitoring and treatment.

As with malignant lymphoma, treatment successful in suppression of uptake in all ^{18}F-FDG PET or PET/CT skeletal FL and sites of EMD prior to initial stem cell transplantation confers superior overall and event-free survival.

Progression of disease on treatment identified by medical imaging is a poor prognostic sign identifying patients in need of immediate intervention.

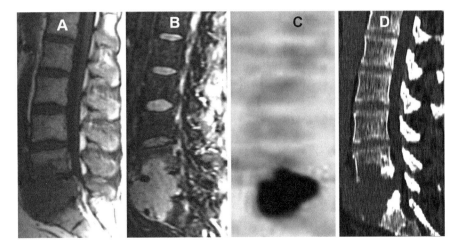

Fig. 2.35 Solitary bone plasmacytoma. Sagittal T1-weighted MRI (**a**), T2-weighted MRI (**b**), ¹⁸F-FDG PET (**c**), and CT (**d**) images of the lumbar spine demonstrate a soft tissue mass at the L5/S1 level with destructive, osteolytic changes involving L5 and S1, with "breakout" into the surrounding tissues.

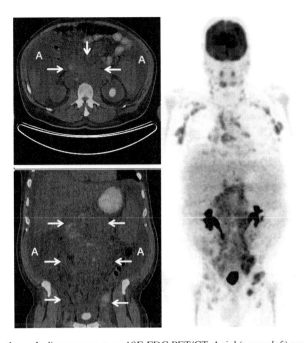

Fig. 2.36 Castleman's disease as seen on 18F-FDG PET/CT. Axial (*upper left*) and coronal (*lower left*) fused PET/CT images with an anterior 3D MIP image (*right*) demonstrate severe adenopathy with increased uptake in the cervical, axillary, lateral thoracic, mediastinal, retroperitoneal, and inguinal regions. The fused PET/CT images also reveal a large amount of malignant ascites (*A*) as well as the conglomerate retroperitoneal nodal mass (*arrows*) in this patient presenting with multicentric Castleman's disease

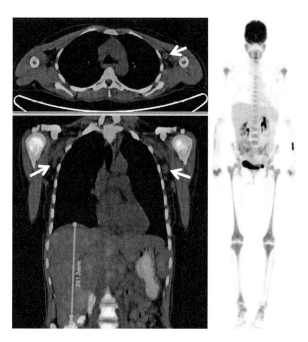

Fig. 2.37 Waldenstrom's macroglobulinemia (WM) as seen on ^{18}F-FDG PET/CT. Axial (*upper left*) and coronal (*lower left*) fused PET/CT images with an anterior whole-body 3D MIP image (*right*) demonstrate abnormally increased uptake throughout the marrow space, extending into the distal tibiae. Adenopathy with increased uptake is also present in the bilateral axillary regions (*arrows*). Hepatomegaly is also present as seen on the coronal image in this patient with intramedullary and extramedullary WM

◀——

Fig. 2.35 (continued) MBS, extensive MRI, and whole-body PET scanning failed to demonstrate additional lesions. Biopsy of the marrow away from the single bone lesion failed to demonstrate evidence of tumor. The patient was treated for a solitary bone plasmacytoma and did well, without progression to MM at last follow-up (Adapted from Walker et al. [50], used with permission)

References

1. Angtuaco EJ, Fassas AB, Walker R, Sethi R, Barlogie B. Multiple myeloma: clinical review and diagnostic imaging. Radiology. 2004;231:11–23.
2. Dankerl A, Liebisch P, Glatting G, et al. Multiple myeloma: molecular imaging with 11C-methionine PET/CT – initial experience. Radiology. 2007;242:498–508.
3. Nanni C, Zamagni E, Cavo M, et al. 11C-choline vs. 18F-FDG PET/CT in assessing bone involvement in patients with multiple myeloma. World J Surg Oncol. 2007;5:68.
4. Pace L, Catalano L, Pinto A, et al. Different patterns of technetium-99m sestamibi uptake in multiple myeloma. Eur J Nucl Med. 1998;25:714–720.
5. Fonti R, Del Vecchio S, Zannetti A, et al. Bone marrow uptake of 99mTc-MIBI in patients with multiple myeloma. Eur J Nucl Med. 2001;28:214–220.

6. Chiu ML, Kronauge JF, Piwnica-Worms D. Effect of mitochondrial and plasma membrane potentials on accumulation of hexakis (2-methoxyisobutylisonitrile) technetium(I) in cultured mouse fibroblasts. J Nucl Med. 1990;31:1646–1653.

7. Tian E, Zhan F, Walker R, et al. The role of the Wnt-signaling antagonist DKK1 in the development of osteolytic lesions in multiple myeloma. N Engl J Med. 2003;349: 2483–2494.

8. Roodman GD. Pathogenesis of myeloma bone disease. Blood Cells Mol Dis. 2004;32: 290–292.

9. Epstein J, Walker R. Myeloma and bone disease: "the dangerous tango". Clin Adv Hematol Oncol. 2006;4:300–306.

10. Nanni C, Rubello D, Zamagni E, et al. 18F-FDG PET/CT in myeloma with presumed solitary plasmocytoma of bone. In Vivo. 2008;22:513–517.

11. Blade J, Kyle RA. Nonsecretory myeloma, immunoglobulin D myeloma, and plasma cell leukemia. Hematol Oncol Clin North Am. 1999;13:1259–1272.

12. Dispenzieri A, Kyle R, Merlini G, et al. International Myeloma Working Group guidelines for serum-free light chain analysis in multiple myeloma and related disorders. Leukemia. 2009;23:215–224.

13. Drayson M, Tang LX, Drew R, Mead GP, Carr-Smith H, Bradwell AR. Serum free light-chain measurements for identifying and monitoring patients with nonsecretory multiple myeloma. Blood. 2001;97:2900–2902.

14. Durie BG, Kyle RA, Belch A, et al. Myeloma management guidelines: a consensus report from the Scientific Advisors of the International Myeloma Foundation. Hematol J. 2003;4:379–398.

15. Orchard K, Barrington S, Buscombe J, Hilson A, Prentice HG, Mehta A. Fluorodeoxyglucose positron emission tomography imaging for the detection of occult disease in multiple myeloma. Br J Haematol. 2002;117:133–135.

16. Schirrmeister H, Bommer M, Buck AK, et al. Initial results in the assessment of multiple myeloma using 18F-FDG PET. Eur J Nucl Med Mol Imaging. 2002;29:361–366.

17. Durie BG, Waxman AD, D'Agnolo A, Williams CM. Whole-body (18)F-FDG PET identifies high-risk myeloma. J Nucl Med. 2002;43:1457–1463.

18. Durie BG, Salmon SE. A clinical staging system for multiple myeloma. Correlation of measured myeloma cell mass with presenting clinical features, response to treatment, and survival. Cancer. 1975;36:842–854.

19. Durie BG. The role of anatomic and functional staging in myeloma: description of Durie/Salmon plus staging system. Eur J Cancer. 2006;42:1539–1543.

20. Edelstyn GA, Gillespie PJ, Grebbell FS. The radiological demonstration of osseous metastases. Experimental observations. Clin Radiol. 1967;18:158–162.

21. Baur-Melnyk A, Reiser M. [Staging of multiple myeloma with MRI: comparison to MSCT and conventional radiography]. Radiologe. 2004;44:874–881.

22. Bartel TB, Haessler J, Brown TL, et al. F18-fluorodeoxyglucose positron emission tomography in the context of other imaging techniques and prognostic factors in multiple myeloma. Blood. September 3, 2009;114(10):2068–2076.

23. Dispenzieri A, Kyle RA, Lacy MQ, et al. POEMS syndrome: definitions and long-term outcome. Blood. 2003;101:2496–2506.

24. Gandhi GY, Basu R, Dispenzieri A, Basu A, Montori VM, Brennan MD. Endocrinopathy in POEMS syndrome: the Mayo Clinic experience. Mayo Clin Proc. 2007;82:836–842.

25. Dispenzieri A. POEMS syndrome. Blood Rev. 2007;21:285–299.

26. Prasad R, Yadav RR, Singh A, Mathur SP, Mangal Y, Singh M.. Case report. Non-secretory multiple myeloma presenting with diffuse sclerosis of affected bones interspersed with osteolytic lesions. Br J Radiol. 2009;82:e29–e31.

27. Ludwig H, Fruhwald F, Tscholakoff D, Rasoul S, Neuhold A, Fritz E. Magnetic resonance imaging of the spine in multiple myeloma. Lancet. 1987;2:364–366.

28. Fruehwald FX, Tscholakoff D, Schwaighofer B, et al. Magnetic resonance imaging of the lower vertebral column in patients with multiple myeloma. Invest Radiol. 1988;23:193–199.

29. Libshitz HI, Malthouse SR, Cunningham D, MacVicar AD, Husband JE. Multiple myeloma: appearance at MR imaging. Radiology. 1992;182:833–837.
30. Moulopoulos LA, Varma DG, Dimopoulos MA, et al. Multiple myeloma: spinal MR imaging in patients with untreated newly diagnosed disease. Radiology. 1992;185:833–840.
31. Rahmouni A, Divine M, Mathieu D, et al. Detection of multiple myeloma involving the spine: efficacy of fat-suppression and contrast-enhanced MR imaging. AJR Am J Roentgenol. 1993;160:1049–1052.
32. Moulopoulos LA, Dimopoulos MA, Smith TL, et al. Prognostic significance of magnetic resonance imaging in patients with asymptomatic multiple myeloma. J Clin Oncol. 1995;13:251–256.
33. Dimopoulos MA, Moulopoulos LA, Datseris I, et al. Imaging of myeloma bone disease – implications for staging, prognosis and follow-up. Acta Oncol. 2000;39:823–827.
34. Tertti R, Alanen A, Remes K. The value of magnetic resonance imaging in screening myeloma lesions of the lumbar spine. Br J Haematol. 1995;91:658–660.
35. Van de Berg BC, Lecouvet FE, Michaux L, et al. Stage I multiple myeloma: value of MR imaging of the bone marrow in the determination of prognosis. Radiology. 1996;201: 243–246.
36. Walker R, Barlogie B, Haessler J, et al. Magnetic resonance imaging in multiple myeloma: diagnostic and clinical implications. J Clin Oncol. 2007;25:1121–1128.
37. Talamo G, Angtuaco E, Walker RC, et al. Avascular necrosis of femoral and/or humeral heads in multiple myeloma: results of a prospective study of patients treated with dexamethasone-based regimens and high-dose chemotherapy. J Clin Oncol. 2005;23: 5217–5223.
38. Garcia-Ferrer L, Bagan JV, Martinez-Sanjuan V, et al. MRI of mandibular osteonecrosis secondary to bisphosphonates. AJR Am J Roentgenol. 2008;190:949–955.
39. Bisdas S, Chambron Pinho N, Smolarz A, Sader R, Vogl TJ, Mack MG. Bisphosphonate-induced osteonecrosis of the jaws: CT and MRI spectrum of findings in 32 patients. Clin Radiol. 2008;63:71–77.
40. Agarwal R, Brunelli SM, Williams K, Mitchell MD, Feldman HI, Umscheid CA. Gadolinium-based contrast agents and nephrogenic systemic fibrosis: a systematic review and meta-analysis. Nephrol Dial Transplant. 2009;24:856–863.
41. Broome DR. Nephrogenic systemic fibrosis associated with gadolinium based contrast agents: a summary of the medical literature reporting. Eur J Radiol. 2008;66:230–234.
42. Chrysochou C, Buckley DL, Dark P, Cowie A, Kalra PA. Gadolinium-enhanced magnetic resonance imaging for renovascular disease and nephrogenic systemic fibrosis: Critical review of the literature and UK experience. J Magn Reson Imaging. 2009;29:887–894.
43. Zamagni E, Nanni C, Patriarca F, et al. A prospective comparison of 18F-fluorodeoxyglucose positron emission tomography-computed tomography, magnetic resonance imaging and whole-body planar radiographs in the assessment of bone disease in newly diagnosed multiple myeloma. Haematologica. 2007;92:50–55.
44. Weininger M, Lauterbach B, Knop S, et al. Whole-body MRI of multiple myeloma: comparison of different MRI sequences in assessment of different growth patterns. Eur J Radiol. 2009;69:339–345.
45. Baur-Melnyk A, Buhmann S, Becker C, et al. Whole-body MRI versus whole-body MDCT for staging of multiple myeloma. AJR Am J Roentgenol. 2008;190:1097–1104.
46. Miceli MH, Jones Jackson LB, Walker RC, Talamo G, Barlogie B, Anaissie EJ. Diagnosis of infection of implantable central venous catheters by [18F]fluorodeoxyglucose positron emission tomography. Nucl Med Commun. 2004;25:813–818.
47. Miceli M, Atoui R, Thertulien R, et al. Deep septic thrombophlebitis: an unrecognized cause of relapsing bacteremia in patients with cancer. J Clin Oncol. 2004;22:1529–1531.
48. Miceli M, Atoui R, Walker R, et al. Diagnosis of deep septic thrombophlebitis in cancer patients by fluorine-18 fluorodeoxyglucose positron emission tomography scanning: a preliminary report. J Clin Oncol. 2004;22:1949–1956.

49. Mahfouz T, Miceli MH, Saghafifar F, et al. 18F-fluorodeoxyglucose positron emission tomography contributes to the diagnosis and management of infections in patients with multiple myeloma: a study of 165 infectious episodes. J Clin Oncol. 2005;23:7857–7863.
50. Walker R, Jones-Jackson L, Rasmussen E, et al. PET and PET/CT imaging in multiple myeloma, solitary plasmacytoma, MGUS and other plasma cell dyscrasias. In: Valk PE, Delbeke D, Bailey DL, Townsend DW, Maisey MN, eds. Positron Emission Tomography: Clinical Practice. 2nd ed. Vol. 2. London, UK: Springer-Verlag London Limited; 2006:475p.
51. Delbeke D, Coleman RE, Guiberteau MJ, et al. Procedure guideline for tumor imaging with 18F-FDG PET/CT 1.0. J Nucl Med. 2006;47:885–895.
52. Cohade C, Osman M, Pannu HK, Wahl RL. Uptake in supraclavicular area fat ("USA-Fat"): description on 18F-FDG PET/CT. J Nucl Med. 2003;44:170–176.
53. Cohade C, Mourtzikos KA, Wahl RL. "USA-Fat": prevalence is related to ambient outdoor temperature-evaluation with 18F-FDG PET/CT. J Nucl Med. 2003;44:1267–1270.
54. Baba S, Tatsumi M, Ishimori T, Lilien DL, Engles JM, Wahl RL. Effect of nicotine and ephedrine on the accumulation of 18F-FDG in brown adipose tissue. J Nucl Med. 2007;48:981–986.
55. Parysow O, Mollerach AM, Jager V, Racioppi S, San Roman J, Gerbaudo VH. Low-dose oral propranolol could reduce brown adipose tissue F-18 FDG uptake in patients undergoing PET scans. Clin Nucl Med. 2007;32:351–357.
56. Basu S. Functional imaging of brown adipose tissue with PET: can this provide new insights into the pathophysiology of obesity and thereby direct antiobesity strategies? Nucl Med Commun. 2008;29:931–933.
57. Williams G, Kolodny GM. Method for decreasing uptake of 18F-FDG by hypermetabolic brown adipose tissue on PET. AJR Am J Roentgenol. 2008;190:1406–1409.
58. el-Shirbiny AM, Yeung H, Imbriaco M, Michaeli J, Macapinlac H, Larson SM. Technetium-99m-MIBI versus fluorine-18-FDG in diffuse multiple myeloma. J Nucl Med. 1997;38:1208–1210.
59. Blocklet D, Schoutens A, Kentos A, Feremans W. Bone marrow uptake of 99mTc-MIBI in patients with multiple myeloma. Eur J Nucl Med. 2001;28:1430–1432.
60. Giovanella L, Taborelli M, Ceriani L, Zucca E, Cavalli F, Delaloye AB.. 99mTc-sestamibi imaging and bone marrow karyotyping in the assessment of multiple myeloma and MGUS. Nucl Med Commun. 2008;29:535–541.
61. Fonti R, Salvatore B, Quarantelli M, et al. 18F-FDG PET/CT, 99mTc-MIBI, and MRI in evaluation of patients with multiple myeloma. J Nucl Med. 2008;49:195–200.
62. Avva R, Vanhemert RL, Barlogie B, Munshi N, Angtuaco EJ. CT-guided biopsy of focal lesions in patients with multiple myeloma may reveal new and more aggressive cytogenetic abnormalities. AJNR Am J Neuroradiol. 2001;22:781–785.
63. Walker R. Jones-Jackson L, Miceli M, et al. FDG PET functional imaging in multiple myeloma: clinically important caveats, pitfalls, and pearls. In: ASH Meeting 2004; San Diego, 2004 (Blood. November 16, 2004;104:11 (abs)).
64. Fletcher JW, Djulbegovic B, Soares HP, et al. Recommendations on the use of 18F-FDG PET in oncology. J Nucl Med. 2008;49:480–508.
65. Suzuki C, Jacobsson H, Hatschek T, et al. Radiologic measurements of tumor response to treatment: practical approaches and limitations. Radiographics. 2008;28:329–344.
66. Michaelis LC, Ratain MJ. Measuring response in a post-RECIST world: from black and white to shades of grey. Nat Rev Cancer. 2006;6:409–414.
67. Ratain MJ, Eckhardt SG. Phase II studies of modern drugs directed against new targets: if you are fazed, too, then resist RECIST. J Clin Oncol. 2004;22:4442–4445.
68. Bogaerts J, Ford R, Sargent D, et al. Individual patient data analysis to assess modifications to the RECIST criteria. Eur J Cancer. 2009;45:248–260.
69. Eisenhauer EA, Therasse P, Bogaerts J, et al. New response evaluation criteria in solid tumours: revised RECIST guideline (version 1.1). Eur J Cancer. 2009;45:228–247.
70. Schwartz LH, Bogaerts J, Ford R, et al. Evaluation of lymph nodes with RECIST 1.1. Eur J Cancer. 2009;45:261–267.

71. Verweij J, Therasse P, Eisenhauer E. Cancer clinical trial outcomes: any progress in tumour-size assessment? Eur J Cancer. 2009;45:225–227.

72. Wahl RL Jacene H, Kasamon Y, Lodge MA. From RECIST to PERCIST: Evolving considerations for PET response criteria in solid tumors. J Nucl Med. 2009;50:122S–150S.

73. Callander NS, Roodman GD. Myeloma bone disease. Semin Hematol. 2001;38: 276–285.

74. Barlogie B, Shaughnessy J, Tricot G, et al. Treatment of multiple myeloma. Blood. 2004;103:20–32.

75. Chim CS, Ooi GC, Loong F, Liang R. Unusual presentations of hematologic malignancies: CASE 1. Solitary bone plasmacytoma: role of magnetic resonance imaging and positron emission tomography. J Clin Oncol. 2004;22:1328–1330.

76. Liebross RH, Ha CS, Cox JD, Weber D, Delasalle K, Alexanian R. Solitary bone plasmacytoma: outcome and prognostic factors following radiotherapy. Int J Radiat Oncol Biol Phys. 1998;41:1063–1067.

77. Moulopoulos LA, Dimopoulos MA, Weber D, Fuller L, Libshitz HI, Alexanian R. Magnetic resonance imaging in the staging of solitary plasmacytoma of bone. J Clin Oncol. 1993;11:1311–1315.

78. Schirrmeister H, Buck AK, Bergmann L, Reske SN, Bommer M. Positron emission tomography (PET) for staging of solitary plasmacytoma. Cancer Biother Radiopharm. 2003;18:841–845.

79. Weber DM. Solitary bone and extramedullary plasmacytoma. Hematol Am Soc Hematol Educ Program. 2005;45:373–376.

80. Soutar R, Lucraft H, Jackson G, et al. Guidelines on the diagnosis and management of solitary plasmacytoma of bone and solitary extramedullary plasmacytoma. Br J Haematol. 2004;124:717–726.

81. Schomburg A, Bender H, Reichel C, et al. Standardized uptake values of fluorine-18 fluorodeoxyglucose: the value of different normalization procedures. Eur J Nucl Med. 1996;23:571–574.

82. Shortt CP, Gleeson TG, Breen KA, et al. Whole-Body MRI versus PET in assessment of multiple myeloma disease activity. AJR Am J Roentgenol. 2009;192:980–986.

83. Kubota R, Yamada S, Kubota K, Ishiwata K, Tamahashi N, Ido T. Intratumoral distribution of fluorine-18-fluorodeoxyglucose in vivo: high accumulation in macrophages and granulation tissues studied by microautoradiography. J Nucl Med. 1992;33:1972–1980.

84. Higashi K, Clavo AC, Wahl RL. In vitro assessment of 2-fluoro-2-deoxy-D-glucose, L-methionine and thymidine as agents to monitor the early response of a human adeno-carcinoma cell line to radiotherapy. J Nucl Med. 1993;34:773–779.

85. Naumann R, Vaic A, Beuthien-Baumann B, et al. Prognostic value of positron emission tomography in the evaluation of post-treatment residual mass in patients with Hodgkin's disease and non-Hodgkin's lymphoma. Br J Haematol. 2001;115:793–800.

86. Weihrauch MR, Re D, Scheidhauer K, et al. Thoracic positron emission tomography using 18F-fluorodeoxyglucose for the evaluation of residual mediastinal Hodgkin disease. Blood. 2001;98:2930–2934.

87. Walker RC, Jones-Jackson LB, Martin W, Habibian MR, Delbeke D. New imaging tools for the diagnosis of infection. Future Microbiol. 2007;2:527–554.

88. Migliorati CA. Bisphosphonates and oral cavity avascular bone necrosis. J Clin Oncol. 2003;21:4253–4254.

89. Leung AN, Gosselin MV, Napper CH, et al. Pulmonary infections after bone marrow transplantation: clinical and radiographic findings. Radiology. 1999;210:699–710.

90. Mulligan ME, Badros AZ. PET/CT and MR imaging in myeloma. Skeletal Radiol. 2007;36:5–16.

91. Dimopoulos M, Terpos E, Comenzo RL, et al. International myeloma working group consensus statement and guidelines regarding the current role of imaging techniques in the diagnosis and monitoring of multiple Myeloma. Leukemia. 2009;23:1545–1556.

92. Nelis GF. An unusual case of myeloma. Non-secretory IgD-kappa myeloma with de-differentiation of kappa myeloma evolving from solitary plasmocytoma. Acta Med Scand. 1982;211:141–144.

93. Volberding PA, Baker KR, Levine AM. Human immunodeficiency virus hematology. Hematol Am Soc Hematol Educ Program. 2003;294–313.

94. Roca B, Torres V. Castleman's disease presenting as fever of unknown origin: diagnostic value of fluorodeoxyglucose-positron emission tomography/computed tomography. Am J Med Sci. 2009;337:295–296.

95. Roca B.. Castleman's disease. A review. AIDS Rev. 2009;11:3–7.

96. Powles T, Stebbing J, Bazeos A, et al. The role of immune suppression and HHV-8 in the increasing incidence of HIV-associated multicentric Castleman's disease. Ann Oncol. 2009;20:775–779.

97. Ghobrial IM, Gertz MA, Fonseca R.. Waldenstrom macroglobulinaemia. Lancet Oncol. 2003;4:679–685.

98. Blade J, Samson D, Reece D, et al. Criteria for evaluating disease response and progression in patients with multiple myeloma treated by high-dose therapy and haemopoietic stem cell transplantation. Myeloma Subcommittee of the EBMT. European Group for Blood and Marrow Transplant. Br J Haematol. 1998;102:1115–1123.

99. Durie BG, Harousseau JL, Miguel JS, et al. International uniform response criteria for multiple myeloma. Leukemia. 2006;20:1467–1473.

100. Okada J, Yoshikawa K, Imazeki K, et al. The use of FDG-PET in the detection and management of malignant lymphoma: correlation of uptake with prognosis. J Nucl Med. 1991;32:686–691.

101. Kostakoglu L, Goldsmith SJ.. 18F-FDG PET evaluation of the response to therapy for lymphoma and for breast, lung, and colorectal carcinoma. J Nucl Med. 2003;44:224–239.

102. Juweid ME. Utility of positron emission tomography (PET) scanning in managing patients with Hodgkin lymphoma. Hematol Am Soc Hematol Educ Program. 2006;2006(1):259–265.

103. Juweid ME, Stroobants S, Hoekstra OS, et al. Use of positron emission tomography for response assessment of lymphoma: consensus of the Imaging Subcommittee of International Harmonization Project in Lymphoma. J Clin Oncol. 2007;25:571–578.

104. Haessler J, Shaughnessy JD Jr, Zhan F, et al. Benefit of complete response in multiple myeloma limited to high-risk subgroup identified by gene expression profiling. Clin Cancer Res. 2007;13:7073–7079.

Chapter 3
Biochemical Markers of Bone Remodeling in Multiple Myeloma

Evangelos Terpos

Abstract Osteolytic bone disease is a frequent complication of multiple myeloma which results in significant skeletal morbidity. A characteristic feature of myeloma bone disease is that the lesions rarely heal and bone scans are often negative in myeloma patients who have extensive lytic lesions, offering very little in the follow-up of bone disease. X-rays are also of limited value in monitoring bone destruction during anti-myeloma or anti-resorptive treatment. Biochemical markers of bone resorption, such as N- and C-terminal cross-linking telopeptide of type I collagen and markers of bone formation, such as bone-specific alkaline phosphatase and osteocalcin, provide information on bone dynamics that in turn may reflect disease activity in bone. These markers have been investigated as tools for evaluating the extent of bone disease, risk of skeletal morbidity, and response to anti-resorptive treatment in myeloma. Several studies have shown that the majority of biochemical markers of bone resorption are elevated in myeloma patients with lytic bone lesions, thus reflecting changes in bone metabolism associated with tumor growth. There is also a growing body of evidence that markers of bone resorption correlate with the risk of skeletal complications, disease progression, and survival. In addition, bone markers could potentially be used as a tool for early diagnosis of bone lesions. This chapter summarizes the existing data for the role of bone markers in assessing the extent of bone destruction in myeloma and monitoring bone turnover during specific anti-myeloma therapies, while it gives information for novel markers that may be of particular interest in the near future.

Keywords Myeloma · Bone markers · N-terminal cross-linking telopeptide of type I collagen (NTX) · C-terminal cross-linking telopeptide of type I collagen (CTX) · C-terminal cross-linking telopeptide of type I collagen generated

E. Terpos (✉)
Department of Clinical Therapeutics, University of Athens School of Medicine, Alexandra Hospital, 80 Vas. Sofias Av., Athens 115-28, Greece
e-mail: eterpos@med.uoa.gr

G.D. Roodman (ed.), *Myeloma Bone Disease*, Current Clinical Oncology,
DOI 10.1007/978-1-60761-554-5_3, © Springer Science+Business Media, LLC 2010

by MMPs (ICTP) · Pyridinoline · Deoxypyridinoline · Bone-specific alkaline phosphatase · Osteocalcin · Tartrate-resistant acid phosphatase isoform 5b · Receptor
activator of nuclear factor kB-ligand (RANKL) · Osteoprotegerin · Bone-specific
alkaline phosphatase · Osteocalcin · Dickkopf-1

3.1 Introduction

Multiple myeloma (MM) is a B-cell malignancy characterized by the accumulation of clonal plasma cells in the bone marrow. Patients with MM typically
develop osteolytic bone lesions that result in debilitating skeletal complications
such as pathologic fractures, severe bone pain, and hypercalcemia. As a result,
these patients often require analgesics, palliative radiation therapy, and surgery
to bone. In the absence of effective bisphosphonate therapy, more than 50% of
patients with Durie–Salmon stage III MM will experience at least one skeletal-
related event (SRE) over 2 years [1]. The development of lytic bone lesions is
related not only to increased osseous breakdown but also to the uncoupling of the
normal process of bone remodeling [2]. This disrupted process involves increased
osteoclast-mediated bone resorption accompanied by a reduction in new bone formation [3]. These consequences of myeloma bone disease result in rapid bone loss
and development of lytic lesions that rarely heal even when the patients are in
complete remission [4]. This finding is in keeping with the observation that bone
scans are often negative in myeloma patients who have extensive lytic lesions and
offer very little in the follow-up of bone disease in these patients [5]. Furthermore,
sequential measurement of bone mineral density (BMD) using DXA scans produced heterogeneous local BMD changes and the available data do not support
routine use of sequential DXA scans in MM [6]. The bone disease in MM is usually
assessed by plain radiographs that show radiolucent lesions without calcification
known as "punched-out" lesions. Although radiographs are useful in diagnosing
osteolytic lesions, they do not provide information about ongoing bone remodeling
[7]. Biochemical markers of bone remodeling have been used to assess the rate of
bone turnover in patients with MM and to improve monitoring of bone destruction
in MM.

In addition, strategies that target osteoclast activation and proliferation represent an important approach to the management of myeloma bone disease.
Bisphosphonates consist of a heterogeneous group of agents that affect bone
metabolism and regulation of calcium homeostasis, mainly through an inhibitory
effect on osteoclasts. Several studies have demonstrated their efficacy in myeloma
bone disease, and therefore they are included in all therapeutic regimens for
symptomatic myeloma patients with bone disease [8]. Novel anti-myeloma agents
including proteasome inhibitor bortezomib have shown a strong anabolic effect on
myeloma along with an inhibitory effect on osteoclasts [9]. Biochemical markers

of bone resorption and formation have also been used to follow up myeloma bone disease during administration of bisphosphonates or bortezomib-based regimens. This chapter summarizes the existing data for the role of markers of bone remodeling in assessing the extent of bone destruction in myeloma and monitoring bone turnover during specific anti-myeloma therapies or bisphosphonates administration, while it presents novel markers that may be of particular interest in the near future.

3.2 Markers of Bone Remodeling

Throughout life bone undergoes continuous remodeling with removal of old bone and replacement with new bone. Bone turnover is always initiated by osteoclasts eroding a mineralized surface. This process is followed by the recruitment of successive teams of osteoblasts to the outer edge of the erosion cavity that secrete new bone matrix and gradually fill in the resorption cavity [10]. Resorption of old bone and formation of new bone are balanced under normal conditions. In MM, there is a pronounced imbalance in these processes: increased activation of osteoclasts and suppression of osteoblast function [2–4].

Over the past two decades, the isolation and characterization of cellular and extracellular components of the skeletal matrix have resulted in the development of biochemical markers that specifically reflect either bone formation or bone resorption. Most of the traditional and new markers of bone resorption measure the collagen degradation products from osteoclast activity and include urinary hydroxyproline, hydroxylysine glycosides, total or free pyridinoline cross-links, and cross-linked N- or C-telopeptides [11]. Serum tartrate-resistant acid phosphatase isoform type 5b (TRACP-5b) which is an enzyme secreted by activated osteoclasts and bone sialoprotein (BSP), a non-collagenous protein also reflect bone resorptive processes [12, 13].

The formation markers are direct or indirect products of active osteoblasts that enter into the circulation (Fig. 3.1). These include serum bone-specific alkaline phosphatase, osteocalcin, and type I procollagen peptides [14]. Markers of resorption and formation are depicted in Tables 3.1 and 3.2. Fasting urinary calcium, used by some researchers to measure bone resorption, is not discussed here as it has limited value in MM bone disease.

Bone markers are non-invasive, comparatively inexpensive, and, when applied and interpreted correctly, helpful tools in the assessment of bone diseases. However, factors that affect their levels, including circadian rhythmicity, diet, age, gender, renal function, and drugs, should be clearly defined and appropriately adjusted whenever possible. Another important issue is that biochemical indices reflect the total bone turnover and give little information about the function of individual groups of osteoclasts. All these issues are discussed below.

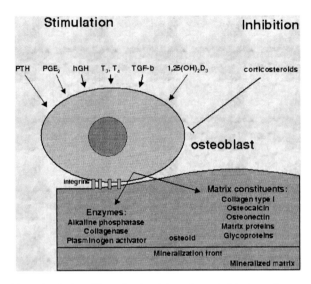

Fig. 3.1 Osteoblast stimulation. Through stimulators, the osteoblasts produce enzymes, such as ALP and matrix constituents, such as collagen type I and osteocalcin. Bone ALP, osteocalcin, and degradation products of procollagen type I can be measured in urine and serum and are considered as sensitive markers of bone formation

Table 3.1 Markers of bone resorption

Marker	Abbreviation[a]	Tissue of origin	Analytical method	Analytical specimen
Hydroxyproline	Hyp	All tissues and all genetic types of collagen	Colorimetric, assay, HPLC	Urine
Hydroxylysine	Hyl	All tissues and all genetic types of collagen	Reversed-phase HPLC	Urine
Galactosyl-hydroxylysine	Gal-Hyl	Both Gal-Hyl and Glc-Gal-Hyl appear to be specific for bone collagen degradation	Reversed-phase HPLC	Urine
Glucosyl-galactosyl-hydroxylysine	Glc-Gal-Hyl			
Pyridinoline	PYD	Bone, cartilage, tendon, blood vessels	HPLC, ELISA	Urine

Table 3.1 (continued)

Marker	Abbreviation[a]	Tissue of origin	Analytical method	Analytical specimen
Deoxy pyridinoline	DPD	Bone, dentin	RIA	Urine (free DPD can be also measured in serum or plasma)
N-terminal cross-linking telopeptide of type I collagen	NTX	All tissues containing type I collagen	ELISA, RIA	Urine, serum
C-terminal cross-linking telopeptide of type I collagen	CTX	All tissues containing type I collagen	ELISA, RIA	Urine, serum (β-form only)
C-terminal cross-linking telopeptide of type I collagen generated by MMPs	CTX-MMP or ICTP	All tissues containing type I collagen	RIA	Serum
Tartrate-resistant acid phosphatase isoform 5b	TRACP-5b	Bone (osteoclasts)	Colorimetric RIA, ELISA	Serum, plasma
Bone sialoprotein	BSP	Bone, dentin, hypertrophic cartilage, cancer cells	RIA, ELISA	Serum

[a]According to the Bone Marker Nomenclature by the Committee of Scientific Advisors of the International Osteoporosis Foundation [15].

3.3 Biochemistry of Bone Markers

3.3.1 Bone Resorption Markers

Hydroxyproline and Hydroxylysine: Hydroxyproline (Hyp) is formed in the cell from the post-translational hydroxylation of proline. Hyp is the predominant amino acid of collagens, comprising about 13% of these proteins. Hydroxylysine (Hyl) is another amino acid essentially unique to collagenous proteins. Bone is the primary store of collagen in the body, but both Hyp and Hyl are present in essentially all tissues and all genetic types of collagen. The Hyp released during collagen degradation is primarily metabolized in the liver and subsequently excreted in the urine. However, only about 10% of Hyp-containing products from collagen breakdown are excreted in the urine [10]. The small pool of urinary Hyp originates from the

Table 3.2 Markers of bone formation

Marker	Abbreviation[a]	Tissue of origin	Analytical method	Analytical specimen
Osteocalcin (or bone gla-protein)	OC	Bone, platelets	RIA, ELISA, IRMA	Serum
Bone alkaline phosphatase	Bone ALP	Bone	ELISA, IRMA, colorimetric assay	Serum
Procollagen type I N propeptide	PINP	Bone, soft tissue, skin	RIA, ELISA	Serum
Procollagen type I C propeptide	PICP	Bone, soft tissue, skin	RIA, ELISA	Serum

[a] According to the Bone Marker Nomenclature by the Committee of Scientific Advisors of the International Osteoporosis Foundation [15].

N-propeptide of type I collagen. Normal ingestion of gelatin or collagen-rich foods such as meat can increase the level of urinary Hyp, and the urinary peptides containing Hyp from endogenous collagen breakdown are indistinguishable from the dietary peptides [16]. This is a major disadvantage for the use of this marker as a specific index of bone resorption.

Hyl is glycosylated and two glycosides are formed, galactosyl hydroxylysine (Gal-Hyl) and glucosyl galactosyl hydroxylysine (Glc-Gal-Hyl), which also appear in the urine. While Hyl and its glycosides are less abundant than Hyp in bone collagen, certain properties make Hyl theoretically a better marker of bone turnover than urinary Hyp. Gal-Hyl is not metabolized and not influenced by dietary factors. In normal urine, 80% of the total Hyl is in the form of Hyl, 10% is free and unglycosylated, and the remainder is peptide-bound, which suggests that free Hyl is largely metabolized and not excreted. However, in addition to all structural collagens, both Hyp and Hyl are also found in certain serum proteins, such as the C1q component of complement. This disadvantage, in combination with the effect of age and the circadian rhythm (both have their peak excretion after midnight), makes them less specific indices of bone resorption, and therefore they have been largely replaced by newer markers [17, 18].

Pyridinoline and Deoxypyridinoline Cross-links of Type I Collagen: In the decade of 1990s, collagen cross-links have evolved as promising markers of bone resorption. Pyridinoline (PYD) and deoxypyridinoline (DPD) are formed by the enzymatic action of lysyl oxidase on lysine and Hyl. Newly deposited collagen fibrils in the extracellular matrix are stabilized by cross-links formed by the action of lysyl oxidase on lysine and Hyl residues in telopeptide domains of the collagen molecules. The resulting aldehydes condense with Hyl or lysyl residues on

Fig. 3.2 Fibrils of collagen showing the N- and C-terminal ends bonding to helical areas of adjacent fibrils by PYD and DPD

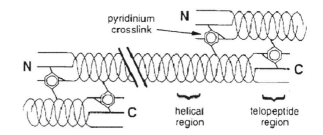

adjacent collagen molecules to form divalent cross-links, which can mature by further condensation with telopeptide aldehydes to the trivalent structures DPD and PYD [10]. PYD and DPD act as mature cross-links in type I collagen of all major connective tissues. These include type I collagen of bone, dentin, tendon, vascular walls, muscle, intestine, etc. Figure 3.2 depicts the basic cross-linking of collagen fibrils that construct type I collagen, the protein comprising most of the organic matrix of the bone. Each of the fibrils contains amino-terminal and carboxy-terminal ends that are termed N- or C-terminal cross-linking telopeptides of collagen type I (NTX and CTX), respectively. In type I collagen, these ends are each linked to a helical portion of a nearby molecule by a PYD or DPD cross-link. The pyridinoline cross-links occur essentially at two intermolecular sites in the collagen fibril: two amino-telopeptides are linked to a helical site at or near residue 930 and two carboxy-telopeptides to helical residue 87 [19]. DPD is derived from two hydroxyly sines and one lysine residue, while PYD is derived from three hydroxylysine residues. In all tissues, PYD predominates, while DPD is the minor component. The products of collagen degradation by osteoclasts include NTX and CTX fragments of various sizes, still attached to helical portions of a nearby molecule by a pyridinium cross-link, that insert into the circulation. With additional degradation in the liver and kidney the fragments are finally broken down to their constituent amino acids and the pyridiniums, PYD and DPD. Although it is possible that soft tissues contribute to the normal excretion of DPD and PYD, bone represents the major reservoir of total collagen in the body and turns over faster than most major connective tissues. In contrast to Hyp and Hyl, the measurement of urine DPD and PYD is not influenced by the degradation of newly synthesized collagen fibrils or by dietary collagen intake. The pyridinolines are present in the diet, but unlike Hyp, they are not absorbed. Furthermore, unlike Hyp, the pyridinoline amino acids are fully excreted with no known pathway of metabolic degradation [20].

Amino- and Carboxy-Terminal Cross-linking Telopeptide of Type I Collagen: During collagen type I degradation by osteoclasts, N- and C-terminal peptide fragments are released into the circulation [20]. These fragments represent a spectrum of proteins having different sizes, as shown in Fig. 3.3. The majority of these is relatively small and passes through the glomerulus into the urine. NTX are regarded to be specific for bone tissue breakdown as other tissues comprised of type I collagen, e.g., skin, are not actively metabolized by osteoclasts, and, therefore, different

**Distribution of type I collagen fragments after
osteoclastic degradation**

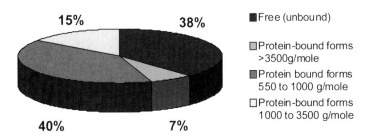

Fig. 3.3 Distribution of type I collagen fragments after osteoclastic degradation

types of fragments are formed during breakdown of non-skeletal tissues [14]. An ELISA method has been developed to recognize a discrete pool of NTX isolated from urine. The monoclonal antibody recognizes the $\alpha2$ chain *N*-telopeptide fragment. This fragment contains the pyridinium cross-links, but this assay does not recognize the PYD and DPD per se. This implies bone specificity since the pyridinoline cross-link in bone primarily involves the $\alpha2$ chain whereas in other tissues the $\alpha1$ chain predominates [21]. NTX contains the cross-linked $\alpha2$ N-telopeptide sequence, QYDGKGVG, which is a product of osteoclastic proteolysis and in which lysine (K) is embodied in a trivalent cross-linkage. Collagen must be broken down to small cross-linked peptides that contain this exact sequence before the antibody can bind to the NTX antigen. This suggests that the NTX peptide is a direct product of osteoclastic proteolysis, does not require further metabolism in the liver or kidney for generation, and is rapidly cleared by the kidney [22].

Other assays have also been developed for the measurement of epitopes associated with the CTX (α-CTX, β-CTX, ICTP) in both serum and urine [23, 24]. Due to bone specificity and their unique characteristics NTX, ICTP, and CTX have almost totally replaced the use of older resorption indices in the diagnostic assessment of bone diseases.

Tartrate-Resistant Acid Phosphatase Isoform Type 5b (TRACP-5b): TRACP-5b is a marker of bone resorption which has been in use over the last 7–8 years with very encouraging results. TRACP is produced by both osteoclasts and activated macrophages and subsequently is secreted into the circulation. Two forms of TRACP circulate in human serum, macrophage-derived TRACP-5a and osteoclast-derived TRACP-5b [25, 26]. The only structural difference between TRACP-5a and TRACP-5b is that the former contains sialic acid residues that are not found in TRACP-5b [27]. In human serum, TRACP-5b circulates in a large complex that contains $\alpha2$-microglobulin and calcium [28]. Osteoclasts secrete TRACP-5b into the blood circulation as a catalytically active enzyme that is inactivated and degraded to fragments in the circulation. Thus, all catalytically active TRACP 5b molecules measured in the serum are freshly liberated from the osteoclasts, providing a sensitive resorptive index [25].

3.3.2 Bone Formation Markers

Bone-Specific Alkaline Phosphatase: Alkaline phosphatase (ALP) is a ubiquitously expressed, cell membrane enzyme. ALP belongs to the category of molecules that are localized to cell membranes through a COOH-terminal glycan-phosphatidylinositol anchor, providing a basis for understanding the generation of different isoforms observed in plasma. Isoforms produced by differential cleavage or preservation of the glycan-phosphatidylinositol anchor originate from different tissues, such as liver, bone, intestine, spleen, kidney, and placenta [29]. Liver and bone (bALP) isoforms account for almost 95% of the total ALP activity in the serum. Bone ALP is produced by osteoblasts and has been demonstrated in matrix vesicles deposited as "buds" derived from the cells membrane. These deposits seem to play an important role in bone formation [14]. Bone ALP is produced in extremely high amounts during bone formation phase of bone turnover, and is, therefore, an excellent indicator of total bone formation activity [29].

Osteocalcin: It is one of the most abundant non-collagenous bone proteins produced by osteoblasts, odontoblasts, and hypertrophic chondrocytes. Most of the circulating osteocalcin is a product of osteoblast activity and thus considered a marker of bone formation. It is a small protein of 49 amino acids and in most species contains three residues (at 17, 21, and 24) of γ-carboxy glutamic acid, a calcium-binding amino acid [30]. This vitamin K-dependent post-translational modification of newly synthesized proteins results in γ-carboxylation of specific glutamate residues. The reaction is comparable to the activation of vitamin K-dependent blood coagulation factors and is inhibited by warfarin [31]. The human osteoblast produces an 11-kDa molecule consisting of a 23-residue hydrophobic signal peptide, a 26-residue propeptide, and the 49-residue mature protein. The pro-region contains a γ-carboxylation recognition site homologous to corresponding regions in the vitamin K-dependent clotting factors. After the hydrophobic regions cleaved by a signal peptidase, pro-osteocalcin is γ-carboxylated. Subsequently, the propeptide is removed and the mature protein is secreted [10]. In serum, osteocalcin is degraded so that both the intact peptide and the fragments coexist in the circulation [32]. Therefore, assays that evaluate both intact osteocalcin and fragments are more accurate for the measurement of serum osteocalcin.

A fraction of newly synthesized osteocalcin is secreted into the circulation, while during bone resorption osteocalcin is also degraded. Thus, there is some question whether osteocalcin should be considered an indicator of osteoblast activity or a marker of bone matrix metabolism or turnover [14].

The human osteocalcin gene is located at the distal long arm of chromosome 1. Various promoter elements contribute to basal expression and osteoblast specificity. The gene is further modulated by vitamin D and glucocorticoid response elements [33]. Although osteocalcin is present in significant amounts in bone, dentin, and calcified cartilage, it has recently also been found in osteosarcomas, prostate, ovarian, lung, and brain cancer [34]. Osteocalcin function has not clearly defined yet. However, it is assumed that much of the newly synthesized protein is incorporated into the bone matrix-binding calcium. Serum levels of osteocalcin are significantly influenced by gender, age, and renal function [32].

Type I Procollagen Propeptides: Collagen type I, a 300-kDa protein, makes up 90% of the organic bone matrix and is synthesized by osteoblasts in the form of procollagen, having a molecular weight (MW) of 450-kDa. Extracellular processing of procollagen before fiber assembly includes cleavage of the N- and C-terminal extension propeptides, that are termed procollagen type I N-propeptide (PINP) or C-propeptide (PICP), having a MW of 35-kDa and 100-kDa, respectively [35]. PINP is cleared via the scavenger endothelial system in the liver and PICP via the mannose receptors on liver endothelial cells [36]. Because these peptides are generated in a stoichiometric 1:1 ratio with newly formed collagen molecules, their levels in serum are considered an index of collagen synthesis and thus of bone formation [37]. Serum levels of the PICP have been demonstrated to correlate with histomorphometric measures of bone formation, and hormone replacement or bisphosphonate therapy leads to a reduction in the circulating concentration of this marker. Most recent studies, however, suggest that the PINP has a greater diagnostic validity than PICP in metastatic bone disease [38].

3.4 Markers of Bone Remodeling and Myeloma Bone Disease

Comparison Between Myeloma Patients and Healthy Individuals and Correlations with the Extent of Myeloma Bone Disease: Markers of both resorption and formation have been used in an attempt to better evaluate the extent of bone disease in multiple myeloma and assess clinical correlations. Table 3.3 summarizes the results of the most important publications regarding the levels of bone markers in myeloma patients compared with healthy individuals and their correlations with clinical data. Markers of bone resorption are increased in the urine or serum of patients with MM compared to healthy individuals [39–56]. Both PYD and DPD, NTX in the urine and CTX, ICTP, and TRACP-5b in the serum are elevated in patients with MM compared to healthy controls and correlate with the extent of bone disease [42, 44, 47–52, 54–56]. NTX urinary levels have been increased even in myeloma patients at the plateau phase of their disease [57], while PYD, DPD, and NTX were also elevated in myeloma patients before autologous transplantation [58, 59]. A histomorphometric study in bone marrow biopsies of 16 myeloma patients has shown that urinary NTX levels have shown the strongest positive correlation with the dynamic histomorphometric indices of bone resorption, followed by serum ICTP and urine DPD, while urine PYD did not correlate with the histomorphometric findings [60]. Moreover, a comparison between these four markers (PYD, DPD, NTX, and ICTP) has revealed that serum ICTP and urine NTX reflected the extent of myeloma bone disease more accurately and could also predict early progression of the bone disease after conventional chemotherapy [6, 50]. However, serum ICTP remained more sensitive than the urinary assays when patients with impaired renal function were excluded from that analysis [50]. Jakob et al. demonstrated that serum ICTP was significantly elevated in MM patients who did not have detectable osteolytic bone lesions by plain radiograph but had abnormal bone magnetic resonance imaging (MRI) scans, suggesting that ICTP is a useful marker for identifying MM patients with skeletal involvement that is not readily detected on plain radiographs [61]. In this study the sensitivity of ICTP for depiction of MRI abnormalities was 79%, while the positive and negative predictive values were 85 and 84%, respectively [61]. NTX urinary levels also correlated with the overall score of skeletal involvement as measured by Tc-99m-MIBI scintigraphy and bone marrow infiltration by plasma cells [62]. Coleman et al. showed in 210 myeloma patients that high or intermediate NTX urinary levels correlated with increased risk for developing a SRE compared with low NTX values (RR 2.25, $p = 0.032$ and RR 1.75, $p = 0.016$, respectively) [53]. High NTX values also correlated with a three-fold increased risk for developing a first SRE (RR 3.01, $p = 0.008$; Fig. 3.4),

Table 3.3 Markers of bone remodeling in myeloma patients and correlations with clinical data

Reference	No. of patients	Parameter studied	Comparison with controls (symbol refers to MM patients)	Correlation with extent of bone disease	Correlation with survival (in multivariate models)
Nawawi et al. [39]	17	DPD	↑	NA	NA
		TRACP	NS		
		OC	NS		
		bALP	NS		
		PICP	NS		
Abildgaard et al. [40]	109	ICTP	↑	NA	Yes
		OC	NS		Yes
		bALP	↑		No
		PICP	NS		No
		PIIINP	↑		No
Withold et al. [41]	15	DPD, PYD	↑	NA	NA
		bALP, PICP	↓		
Carlson et al. [42]	73	DPD	↑	Yes	No
		ICTP	↑	Yes	Yes
		OC	NS	No	No
		PICP	NS	No	No
Woitge et al. [43]	18	PYD	↑	NA	NA
		DPD	↑		
		NTX	↑		
		CTX	↑		
		BSP	↑		
Fonseca et al. [44]	313	ICTP	↑	Yes	Yes
		TRACP	↑	No	No
		OC	↓	No	No
		bALP	NS	Yes	No
		PICP	NS	No	No

Table 3.3 (continued)

Reference	No. of patients	Parameter studied	Comparison with controls (symbol refers to MM patients)	Correlation with extent of bone disease	Correlation with survival (in multivariate models)
Terpos et al. [45]	62	NTX	↑	NA	NA
		OC	↓		
		bALP	↓		
Woitge et al. [46]	43	OC	NS	NA	NA
		bALP	↓		
Corso et al. [47]	52	DPD	↑	Yes	NA
		OC	↓	No	
		bALP	NS	No	
Jakob et al. [48][a]	57	DPD	↑	Yes	No
		NTX	NS	No	$p = 0.05$
		ICTP	↑	Yes	Yes
Alexandrakis et al. [49]	38	PYD	↑	Yes	NA
		DPD	↑	Yes	
		NTX	↑	Yes	
		OC	↑	No	
		bALP	NS	No	
Abildgaard et al. [50]	34	PYD	↑	Yes	NA
		DPD	↑	Yes	
		ICTP	↑	Yes	
		NTX	↑	Yes	
Terpos et al. [51, 52]	121	NTX	↑	Yes	No
		TRACP-5b	↑	Yes	No
		OC	↓	Yes	No
		bALP	↓	No	No
		sRANKL/OPG	↑	Yes	Yes
Coleman et al. [53]	318	NTX	↑	Yes[b]	Yes
Kuliszkiewicz-Janus et al. [54]	75	ICTP	↑	Yes	NA
		OC	NS	No	
Dizdar et al. [55]	25	CTX	↑	Yes	NA
		DPD	↑	Yes	
Jakob et al. [56]	100	ICTP	↑[a]	Yes	Yes

[a] MM compared with MGUS patients.
[b] Correlation with SREs.
NS: non–significant.
NA: not assessed.

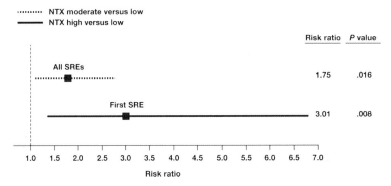

Fig. 3.4 Relative risk for experiencing any skeletal-related event (SRE) and a first SRE for multiple myeloma patients with high levels of N-telopeptide of type I collagen (NTX; ≥100 nM BCE/mM creatinine) or moderate NTX (50–99 nM BCE/mM creatinine) versus patients with low NTX (<50 nM BCE/mM creatinine) treated with zoledronic acid. Length of horizontal lines represents 95% confidence intervals [53, 72]

while there was a trend toward increased risk of osteolytic lesions progression in the high NTX group ($p = 0.08$) [53]. These results suggest that serum ICTP and urinary NTX correlate significantly with the extent of myeloma bone disease, the risk for developing SREs, and possibly with myeloma progression. The measurement of these values may be useful for diagnosing and monitoring bone disease in MM and is feasible in the context of any therapeutic clinical trials.

Markers of bone formation have been used in several studies but the results have been variable [39–42, 44–47, 49, 51, 52]. In some studies, osteocalcin and bALP were elevated in myeloma patients compared with controls, while in others they were either reduced or within normal limits. In the study of Fonseca et al., which includes a large number of myeloma patients ($n = 313$) serum levels of bALP correlated with bone pain, lesions, and fractures even if the mean values were not different from control values; osteocalcin levels were lower in myeloma patients than in controls but they showed no correlation with the extent of bone disease [44]. Furthermore, Coleman et al. showed that myeloma patients with high bALP levels have increased risk for developing a SRE (RR 3.29; 95% CI 2.38–4.55; $p < 0.001$) and for disease progression (RR 2.42; 95% CI 1.53–3.81; $p < 0.001$) [53]. Terpos et al. showed that OC levels were reduced in myeloma patients and correlated with the extent of bone disease, while bALP levels were not [51]. These differences among the different studies may be due to different study population and the different phase of bone turnover in each population. PICP values seem not to predict the extent of myeloma bone disease [39–42, 44]. As shown in Table 3.3, markers of bone formation may be of some value in myeloma but may not necessarily reflect the extent of myeloma bone destruction and thus their clinical utility is doubtful.

Correlations of Bone Markers with Myeloma Activity and Patients' Survival: There are several studies in which markers of bone remodeling have shown strong correlation with the stage of myeloma. Serum levels of ICTP and urinary values of NTX were higher in myeloma stage II/III than stage I disease [40, 44, 49]. Abnormal high DPD urinary levels also correlated with advanced myeloma stage [47, 48]. Terpos et al. has reported in 121 newly diagnosed myeloma patients that stage of the disease correlated with both TRACP-5b and NTX ($p < 0.0001$ and $p = 0.014$, respectively), showing a borderline correlation with OC ($p = 0.046$) but no correlation with bALP ($p = 0.73$) [51]. The association of osteocalcin with stage III myeloma has also been shown in the study of Woitge et al. [46], while two other studies showed no correlation of either osteocalcin or bALP with myeloma stage [44, 47]. Markers of both formation and resorption also correlated with markers of disease activity, such as β2-microglobulin and IL-6 in several studies [44, 47, 51, 60].

However, it is clear that markers of bone resorption and in particular ICTP and NTX correlate with overall survival (OS) in myeloma [40, 42, 44, 48, 63, 64]. Fonseca et al. have shown that the median survival was 4.1 years and 3.5 years for patients with low and high ICTP levels, respectively ($p = 0.02$) [44]. Furthermore, Jakob et al. have shown that ICTP is a prognostic factor for OS ($p < 0.03$), while urinary NTX showed borderline prognostic value ($p = 0.05$) [48]. The same group investigated the prognostic impact of ICTP in combination with myeloma stage (ISS), β2-microglobulin, albumin, deletion of chromosome 13, and high-dose therapy in 100 patients with newly diagnosed symptomatic MM. ISS, β2-microglobulin alone, albumin alone, del(13q14), high-dose therapy, and ICTP were significant prognostic factors for OS. However, in the multivariate analysis, ICTP was the most powerful prognostic factor (log-rank $p < 0.001$, hazard ratio: ninefold increase). ICTP clearly separated two subgroups with a good and a worse prognosis within each of the three ISS stages (ISS I: $p = 0.027$; ISS II: $p = 0.022$, ISS III: $p = 0.013$). Incorporation of ICTP in a combined ICTP-ISS score significantly ($p < 0.001$) separated four risk groups with a 5-year OS rate of 95, 65, 46, and 32%, respectively. These data demonstrate that the inclusion of the collagen-I degradation product ICTP, as a biomarker of bone resorption, adds to the prognostic value of ISS in MM [56]. The significance of ICTP in predicting OS was also demonstrated in a multivariate model in 84 myeloma patients (44 pretreated) in which elevated ICTP (>5 mg/l) correlated with poor outcome (Hazard ratio 2.88, 95% CI 1.11–7.42, $p = 0.029$) [64].

In a study by Terpos et al., urinary NTX levels correlated with OS in patients treated with conventional chemotherapy but this was not confirmed by the multivariate analysis [52]. Abildgaard et al. using sequential measurements of both ICTP and NTX showed that high levels of ICTP and NTX correlated with an increased risk for early progression of bone lesions during standard melphalan–prednisolone treatment [6]. This study suggests that ICTP and NTX are clinically useful for identifying patients with increased risk of early progression of bone disease and therefore of disease progression. In a recent study, Terpos et al. analyzed the effect of urinary NTX on survival in 210 patients participated in a randomized study comparing zoledronic acid with pamidronate. Baseline increased urinary NTX values (≥50 nM BCE/mM creatinine) correlated with an 88% increased risk of death (RR 1.88; $p = 0.026$) and a 67% increased risk of first SRE

(RR 1.67; $p = 0.015$) versus normal NTX values (Fig. 3.5) [65]. Markers of bone formation did not correlate with survival in the majority of studies, although in some studies bone formation markers correlated with survival in the univariate analysis [66].

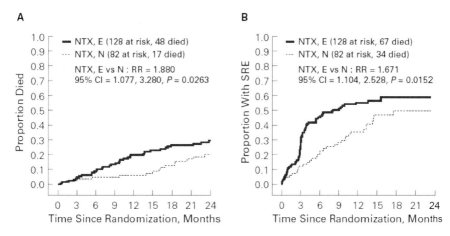

Fig. 3.5 Kaplan–Meier curves for (**a**) survival and (**b**) first on-study SRE by baseline NTX levels in 210 myeloma patients treated with conventional chemotherapy and zoledronic acid [65]. NTX, N-telopeptide of type 1 collagen; E, elevated; N, normal; RR, risk ratio; CI, confidence interval; SRE, skeletal-related event

These data suggest that both serum ICTP and urinary NTX can be of predictive value for disease progression and survival in MM patients and their measurement in clinical trials will reveal their exact prognostic significance mainly in the era of novel anti-myeloma agents.

Bone Markers During Bisphosphonates Therapy: Bisphosphonates are considered as the cornerstone for the management of myeloma bone disease. Oral clodronate and intravenous pamidronate and zoledronic acid significantly reduce bone pain and the incidence of pathologic fractures and other skeletal complications in myeloma patients with lytic bone disease [1, 8]. Biochemical markers of bone turnover have been used in myeloma patients to monitor bisphosphonate treatment in an attempt to identify who will benefit the most from bisphosphonate therapy. Both ICTP and NTX have shown a dramatic reduction post-clodronate, pamidronate, or zoledronic acid administration in myeloma patients with lytic bone disease who also receive anti-myeloma therapies [41, 45, 53, 57, 66–70]. Elomaa et al. have shown that clodronate administration resulted in a significant reduction of ICTP and PINP in 244 myeloma patients compared to the control group; furthermore, high baseline ICTP, PINP, and ALP levels indicated a poor prognosis [66]. Terpos et al. also reported a reduction in biochemical markers of bone metabolism and disease-related pain in MM patients treated with pamidronate. In this study, 62 patients with newly diagnosed MM were randomized to receive both chemotherapy and 90 mg IV pamidronate ($n = 32$) or chemotherapy only ($n = 30$). Biochemical markers of bone metabolism (NTX, bALP, and osteocalcin), disease-related pain, and SREs events were evaluated at the beginning of the study and after 1, 3, 6, 9, 12, and 14 months of treatment. The addition of pamidronate to chemotherapy significantly reduced NTX and disease-related pain compared with patients who only received chemotherapy [45]. Furthermore, in addition to the inhibition of osteoclastic activity, pamidronate in combination with interferon-alpha was shown to induce bone formation in myeloma patients at the plateau phase of their disease [57].

The correlation between bone markers and clinical events has also been studied in a placebo-controlled trial of intravenous ibandronate in patients with advanced MM and measurable bone disease. Patients were randomly assigned to 2 mg IV ibandronate ($n = 99$) or placebo ($n = 99$) in addition to conventional chemotherapy. The effect of ibandronate on bone metabolism was evaluated using serum bALP, osteocalcin, and urinary CTX. Because of patient-to-patient variation in bone markers levels, a post hoc analysis was performed based on mean relative decrease (MRD) from baseline for each of these markers. Among patients who had an MRD $\geq 30\%$ in osteocalcin and $\geq 50\%$ in CTX ($n = 20$), the mean annual incidence of SREs was 0.14 event/year compared with 1.97 events/year in patients who did not achieve an MRD in these markers ($p < 0.0001$). These data suggest that serum osteocalcin and urinary CTX may be useful for monitoring the efficacy of bisphosphonates in individual MM patients and that reduction in these markers below a threshold is associated with a lower risk of skeletal complications [69].

Terpos et al. compared the effect of pamidronate and ibandronate on markers of bone metabolism in myeloma patients. Forty-four patients with advanced MM were randomized to receive either 90 mg IV pamidronate ($n = 23$) or 4 mg IV ibandronate ($n = 21$) in addition to conventional chemotherapy. Both treatment groups showed significant reductions of NTX and TRACP-5b, but no effect on bone formation markers. However, pamidronate produced a greater reduction in NTX and TRACP-5b compared with ibandronate [52, 70]. In a large, randomized study comparing 4 mg zoledronic acid with 90 mg pamidronate every 3–4 weeks in patients with bone metastases from breast cancer or with lytic bone lesions from MM, urinary NTX was dramatically suppressed up to 64% below baseline in both treatment groups for the duration of the study, while the risk of developing a skeletal complication was comparable in the zoledronic acid and pamidronate groups in myeloma patients [68].

Bone marker data from this and other bisphosphonate studies also clearly demonstrate that there is a subset of patients with myeloma bone disease who do not respond to bisphosphonate therapy or may become refractory to bisphosphonate therapy. For example, CTX was shown to be increased in the majority of patients with relapsed/refractory MM despite the use of zoledronic acid [71]. Patients with persistently elevated bone marker levels are at higher risk for SREs and disease progression compared with patients who respond to bisphosphonate therapy and have normalized bone resorption. Lipton et al. examined the correlation between urinary NTX and clinical outcomes in a large database from the randomized trial of intravenous zoledronic acid vs. pamidronate in patients with breast cancer or MM [68].

Results from this exploratory analysis showed that among patients ($n = 170$) who had high baseline NTX ($\geq$64 nM BCE/mM creatinine), patients with persistently elevated NTX levels after 3 months of zoledronic acid therapy ($n = 26$, 15%) had a significantly increased risk of developing a first SRE (RR = 1.71; $p = 0.035$) and shorter SRE-free survival (RR = 1.65; $p = 0.039$) compared with patients with normalized NTX ($n - 137$, 81%) [72]. Therefore, normalization of elevated NTX levels after 3 months of zoledronic acid appears to correlate well with a reduced risk of SREs and a delay in time to first SRE. These findings suggest that normalization of bone resorption is an indicator of good prognosis. In this study, among patients with high NTX at baseline, 15% treated with zoledronic acid and 30% treated with pamidronate did not have normalized NTX after 3 months of bisphosphonate therapy. However, seven (4.1%) and five (3.5%) of patients had died before the 3-month assessment in the zoledronic acid and pamidronate groups, respectively. This subset of patients who did not improve may have an osteoclast-independent mechanism of bone resorption and may benefit from additional therapies [72].

3.5 Novel Markers of Bone Remodeling and Myeloma Bone Disease

Receptor Activator of Nuclear Factor-κB Ligand (RANKL) and Osteoprotegerin (OPG): RANKL and OPG play a crucial role in the development of myeloma bone disease as it has been demonstrated that the ratio of RANKL/OPG is in favor of RANKL in the myeloma microenvironment leading to increased osteoclastogenesis and subsequently increased bone resorption [2–4]. OPG serum levels were reduced in myeloma patients, while the ratio of sRANKL/OPG was increased [59, 73–75]. Our group and others have shown that the ratio of sRANKL/OPG correlates with the extent of bone disease, markers of bone resorption, such as NTX and TRACP-5b, and myeloma stage [59, 75]. The administration of zoledronic acid in patients with asymptomatic myeloma increased serum OPG and thus reduced RANKL/OPG ratio accounting for an effect of zoledronic acid on osteoblast and/or bone marrow stromal cells together with the direct effect on osteoclasts [76]. Terpos et al. showed that the ratio of sRANKL/OPG had an independent predictive value for OS in myeloma patients who received conventional chemotherapy [59] and in patients with relapsed/refractory disease who received the combination of bortezomib, melphalan, dexamethasone, and intermittent thalidomide [77]. However, other researchers have failed to show any significant correlations between serum RANKL and clinical features of myeloma patients [64, 78]. This may be due to the different patient population and different therapies administered. Further studies are needed before we recommend the use of serum RANKL and OPG in the everyday clinical setting. The development of novel therapies targeting the RANK/RANKL/OPG pathway may reveal the importance of the measurement of serum RANKL and OPG. However, this has to be proven in clinical studies.

Other Potential Markers Reflecting Bone Destruction in MM: Bone sialoprotein (BSP) is a phosphorylated 70–80 kDa glycoprotein that accounts for 5–10% of the non-collagenous bone matrix. The protein is a major synthetic product of active osteoclasts and odontoblasts. In bone remodeling BSP is involved in the adhesion of bone resorbing cells to the extracellular bone matrix [79]. BSP levels were associated with skeletal involvement and tumor cell burden and survival in MM patients [13]. The quantification of serum BSP may be a non-invasive method for the diagnosis and follow-up and may improve the prognostic value of conventional staging in myeloma.

Dickkopf-1 (Dkk-1) protein is a wingless type (Wnt) pathway inhibitor which is crucial for osteoblast stimulation. In myeloma patients, Tian et al. first described that there is increased expression of Dkk-1 in plasma cells which correlates with the presence of lytic lesions both in plain radiography and in MRI [80]. Dkk-1 was elevated in the bone marrow plasma of MM patients and associated with the concentrations of Dkk-1 in peripheral blood, the levels of Dkk-1 transcripts in myeloma cells, and the presence of osteolytic lesions [80–82]. Studies on gene expression in 171 newly diagnosed MM patients showed that overexpression of Dkk-1 correlated to the degree of osteolytic bone disease [83]. Similarly, serum Dkk-1 was elevated in myeloma patients with lytic bone disease compared to those without lytic lesions in conventional radiography, but it also correlated with the number of bone lesions [81]. On the contrary, MGUS patients had lower serum levels of Dkk-1 compared with MM patients and did not differ from controls values, supporting the notion that osteoblast function may not been altered in MGUS, at least through the Dkk-1 pathway. Furthermore, serum Dkk-1 concentrations correlate with ISS stage; patients with stage 2 and stage 3 disease had higher values of Dkk-1 than patients with stage 1 disease [81]. The Arkansas group has reported that Dkk-1-negative myeloma cells in trephine biopsies had more aggressive features and plasmablastic morphology, while Dkk-1 was rarely expressed by plasma cells of myeloma patients who have end-stage disease or secondary plasma cell leukemia, suggesting that Dkk-1 expression is restricted to a specific stage of myeloma [84].

3.6 The Effect of Novel Anti-myeloma Agents on Markers of Bone Remodeling

Immunomodulatory drugs (IMiDs) and proteasome inhibitors, such as bortezomib, are used for the management of myeloma patients during the last decade. Thalidomide, lenalidomide, and bortezomib are very effective in both newly diagnosed and relapsed/refractory myeloma patients. The role of these drugs in bone metabolism has been evaluated in several studies.

Immunomodulatory Drugs: Two clinical, phase II trials have studied the effect of thalidomide on bone metabolism of patients with MM (Table 3.4). In the first study, Terpos et al. showed in relapsed/refractory MM patients that the combination of intermediate dose of thalidomide (200 mg/day) with dexamethasone produced a significant reduction of serum markers of bone resorption (CTX and TRACP-5b) at the third month post-initiation of treatment, which continued at the sixth month of the study. The combined treatment also reduced sRANKL levels and sRANKL/OPG ratio at 6 months posttreatment initiation. Furthermore, there was a strong correlation between changes of sRANKL/OPG ratio and changes of TRACP-5b and CTX, suggesting that the reduction of bone resorption by thalidomide is, at least partially, due to the reduction of RANKL levels. Despite the reduction of bone resorption, intermediate doses of thalidomide and dexamethasone showed no effect on bone formation, as assessed by serum levels of bALP and OC [85]. In the second study, Tosi et al. showed in newly diagnosed MM patients that the combination of thalidomide (100 mg/day for 2 weeks and then 200 mg/day), dexamethasone, and zoledronic acid for 4 months produced a significant reduction in markers of bone resorption (urinary NTX and serum CTX), but only in responders. This reduction was accompanied by a reduction in bone pain in 60% of the patients. However, markers of bone formation (bALP and OC) were also reduced in all patients (responders and refractory), suggesting that the combined regimen may have a negative effect on the already exhausted osteoblasts of newly diagnosed patients, possibly due to the concomitant use of dexamethasone [86].

Table 3.4 Clinical studies for the effect of novel anti-myeloma agents on bone metabolism

Agent	MM study population	No. of patients	Results	Subpopulation analysis
Thalidomide (+Dexa)				
Tosi et al. [86][a]	Newly diagnosed	40	↓ Bone resorption markers (CTX and NTX)	In responders
			↓ Bone formation markers (bALP and OC)	In all patients
Terpos et al. [85][a]	Refractory/relapsed	35	↓ Bone resorption markers (CTX and TRACP-5b)	In all patients
			↓ Osteoclast stimulators (sRANKL, sRANKL/OPG ratio)	In all patients
			↔ Bone formation markers (bALP and OC)	In all patients
Lenalidomide				
Breitkreutz et al. [87]	Refractory/relapsed	11	↓ Osteoclast numbers	ND
			↓ Osteoclast differentiation	
			↓ Bone resorption	
Bortezomib (± Dexa)				

Table 3.4 (continued)

Agent	MM study population	No. of patients	Results	Subpopulation analysis
Heider et al. [90][a]	Refractory/relapsed	58	↑ Bone formation markers (bALP and OC)	In all patients
Terpos et al. [92][a]	Refractory/relapsed	34	↓ Bone resorption markers (CTX and TRACP-5b)	In all patients
			↓ Osteoclast stimulators (sRANKL, sRANKL/OPG ratio)	In all patients
			↑ Bone formation markers (bALP and OC)	In responders[b]
			↓ Osteoblast inhibitors (Dkk-1)	In all patients
			↓ Osteoclast stimulators (sRANKL, sRANKL/OPG ratio)	In all patients
Giuliani et al. [91][a]	Refractory/relapsed	21	↓ Bone resorption markers (CTX)	In all patients[c]
			↑ Osteoblast numbers	In responders
Terpos et al. [77][a] (VMDT regimen)	Refractory/relapsed	62	↓ Bone resorption markers (CTX and TRACP-5b)	In all patients
			↓ Osteoclast stimulators (sRANKL, sRANKL/OPG, MIP-1α)	In all patients
			↔ Bone formation markers (bALP and OC)	In all patients
			↓ Osteoblast inhibitors (Dkk-1)	In all patients

[a] Concomitant bisphosphonates administration in the majority of patients.
[b] bALP was increased only in responders while OC was elevated in all patients.
[c] This reduction did not reach statistical significance.

There are very limited data on the effect of lenalidomide on bone remodeling in myeloma patients. In a small study, lenalidomide reduced serum RANKL and increased serum OPG leading to a reduction of the serum RANKL/OPG ratio [87]. In conclusion, it seems that thalidomide reduces bone resorption either directly through the inhibition of osteoclast formation or indirectly through the reduction of tumor burden, and therefore it seems to have a beneficial effect on the altered bone remodeling in MM. For lenalidomide, this has to be confirmed by further clinical studies. However, IMiDs may have no effect on osteoblast function and bone formation.

Bortezomib: An increasing number of studies are reporting the effects of borte-zomib on bone formation in the clinical setting, confirming preclinical observations. The first indications that bortezomib may have a positive effect on bone formation came from Zangari et al., who observed a significant increase in serum ALP lev-els in patients who responded to bortezomib [88, 89]. Osteoblast stimulation by bortezomib was also reported by Heider et al., who measured changes in bALP and OC, in patients who received bortezomib $\pm$ dexamethasone ($n = 25$) and in a control group of patients who received adriamycin/dexamethasone, melpha-lan/prednisone, or thalidomide-containing regimens ($n = 58$). Significant increases in bALP and OC following bortezomib treatment were observed in both respon-ders and non-responders, irrespective of whether dexamethasone was included in the treatment regimen. Conversely, in the control group of patients, who did not receive bortezomib, no increase in osteoblast markers was seen, suggesting that the effect on osteoblasts is unique to the proteasome inhibitor [90]. These results are in accordance with those by Giuliani et al. who found significant increases in the number of osteoblasts/mm^2 of bone tissue and Runx2/Cbfa1-positive osteoblasts in the trephine biopsies of responding patients to bortezomib, but not in those who did not respond [91]. Furthermore, Terpos et al. investigated the effect of bortezomib monotherapy on bone turnover in 34 patients with relapsed MM [92]. Bortezomib administration resulted in a significant reduction in Dkk-1 and RANKL levels, with concomitant reduction in osteoclast function and bone resorption, as assessed by TRACP-5b and CTX serum levels. These reductions occurred irrespective of response to therapy. In addition, bortezomib significantly increased levels of bALP and OC (Table 3.4). Patients who achieved a complete (CR) or a very good partial response to bortezomib had greater elevations of bALP levels. Interestingly, 75% of non-responders had also an increase in bALP levels following four cycles of borte-zomib monotherapy. Although no healing of lytic bone lesions was observed, even in patients who achieved a CR, longer follow-up or prolonged bortezomib therapy may be needed to demonstrate a radiographic improvement after increased bone formation [92]. However, when bortezomib is combined with other anti-myeloma agents, such as melphalan, dexamethasone, and intermittent thalidomide (VMDT regimen) the reduction of Dkk-1, sRANKL, sRANKL/OPG ratio, MIP-1α, and CTX was not accompanied by an increase in bALP and OC [77]. This observation may suggest that bortezomib in combination with other anti-myeloma agents may lose its beneficial effect on osteoblasts. Indeed, Heider et al. found a lower increase in bALP in patients who received the combination of bortezomib with dexamethasone compared with patients who received bortezomib alone [90].

At this point, it is crucial to mention that different effective anti-myeloma reg-imens in combination with bisphosphonates also reduce bone resorption through the reduction of tumor burden and the inhibition of osteoclast function [59]. It is very difficult to distinguish in the previously mentioned clinical studies whether the reduction of bone resorption is due to a direct effect of bortezomib on osteoclasts, due to an indirect effect through reduction of tumor burden, or due to both. Thus, randomized trials are needed to explore whether bortezomib alone or in combina-tion with other agents, including bisphosphonates, can inhibit bone resorption more effectively.

3.7 Conclusions

Biochemical markers of bone remodeling are potentially useful tools for the evaluation of the extent of bone disease and the follow-up of anti-resorptive treatment in MM patients. In patients with established bone lytic lesions, most bone markers are abnormal, indicating that these parameters faithfully reflect changes in bone metabolism associated with the malignant process. Serum ICTP and urinary NTX seem to be more accurate than other resorption markers in reflecting both the severity of bone destruction and the efficacy of bisphosphonate treatment in myeloma. TRACP-5b also seems to be a useful marker but needs further evaluation. Although it is unlikely that a single marker of bone remodeling has sufficient diagnostic or prognostic value in myeloma bone disease, the combination of these markers with other laboratory tests and imaging techniques is likely to improve the clinical assessment of patients with myeloma.

There is a correlation between serum ICTP and urinary NTX with an increased risk of progressive bone disease, development of SREs, and OS. Patients with smoldering myeloma and patients with normal radiographs are subgroups in which resorption markers might be particularly useful. Elevated ICTP or NTX may support a decision to initiate anti-myeloma therapy in patients with smoldering myeloma or to start bisphosphonate treatment in patients without lytic bone disease. In the present era where new anti-resorptive agents (denosumab, other anti-RANKL agents) or new drugs that enhance osteoblast function (anti-Dkk-1 agents) are in development these assays might be of particular value. However, further trials are needed to establish the predictive value of these markers before introducing them into routine use.

References

1. Coleman RE. Bisphosphonates: clinical experience. Oncologist. 2004;9(Suppl 4): 14–27.
2. Terpos E, Dimopoulos MA. Myeloma bone disease: pathophysiology and management. Ann Oncol. 2005;16:1223–1231.
3. Roodman GD. Pathogenesis of myeloma bone disease. Leukemia. 2009;23:435–441.
4. Callander NS, Roodman GD. Myeloma bone disease. Semin Hematol. 2001;38:276–285.
5. Mileshkin L, Blum R, Seymour JF, et al. A comparison of fluorine-18 fluoro-deoxyglucose PET and technetium-99m sestamibi in assessing patients with multiple myeloma. Eur J Haematol. 2004;72:32–37.
6. Abildgaard N, Brixen K, Eriksen EF, et al. Sequential analysis of biochemical markers of bone resorption and bone densitometry in multiple myeloma. Haematologica. 2004;89: 567–577.
7. Winterbottom AP, Shaw AS. Imaging patients with myeloma. Clin Radiol. 2009;64:1–11.
8. Kyle RA, Yee GC, Somerfield MR, et al. American Society of Clinical Oncology 2007 clinical practice guideline update on the role of bisphosphonates in multiple myeloma. J Clin Oncol. 2007;25:2464–2472.
9. Terpos E, Sezer O, Croucher P, Dimopoulos MA. Myeloma bone disease and proteasome inhibition therapies. Blood. 2007;110:1098–1104.

10. Calvo MS, Eyre DR, Gundberg CM. Molecular basis and clinical application of biological markers of bone turnover. Endocrine Rev. 1996;17:333–368.
11. Hannon RA, Eastell R. Biochemical markers of bone turnover and fracture prediction. J Br Menopause Soc. 2003;9:10–15.
12. Hannon RA, Clowes JA, Eagleton AC, et al. Clinical performance of immunoreactive tartrate-resistant acid phosphatase isoform 5b as a marker of bone resorption. Bone. 2004;34: 187–194.
13. Woitge HW, Pecherstorfer M, Horn E, et al. Serum bone sialoprotein as a marker of tumour burden and neoplastic bone involvement and as a prognostic factor in multiple myeloma. Br J Cancer. 2001;84:344–351.
14. Seibel MJ. Biochemical markers of bone turnover: part I: biochemistry and variability. Clin Biochem Rev. 2005;26:97–122.
15. Delmas PD. Bone marker nomenclature. Bone. 2001;28:575–576.
16. Prockop DJ, Keiser HR, Sjoerdsma A. Gastrointestinal absorption and renal excretion of hydroxyproline peptides. Lancet. 1962;2:527–528.
17. Al-Dehaimi AW, Blumsohn A, Eastell R. Serum galactosyl hydroxylysine as a biochemical marker of bone resorption. Clin Chem. 1999;45:676–681.
18. Leigh SD, Ju HS, Lundgard R, et al. Development of an immunoassay for urinary galactosyl-hydroxylysine. J Immunol Methods. 1998;220:169–178.
19. Eyre DR, Paz MA, Gallop PM. Cross-linking in collagen and elastin. Annu Rev Biochem. 1984;53:717–748.
20. Knott L, Bailey AJ. Collagen cross-links in mineralizing tissues: a review of their chemistry, function, and clinical relevance. Bone. 1998;22:181–187.
21. Hanson DA, Weis MA, Bollen AM, et al. A specific immunoassay for monitoring human bone resorption: quantitation of type I collagen cross-linked N-telopeptides in urine. J Bone Miner Res. 1992;7:1251–1258.
22. Apone S, Lee MY, Eyre DR. Osteoclasts generate cross-linked collagen N-telopeptides (NTx) but not free pyridinolines when cultured on human bone. Bone. 1997;21:129–136.
23. Bonde M, Garnero P, Fledelius C, et al. Measurement of bone degradation products in serum using antibodies reactive with an isomerized form of an 8 amino acid sequence of the C-telopeptide of type I collagen. J Bone Miner Res. 1997;12:1028–1034.
24. Rosenquist C, Fledelius C, Christgau S, et al. Serum CrossLaps One Step ELISA. First application of monoclonal antibodies for measurement in serum of bone-related degradation products from C-terminal telopeptides of type I collagen. Clin Chem. 1998;44:2281–2289.
25. Janckila AJ, Takahashi K, Sun SZ, Yam LT. Tartrate-resistant acid phosphatase isoform 5b as serum marker for osteoclastic activity. Clin Chem. 2001;47:74–80.
26. Janckila AJ, Neustadt DH, Nakasato YR, et al. Serum tartrate-resistant acid phosphatase isoforms in rheumatoid arthritis. Clin Chim Acta. 2002;320:49–58.
27. Lam WK, Eastlund DT, Li CY, Yam LT. Biochemical properties of tartrate-resistant acid phosphatase in serum of adults and children. Clin Chem. 1978;24:1105–1108.
28. Ylipahkala H, Halleen JM, Kaija H, et al. Tartrate-resistant acid phosphatase 5B circulates in human serum in complex with alpha2-macroglobulin and calcium. Biochem Biophys Res Commun. 2003;308:320–324.
29. Moss DW. Perspectives in alkaline phosphatase research. Clin Chem. 1992;38:2486–2492.
30. Gallop PM, Lian JB, Hauschka PV. Carboxylated calcium-binding proteins and vitamin K. N Engl J Med. 1980;302:1460–1466.
31. Nelsestuen GL, Shah AM, Harvey SB. Vitamin K-dependent proteins. Vitam Horm. 2000;58:355–389.
32. Young MF, Kerr JM, Ibaraki K, et al. Structure, expression, and regulation of the major noncollagenous matrix proteins of bone. Clin Orthop. 1992;281:275–294.
33. Sierra J, Villagra A, Paredes R, et al. Regulation of the bone-specific osteocalcin gene by p300 requires Runx2/Cbfa1 and the vitamin D3 receptor but not p300 intrinsic histone acetyltransferase activity. Mol Cell Biol. 2003;23:3339–3351.

34. Koeneman KS, Kao C, Ko SC, et al. Osteocalcin-directed gene therapy for prostate-cancer bone metastasis. World J Urol. 2000;18:102–110.
35. Christenson RH. Biochemical markers of bone metabolism: an overview. Clin Biochem. 1997;30:573–593.
36. Smedsrod B, Melkko J, Risteli L, Risteli J. Circulating C-terminal propeptide of type I procollagen is cleared mainly via the mannose receptor in liver endothelial cells. Biochem J. 1990;271:345–350.
37. Risteli J, Risteli L. Assays of type I procollagen domains and collagen fragments: problems to be solved and future trends. Scand J Clin Lab Invest Suppl. 1997;227:105–113.
38. Fohr B, Dunstan CR, Seibel MJ. Clinical review 165: Markers of bone remodeling in metastatic bone disease. J Clin Endocrinol Metab. 2003;88:5059–5075.
39. Nawawi H, Samson D, Apperley J, Girgis S. Biochemical bone markers in patients with multiple myeloma. Clin Chim Acta. 1996;253:61–77.
40. Abildgaard N, Bentzen SM, Nielsen JL, Heickendorff L. Serum markers of bone metabolism in multiple myeloma: prognostic value of the carboxy-terminal telopeptide of type I collagen (ICTP). Br J Haematol. 1997;96:103–110.
41. Withold W, Arning M, Schwarz M, et al. Monitoring of multiple myeloma patients by simultaneously measuring marker substances of bone resorption and formation. Clin Chim Acta. 1998;269:21–30.
42. Carlson L, Larsson A, Simonsson B, et al. Evaluation of bone disease in multiple myeloma: a comparison between the resorption markers urinary deoxypyridinoline/creatinine (DPD) and serum ICTP, and an evaluation of the DPD/osteocalcin and ICTP/osteocalcin ratios. Eur J Haematol. 1999;62:300–306.
43. Woitge HW, Pecherstorfer M, Li Y, et al. Novel serum markers of bone resorption: clinical assessment and comparison with established urinary indices. J Bone Miner Res. 1999;14:792–801.
44. Fonseca R, Trendle MC, Leong T, et al. Prognostic value of serum markers of bone metabolism in untreated multiple myeloma patients. Br J Haematol. 2000;109:24–29.
45. Terpos E, Palermos J, Tsionos K, et al. Effect of pamidronate administration on markers of bone turnover and disease activity in multiple myeloma. Eur J Haematol. 2000;65:331–336.
46. Woitge HW, Horn E, Keck AV, et al. Biochemical markers of bone formation in patients with plasma cell dyscrasias and benign osteoporosis. Clin Chem. 2001;47:686–693.
47. Corso A, Arcaini L, Mangiacavalli S, et al. Biochemical markers of bone disease in asymptomatic early stage multiple myeloma. A study on their role in identifying high risk patients. Haematologica. 2001;86:394–398.
48. Jakob C, Zavrski I, Heider U, et al. Bone resorption parameters [carboxy-terminal telopeptide of type-I collagen (ICTP), amino-terminal collagen type-I telopeptide (NTx), and deoxypyridinoline (Dpd)] in MGUS and multiple myeloma. Eur J Haematol. 2002;69:37–42.
49. Alexandrakis MG, Passam FH, Malliaraki N, et al. Evaluation of bone disease in multiple myeloma: a correlation between biochemical markers of bone metabolism and other clinical parameters in untreated multiple myeloma patients. Clin Chim Acta. 2002;325:51–57.
50. Abildgaard N, Brixen K, Kristensen JE, et al. Comparison of five biochemical markers of bone resorption in multiple myeloma: elevated pre-treatment levels of S-ICTP and U-Ntx are predictive for early progression of the bone disease during standard chemotherapy. Br J Haematol. 2003;120:235–242.
51. Terpos E, Szydlo R, Apperley JF, et al. Soluble receptor activator of nuclear factor kappaB ligand-osteoprotegerin ratio predicts survival in multiple myeloma: proposal for a novel prognostic index. Blood. 2003;102:1064–1069.
52. Terpos E, de la Fuente J, Szydlo R, et al. Tartrate-resistant acid phosphatase isoform 5b: a novel serum marker for monitoring bone disease in multiple myeloma. Int J Cancer. 2003;106:455–457.

53. Coleman RE, Major P, Lipton A, et al. Predictive value of bone resorption and formation markers in cancer patients with bone metastases receiving the bisphosphonate zoledronic acid. J Clin Oncol. 2005;23:4925–4935.
54. Kuliszkiewicz-Janus M, Małecki R, Zółtaszek A, Zastawny M. The significance of carboxy-terminal telopeptide of type I collagen (ICTP) and osteocalcin (OC) in assessment of bone disease in patients with multiple myeloma. Leuk Lymphoma. 2005;46:1749–1753.
55. Dizdar O, Barista I, Kalyoncu U, et al. Biochemical markers of bone turnover in diagnosis of myeloma bone disease. Am J Hematol. 2007;82:185–191.
56. Jakob C, Sterz J, Liebisch P, et al. Incorporation of the bone marker carboxy-terminal telopeptide of type-1 collagen improves prognostic information of the International Staging System in newly diagnosed symptomatic multiple myeloma. Leukemia. 2008;22:1767–1772.
57. Terpos E, Palermos J, Viniou N, et al. Pamidronate increases markers of bone formation in patients with multiple myeloma in plateau phase under interferon-alpha treatment. Calcif Tissue Int. 2001;68:285–290.
58. Clark RE, Flory AJ, Ion EM, et al. Biochemical markers of bone turnover following high-dose chemotherapy and autografting in multiple myeloma. Blood. 2000;96:2697–2702.
59. Terpos E, Politou M, Szydlo R, et al. Autologous stem cell transplantation normalizes abnormal bone remodeling and sRANKL/osteoprotegerin ratio in patients with multiple myeloma. Leukemia. 2004;18:1420–1426.
60. Abildgaard N, Glerup H, Rungby J, et al. Biochemical markers of bone metabolism reflect osteoclastic and osteoblastic activity in multiple myeloma. Eur J Haematol. 2000;64: 121–129.
61. Jakob C, Zavrski I, Heider U, et al. Serum levels of carboxy-terminal telopeptide of type-I collagen are elevated in patients with multiple myeloma showing skeletal manifestations in magnetic resonance imaging but lacking lytic bone lesions in conventional radiography. Clin Cancer Res. 2003;9:3047–3051.
62. Alexandrakis MG, Kyriakou DS, Passam FH, et al. Urinary N-telopeptide levels in multiple myeloma patients, correlation with Tc-99m-sestaMIBI scintigraphy and other biochemical markers of disease activity. Hematol Oncol. 2003;21:17–24.
63. Turesson I, Abildgaard N, Ahlgren T, et al. Prognostic evaluation in multiple myeloma: an analysis of the impact of new prognostic factors. Br J Haematol. 1999;106: 1005–1012.
64. Schütt P, Rebmann V, Brandhorst D, et al. The clinical significance of soluble human leukocyte antigen class-I, ICTP, and RANKL molecules in multiple myeloma patients. Hum Immunol. 2008;69:79–87.
65. Terpos E, Berenson J, Lipton A, et al. High baseline NTX predicts for inferior survival and shorter time to first SRE in Multiple Myeloma. Clin Lymphoma Myeloma. 2009;9(Suppl 1):50–51.
66. Elomaa I, Risteli L, Laakso M, et al. Monitoring the action of clodronate with type I collagen metabolites in multiple myeloma. Eur J Cancer. 1996;32A:1166–1170.
67. Berenson JR, Rosen LS, Howell A, et al. Zoledronic acid reduces skeletal-related events in patients with osteolytic metastases. Cancer. 2001;91:1191–1200.
68. Rosen LS, Gordon D, Kaminski M, et al. Zoledronic acid versus pamidronate in the treatment of skeletal metastases in patients with breast cancer or osteolytic lesions of multiple myeloma: a phase III, double-blind, comparative trial. Cancer J. 2001;7:377–387.
69. Menssen HD, Sakalova A, Fontana A, et al. Effects of long-term intravenous ibandronate therapy on skeletal-related events, survival, and bone resorption markers in patients with advanced multiple myeloma. J Clin Oncol. 2002;20:2353–2359.
70. Terpos E, Viniou N, de la Fuente J, et al. Pamidronate is superior to ibandronate in decreasing bone resorption, interleukin-6 and beta 2-microglobulin in multiple myeloma. Eur J Haematol. 2003;70:34–42.

71. Terpos E, Mihou D, Szydlo R, et al. The combination of intermediate doses of thalido-mide with dexamethasone is an effective treatment for patients with refractory/relapsed multiple myeloma and normalizes abnormal bone remodeling, through the reduction of sRANKL/osteoprotegerin ratio. Leukemia. 2005;19:1969–1976.

72. Lipton A, Cook RJ, Coleman RE, et al. Clinical utility of biochemical markers of bone metabolism for improving the management of patients with advanced multiple myeloma. Clin Lymphoma Myeloma. 2007;7:346–353.

73. Seidel C, Hjertner O, Abildgaard N, et al. Serum osteoprotegerin levels are reduced in patients with multiple myeloma with lytic bone disease. Blood. 2001;98:2269–2271.

74. Lipton A, Ali SM, Leitzel K, et al. Serum osteoprotegerin levels in healthy controls and cancer patients. Clin Cancer Res. 2002;8:2306–2310.

75. Goranova-Marinova V, Goranov S, Pavlov P, Tzvetkova T. Serum levels of OPG, RANKL and RANKL/OPG ratio in newly-diagnosed patients with multiple myeloma. Clinical correlations. Haematologica. 2007;92:1000–1001.

76. Martini G, Gozzetti A, Gennari L, et al. The effect of zoledronic acid on serum osteoprotegerin in early stage multiple myeloma. Haematologica. 2006;91:1720–1721.

77. Terpos E, Kastritis E, Roussou M, et al. The combination of bortezomib, melphalan, dex-amethasone and intermittent thalidomide is an effective regimen for relapsed/refractory myeloma and is associated with improvement of abnormal bone metabolism and angiogenesis. Leukemia. 2008;22:2247–2256.

78. Kraj M, Owczarska K, Sokołowska U, et al. Correlation of osteoprotegerin and sRANKL concentrations in serum and bone marrow of multiple myeloma patients. Arch Immunol Ther Exp. 2005;53:454–464.

79. Nanci A. Content and distribution of noncollagenous matrix proteins in bone and cementum: relationship to speed of formation and collagen packing density. J Struct Biol. 1999;126: 256–269.

80. Tian E, Zhan F, Walker R, et al. The role of the Wnt-signaling antagonist DKK1 in the development of osteolytic lesions in multiple myeloma. N Engl J Med. 2003;349: 2483–2494.

81. Politou MC, Heath DJ, Rahemtulla A, et al. Serum concentrations of Dickkopf-1 protein are increased in patients with multiple myeloma and reduced after autologous stem cell transplantation. Int J Cancer. 2006;119:1728–1731.

82. Kaiser M, Mieth M, Liebisch P, et al. Serum concentrations of DKK-1 correlate with the extent of bone disease in patients with multiple myeloma. Eur J Hematol. 2008;80:490–494.

83. Haaber J, Abildgaard N, Knudsen LM, et al. Myeloma cell expression of 10 candidate genes for osteolytic bone disease. Only overexpression of DKK1 correlates with clinical bone involvement at diagnosis. Br J Haematol. 2008;140:25–35.

84. Yaccoby S, Ling W, Zhan F, et al. Antibody-based inhibition of DKK1 suppresses tumor-induced bone resorption and multiple myeloma growth in vivo. Blood. 2007;109:2106–2111.

85. Terpos E, Mihou D, Szydlo R, et al. The combination of intermediate doses of thalido-mide with dexamethasone is an effective treatment for patients with refractory/relapsed multiple myeloma and normalizes abnormal bone remodeling, through the reduction of sRANKL/osteoprotegerin ratio. Leukemia. 2005;19:1969–1976.

86. Tosi P, Zamagni E, Cellini C, et al. First-line therapy with thalidomide, dexamethasone and zoledronic acid decreases bone resorption markers in patients with multiple myeloma. Eur J Haematol. 2006;76:399–404.

87. Breitkreutz I, Raab MS, Vallet S, et al. Lenalidomide inhibits osteoclastogenesis, sur-vival factors and bone-remodeling markers in multiple myeloma. Leukemia. 2008;22: 1925–1932.

88. Zangari M, Esseltine D, Lee CK, et al. Response to bortezomib is associated to osteoblastic activation in patients with multiple myeloma. Br J Haematol. 2005;131:71–73.

89. Zangari M, Yaccoby S, Cavallo F, et al. Response to bortezomib and activation of osteoblasts in multiple myeloma. Clin Lymphoma Myeloma. 2006;7:109–114.

90. Heider U, Kaiser M, Muller C, et al. Bortezomib increases osteoblast activity in myeloma patients irrespective of response to treatment. Eur J Haematol. 2006;77:233–238.
91. Giuliani N, Morandi F, Tagliaferri S, et al. The proteasome inhibitor bortezomib affects osteoblast differentiation in vitro and in vivo in multiple myeloma patients. Blood. 2007;110:334–338.
92. Terpos E, Heath DJ, Rahemtulla A, et al. Bortezomib reduces serum dickkopf-1 and receptor activator of nuclear factor-kappaB ligand concentrations and normalises indices of bone remodelling in patients with relapsed multiple myeloma. Br J Haematol. 2006;135:688–692.

Chapter 4
Radiation Therapy in Multiple Myeloma

Joel S. Greenberger

Abstract Radiation oncology continues to play an important role in the care of patients with multiple myeloma. Curative therapy of localized bone lesions has been enhanced by the advent of intensity modulated radiotherapy and conformal stereotactic radiation therapy techniques that deliver radiocontrolling doses to small volumes and minimize normal tissue damage. New techniques for total body irradiation and the increasing availability of normal tissue radioprotective agents, allow the radiation oncologist to prepare patients for bone marrow transplantation with further reduction in normal tissue side effects. A major challenge in the total body irradiation patient remains the minimization of pulmonary toxicity. Selective pulmonary radioprotection by inhalation-specific delivery of radioprotectants to the lung could allow bone marrow in ribs, vertebral bodies, sternum, and clavicles to be target of therapeutic irradiation. These new modalities may facilitate improvement in both cure and the quality of life for multiple myeloma patients.

Keywords Radiation · Bone marrow injury · Apoptosis · Palliation · Myeloma

4.1 Introduction

The spectrum of plasma cell malignancies ranges from solitary plasmacytoma to multiple myeloma and challenges the radiation oncologist to apply the basic principles of radiation biology to each clinical presentation. Radiocontrolling doses for the treatment of a solitary plasmacytoma lesion require field size and fractionation considerations specific to this disease. For lesions in critical or weight-bearing skeletal structures such as the cervical or thoracic spine, challenges remain as to

J.S. Greenberger (✉)
Professor and Chairman, Department of Radiation Oncology,
University of Pittsburgh Cancer Institute, Pittsburgh, PA, 15213, USA
e.mail: greenbergerjs@upmc.edu

G.D. Roodman (ed.), *Myeloma Bone Disease*, Current Clinical Oncology,
DOI 10.1007/978-1-60761-554-5_4, © Springer Science+Business Media, LLC 2010

the effectiveness of new specialized radiotherapy technologies such as frameless stereotactic radiosurgery compared to specialized surgical procedures. Palliation of symptoms from the bone destroying sequelae of multiple myeloma demands careful attention to normal tissue tolerance and the frequent requirement for retreatment of anatomic sites that suffer local recurrence particularly those in close proximity to sensitive normal tissues such as heart, lung, spinal cord, and brainstem. Finally, the availability of new chemotherapeutic agents and advances in bone marrow stem cell transplantation continue to challenge the radiation oncologist to apply total body radiation therapy techniques and boost "field within a field" treatment plans in patients who are candidates for potentially curative bone marrow transplantation. In each of these applications of radiation therapy, the radiation oncologist must pay careful attention to normal tissue tolerance and how normal tissue responses are modified by novel chemotherapeutic agents, biological therapies, and the disease itself.

4.2 Considerations in the Radiation Therapy of Plasma Cell Malignancies

Basic radiation biology follows the principle of the four Rs (reoxygenation, repopulation, redistribution, and repair) [1]. In tumor cells as well as normal tissues, increased cellular oxygen provides the availability of oxygen molecules for interaction with high-energy photons or particle beams producing oxygen radicals and other radical oxygen species (ROS) [2]. These ROS are associated with increased radiosensitivity in vitro of well oxygenated compared to hypoxic cells. Between treatments during fractionated radiotherapy, *reoxygenation* plays a central role in the tumor response. The cell cycle effects of ionizing irradiation also control the relatively increased responsiveness of cells in the mitotic phase (M) or late second gap G2 (resting phase after DNA synthetic phase, before mitotis). Cells in M or G2 are more sensitive than cells in the other phases of the cell cycle. Thus, *redistribution* of cells into these sensitive G2/M phases through the process of the cell cycle brings more cells into the relatively radiosensitive phases [1].

Cell populations in relatively poorly oxygenated areas/hypoxic areas within tumors, and those in nondividing or resting phase (that are not cycling) are known to re-enter the cell cycle after several fractions of radiotherapy, which kills dividing cells and produces space in the tumor volume, as well as revascularizing areas within the tumor. Both of which stimulate cell growth. This *repopulation* response or recruitment of resting/noncycling cells into the cell cycle is another phenomenon known to affect the radiation responsiveness of tumors. Finally, DNA *repair* genes, conserved in all biological organisms from bacteria, yeast, multicellular organisms, to humans, when activated by irradiated ROS-induced single- and double-strand DNA breaks facilitate tumor cell repair. Both normal tissue and tumor cell populations from individuals with variants in a DNA repair gene pathway may show altered radiation responsiveness [1].

Equally important to the radiation oncology approach in the treatment of patients with multiple myeloma are the basic clinical principles of clinical radiation oncology. Radiotherapy side effects as well as tumor responsiveness are critically and directly dependent upon three parameters: (1) *total radiation dose* delivered (measured in ergs per milligram, joules per gram in the Physics laboratory, or as rad or cGy in the clinical realm); (2) *fraction size* (dose delivered per day in a multiday or multiweek course of radiotherapy), and (3) *overall treatment time* measured in days or weeks for the treatment course. The basic principles of clinical radiation therapy also involve a critical awareness of the normal tissue radiosensitization capacity of chemotherapeutic drugs to radiosensitized tumor cells but which also can have deleterious effects on normal tissue responses resulting in increased toxicity [1].

This chapter will address considerations in the use of modern radiotherapy techniques and equipment to care for patients with multiple myeloma. A new concept of the four Ss will be applied to the multiple myeloma protocol (stage, sensitization, symptoms, survival). The radiation oncologist who is consulted to see a patient with solitary plasmacytoma, multiple plasmacytomas, or multiple myeloma must pay attention to both sets of principles (Rs and Ss) to ensure safe and effective care of the patient.

4.3 Considerations in Staging of Patients with Multiple Myeloma

Radiographic diagnosis of solitary lesions of bone includes a long list of differential diagnosis usually all leading to a bone biopsy. The *stage* of disease must be known. Bence–Jones, protein in urine, and other "classic" peripheral blood markers of plasma cell dyscrasias, may target plasmacytoma as the bone lesion; however, other diagnoses are also common depending on the age of the patient and the location of the lesion. Considerations in the differential diagnosis include: Giant cell tumor/Osteoclastoma, Histiocytosis X (solitary granuloma), Lymphoma of bone, and lytic metastasis from a previous or silent primary cancer [3]. Careful evaluation of the total skeleton for other sites of lytic disease using CAT scan, Bone scan, and in some cases MRI scan should be carried out to ensure that a solitary lesion is indeed the presenting phenomenon. Biopsy of rib, pelvis, or long bones may facilitate rapid diagnosis. Close interaction with the hematopathologist and/or bone pathologist including the use of special stains is required to confirm the diagnosis. In some cases with solitary lesions near the cervical or thoracic spine, a neurosurgical approach to biopsy should be considered.

Radiotherapy of solitary lesions of plasmacytoma requires a lower dose than that usually required for primary bone tumors or metastatic lesions. Fractionation size of 1.8–2.0 Gy can be utilized [3]. A treatment course of 10 fractions of 1.8 Gy (or depending on location higher fraction size of these fractions of 4.0 Gy over three successive days) may prove adequate to locally control disease. Careful interaction is required with medical oncologists/hematologists to determine whether use of concomitant chemotherapy is contemplated or should occur prior to initiation of radiotherapy. In specific cases, surgical excision of a solitary lesion may prove a more effective therapy such as that associated with a weight-bearing bone in which pending fracture and placement of a prosthesis may be a better and safer alternative. Postoperative radiation may then be added. In the elderly, osteoporosis/osteomalasia may be a concomitant comorbid disease process. Radiotherapy should follow an orthopedic surgery consultation to consider preparation for internal or external fixation which may prove to be of advantage to the patient. For example, in a solitary tumor of the acetabulum, radiotherapy is known to relieve pain, and as such weight bearing may be increased as painful guarding decreases. This result can paradoxically lead to fracture. Multiple plasmacytoma lesions are usually the harbinger of a requirement to consider systemic chemotherapy. This being the case, radiotherapy should be reserved for those lesions unresponsive to chemotherapy, or in a critical weight-bearing site where cortical bone strength is still judged to be effective, but the danger of further bone destruction is impending. In these situations, prophylactic radiotherapy to preserve bone integrity (and obviate the need for surgical fixation) may be of benefit to the patient. Careful staging is critical before initiating a course of radiotherapy.

4.4 Considerations in Use of Radiotherapy for Treatment of Multiple Myeloma

The mainstay of treatment in patients with multiple myeloma is chemotherapy [4–8]. Patients presenting with painful or structurally damaging bone lesions may require concomitant radiotherapy. The concept of normal tissue *sensitization* by chemotherapeutic drugs must be considered before starting a course of radiotherapy.

For example, a patient presenting with multiple myeloma who has multiple spine lesions may require radiation therapy. Before embarking on a course of spine or pelvis stabilizing radiotherapy, attention to the combination and doses of chemotherapeutic agents must be known. Radiation therapy fraction size and total dose may be adjusted if the patient is receiving a chemotherapeutic drug known to sensitize a critical tissue in the target volume or transit volume. Protracted fractionation, with lower dose per fraction, a greater number of fractions over a longer interval, or using multiple small fields rather than one large field that includes intervening disease-free areas may be advisable in patients who are receiving concomitant chemotherapy using radiosensitizing drugs. For the same anatomic lesion in another patient not receiving chemotherapy (perhaps with solitary plasmacytoma), a different approach may be advisable: here larger fraction sizes and shortened treatment course could be considered. For this reason, radiation oncology residents spend a greater portion of time in their training learning about complications from normal tissue damage as these considerations apply in such cases. The availability of intensity modulated radiotherapy techniques (IMRT) [9] as well as frameless stereotactic radiosurgical techniques including CyberKnife, Trilogy, and Synergy can provide another resource for treatment of lesions in weight-bearing bones or symptomatic areas in patients receiving concomitant chemotherapy. Use of these techniques (if available) allows high fraction size delivery over a shortened treatment course, but with minimal transit volume and minimal damage to normal tissue.

4.5 Considerations in Palliative Radiotherapy of Multiple Myeloma Patients

Patients referred for management of radiographic bone lesions in multiple myeloma must be carefully examined, and treatment decisions based upon symptomatology. *Symptoms* provide the main focus for palliative radiotherapy. A lesion on an x-ray of nonweight-bearing bone that does not threaten to compromise the patient's quality of life if unirradiated (and observed during induction of a new combination chemotherapy regimen) may be one which will heal and in which radiotherapy can be avoided. Alternatively, a lesion in a nonweight-bearing bone, in a structurally silent area which is found on physical examination to be causing pain and which by careful history is one which is causing the patient significant discomfort, is a lesion that could be treated with palliative radiotherapy immediately.

Radiotherapy of plasmacytoma of bone requires a lower total dose, lower fraction size, and can be treated with a shortened treatment course (Table 4.1). This is particularly important for outpatients in whom the number of visits to the Radiation Oncology Department should be minimized. The goal of palliative radiotherapy is to relieve the symptoms and secondarily local control. Bone pain is caused by the expansion of tumor foci into the nerve niche of the periosteal region. Some patients describe bone pain as "like that of a fracture"; others describe it as a "dull ache." In a treatment course of four fractions of 4.0 Gy, pain relief is usually achieved within one to two fractions. A full treatment course should still be completed to prevent local recurrence. In a significant number of patients, a full course of radiotherapy does not relieve symptoms. This consequence may underly a different cause of pain such as referred pain from a spinal lesion in another area, nerve damage, nerve root damage, a central nervous system side effect of chemotherapy, or the disease itself.

Table 4.1   Radiotherapy techniques in the multiple myeloma patient

Local lesion	Location	Fractionation	Field
Solitary lesion	Weight-bearing bone	300 cGy × 10	AP-PA or PA
	Nonweight-bearing bone	400 cGy × 4	AP-PA or PA
Multiple local lesions	Skeletal	300 cGy × 10	AP-PA or PA
		200 cGy × 10	
Total body irradiation for marrow transplant	TBI	Fractionated ± lung shielding	110 cGy × d × 3 or 4 d
		Single fraction	800 cGy low-dose rate

4.6 Total Body Irradiation and Bone Marrow Transplantation in Patients with Multiple Myeloma

In patients refractory to first-line chemotherapy, or in those in whom marrow transplantation is felt to be of potential advantage, considerations of the patient's potential improvement and *survival* should be a primary concern. The use of TBI in patients with multiple myeloma has undergone three separate eras of clinical research. In the 1980s [5, 10], fractionated TBI was utilized in preparation of patients for bone marrow stem cell transplantation. Major toxicities included radiation pneumonitis, radiation enteritis, and secondary opportunistic infection [6, 11, 12]. Several applications for use of TBI in the treatment of multiple myeloma from these initial clinical studies are shown in Table 4.1. Alternative regimens to prepare the patient for transplant included busulfan and cyclophosphamide [13]. The consequence of this first series of clinical trials was the realization that multiple myeloma cells are less radiocurable than other bone marrow seeking and proliferating hematopoietic malignancies including lymphoma, Hodgkin's disease, and lymphoid or myeloid leukemia [8, 14, 15].

These clinical trial results produced a paradox since relapse rates were quite high [5, 6, 10, 16, 17]. The paradox was that plasmacytoma cell lines or multiple myeloma-derived cell lines in vitro showed the same radiation survival curves with respect to D_0 and $\bar{n}$, as did cell lines from patients with more radiocurable lymphoma or leukemia [18]. Recent basic science research discoveries have provided some explanations for the resistance of the disease to cure by marrow transplantation [8, 14, 15, 19–22]. The interaction of multiple myeloma cells with bone marrow stromal cells/osteoblast progenitors [14, 15] and cells of the bone marrow vasculature provided several mechanisms of protection from the tumoricidal effects of total body irradiation [23]. The radiation protective capacity of stromal cells, moving myeloma, and other tumor cells into a radioresistant quiescent phase blocked the redistribution and repopulation response [11, 16, 24–26]. Furthermore, elaboration of radioprotective cytokines by irradiated bone marrow stromal cells and endothelial cells provided a second wave of protection [15]. Third, there was evidence for an enhanced DNA repair capacity of irradiated myeloma cells in situ perhaps also explaining the relative inability of TBI to add to the curability of patients receiving marrow transplants [27].

Two other separate areas of the use of TBI in the treatment of multiple myeloma have followed (Table 4.1). The availability of biological response modifiers including those which counteract the protective interaction of stromal cells and endothelial cells with multiple myeloma cells are shown in Table 4.2. The current availability of new targeted therapies again questions whether total body irradiation can be applied to the therapy in these patients.

Basic principles of total body irradiation apply to the multiple myeloma patients as in other patients receiving TBI. A lowered irradiation dose rate, increased fraction size, use of transmission blocks to protect lung, and the potential to utilize normal tissue-specific radioprotective agents (Amifostine) have gained interest in several clinical centers [34–44]. These novel agents using TBI are shown in Table 4.3.

Table 4.2 Biological response modifiers which can interact with radiotherapy in treatment of the multiple myeloma patient

Agent	Radiologic modifier	Reference
Bortozomib	Proteosome inhibition	20–29
Thalidomide	Antiangiogenic agent	21, 6, 30

Table 4.3 Tumor radiosensitizer/normal tissue radioprotectors

Agent	Potential use	Reference
Amifostine	Protect normal marrow hematopoiesis	31
MnSOD-PL	Protects specific organ from transit-volume irradiation toxicity	32–33

4.7 Conclusions

Solitary plasmacytoma, multifocal plasmacytoma, and multiple myeloma pose a challenge for the radiation oncologist. Isolated lesions in weight-bearing bones or near critical structures such as the cervical thoracic spinal cord demand rapid intervention to stabilize the skeleton and prevent further structural and neurological impairment. The treatment of locally recurrent areas, particularly near the spinal cord is facilitated by the availability of IMRT and frameless stereotactic radiosurgical modalities including: CyberKnife, Trilogy, and Synergy devices which allow larger fraction size and fewer treatments to provide radiocontrollability. A major current challenge for the radiation oncologist is the appropriate utilization of total body irradiation in preparing patients for hematopoietic stem cell transplantation in multiple myeloma. The radiation biology of multiple myeloma cells is complex and involves interaction of tumor cells with the hematopoietic microenvironment including bone marrow stromal cells (osteoblast progenitors and in particular adventitial cells and endothelial cells of the bone marrow). With the advent of new chemotherapeutic agents, and targeted therapies, including biological response modifiers, radiosensitizing effects of these modalities must be approached with caution since toxicity to normal tissues may be exacerbated by total body irradiation. The basic principles of total body irradiation must be applied to each particular protocol including consideration of radiation dose rate, number of fractions, fraction size, and the likelihood that transmission block for protection of lung and other radiosensitive organs may prove beneficial to the patient.

References

1. Hall EJ. Radiobiology for the Radiologist. 4th ed. Philadelphia, PA: J.B. Lippincott Inc.; 1999.
2. McCord J. The evolution of free radicals and oxidative stress. Am J Med. 2000;108:652–659.
3. DeVita V, Hellman S, Rosenberg S. In: DePinho R, Weimberg R, eds. Cancer, Principles & Practice of Oncology. Philadelphia, PA: Lippincott Williams & Wilkins; 2005.

4. Weber DM, Chen C, Niesvizky R, Wang M, Belch A, Stadtmauer EA, Siegel D, Borrello I, Rajkumar SV, Chanan-Khan AA, Lonial S, Yu Z, Patin J, Olesnyckyj M, Zeldis JB, Knight RD. Lenalidomide plus Dexamethasone for relapsed multiple myeloma in North America. N. Engl J Med. 2007;357:2133–2142.
5. Ghobrial J, Ghobrial IM, Mitsiades C, Leleu X, Hatjiharissi E, Moreau A-S, Roccaro A-S, Roccaro A, Schlossman R, Hideshima T, Anderson KC, Richardson P. Novel therapeutic avenues in myeloma: changing the treatment paradigm. Oncology. 2007;21:785–790.
6. Kyle RA, Remstein ED, Therrieau TM, Dispenzieri A, Kurtin PJ, Hodnefield JM, Larson DR, Plevak MF, Jelinek DF, Fonseca R, Melton LJ, Rajkumar SV. Clinical course and prognosis of smoldering (asymptomatic) multiple myeloma. N Engl J Med. 2007;356:2582–2590.
7. Suvannasankha A, Fausel C, Juliar BE, Yiannoutsos CT, Fisher WB, Ansari RH, Wood LL, Smith GG, Cripe LD, Abonour R. Final report of toxicity and efficacy of a phase II study of oral cyclophosphamide, thalidomide, and prednisone for patients with relapsed or refractory multiple myeloma: a hoosier oncology group trial, HEM01-21. Oncologist. 2007;12: 99–106.
8. Kyle RA, Rajkumar SV. Multiple myeloma. Blood. 2008;111(6):2962–2969.
9. Hall EJ, Phil D. Intensity-modulated radiation therapy, protons, and the risk of second cancers. Int J Radiat Oncol Biol Phys. 2006;65(1):1–7.
10. Pant S, Copelan EA. Hematopoietic stem cell transplantation in multiple myeloma. Biol Blood Marrow Transplant. 2007;13:877–885.
11. Vanderkerken K, Medicherla S, Coulton L, DeRaeve H, Willems A, Lawson M, Van Camp B, Protter AA, Higgins LS, Menu E, Croucher PI. Inhibition of p38α mitogen-activated protein kinase prevents the development of osteolytic bone disease, reduces tumor burden, and increases survival in murine models of multiple myeloma. Cancer Res. 2007;67:4572–4577.
12. Bruno B, Rotta M, Patriarca F, Mordini N, Allione B, Carnevale-Schianca F, Giaccone L, Sorasio R, Ornede P, Balde I, Bringhen S, Masaya M, Aglietta M, Levis A, Gallamini A, Fanin R, Palumbo A, Storb R, Ciccone G, Boccadora M. A comparison of allografting with autografting for newly diagnosed myeloma. N Engl J Med. 2007;356:1110–1120.
13. Bensinger WI, Buckner CD, Clift RA, Petersen FB, Bianco JA, Singer JW, Appelbaum FR, Dalton W, Beatty P, Fefer A, Storb R, Thomas ED, Hansen JA. Phase I study of busulfan and cyclophosphamide in preparation for allogeneic marrow transplant for patients with multiple myeloma. J Clin Oncol. 1992;10(9):1492–1497.
14. Hideshima T, Bergsagel PL, Kuehl WM, Anderson KC. Advances in biology of multiple myeloma: clinical applications. Blood. 2004;104(3):607–617.
15. Richardson PG, Schlossman R, Hideshima T, Anderson KC. New treatments for multiple myeloma. Oncology. 2005;19:1781–1790.
16. Hideshima T, Mitsiades C, Tonon G, Richardson PG, Anderson KC. Understanding multiple myeloma pathogenesis in the bone marrow to identify new therapeutic targets. Nat Rev Cancer. 2007;7:585–591.
17. Kuruvilla J, Shepherd JD, Sutherland HJ, Nevill TJ, Nitta J, Le A, Forrest DL, Hogge DE, Lavoie JC, Nantel SH, Toze CL, Smith CA, Barnett MJ, Song KW. Long-term outcome of myeloablative allogeneic stem cell transplantation for multiple myeloma. Biol Blood Marrow Transplant. 2007;13:925–931.
18. FitzGerald TJ, Kase K, Daugherty C, Rothstein L, Greenberger JS. Effect of x-irradiation dose rate on the clonogenic survival of human and experimental animal hematopoietic tumor cell lines: evidence for heterogeneity. Int J Radiat Oncol Biol Phys. 1986;12:69–73.
19. Roccaro AM, Hideshima T, Raje N, Kumar S, Ishitsuka K, Yasuri H, Shiraishi N, Ribatti D, Nico B, Vacca A, Dammacco F, Richardson PG, Anderson KC. Bortezomib mediates antiangiogenesis in multiple myeloma via direct and indirect effects on endothelial cells. Cancer Res. 2006;66(1):184–191.
20. Delogu A, Schebesta A, Sun Q, Aschenbrenner K, Perlot T, Busslinger M. Gene repression by Pax5 in B cells is essential for blood cell homeostasis and is reveresed in plasma cells. Immunity. 2006;24:269–281.

21. Richardson PG, Sonneveld P, Schuster MW, Irwin D, Stadtmauer EA, Facon T, Harousseau J-L, Ben-Yehuda D, Lonial S, Goldschmidt H, Reece D, San-Miguel JF, Blade J, Boccadoro M, Cavenagh J, Dalton WS, Boral AL, Esseltine DL, Porter JB, Schenkein D, Anderson KC. Bortezomib or high-dose Dexamethasone for relapsed multiple myeloma. N Engl J Med. 2005;352:2487–2498.
22. Shapiro-Shelef M, Calame K. Regulation of plasma-cell development. Nat Rev Immunol 2005;5:230–239.
23. Attal M, Harousseau J-L, Facon T, Guilhot F, Doyen C, Fuzibet J-G, Monconduit M, Hulin C, Caillot D, Bouabdallah R, Voillat L, Sotto J-J, Grosbois B, Bataille R. Single versus double autologous stem-cell transplantation for multiple myeloma. N Engl J Med. 2003;349: 2495–2502.
24. Annunziata CM, Davis RE, Demchenko Y, Bellamy W, Gabrea A, Zhan F, Lenz G, Hanamura I, Wright G, Xiao W, Dave S, Hurt EM, Tan B, Zhao H, Stephens O, Santra M, Williams DR, Dang L, Barlogie B, Shaughnessy JD, Kuehl WM, Staudt LM. Frequent engagement of the classical and alternative NF-$_K$B pathways by diverse genetic abnormalities in multiple myeloma. Cancer Cell. 2007;12:115–130.
25. Gilmore TD. Multiple myeloma: lusting for NF-$_K$B. Cancer Cell. 2007;12:95–101.
26. Keats JJ, Fonseca R, Chesi M, Schop R, Baker A, Chng W-J, Van Wier S, Tiedemann R, Shi C-X, Sebag M, Braggio E, Henry T, Zhu Y-X, Fogle H, Price-Troska T, Ahmann G, Mancini C, Brents LA, Kumar S, Greipp P, Dispenzier A, Bryant B, Mulligan G, Bruhn L, Barrett M, Valdez R, Trent J, Stewart AK, Carpten J, Bergsagel PL. Promiscuous mutations activate the noncanonical NF-$_K$B pathway in multiple myeloma. Cancer Cell. 2007;12:131–144.
27. Epperly MW, Greenberger EE, Franicola D, Jacobs S, Greenberger JS. Thalidomide radiosensitization of normal murine hematopoietic but not squamous cell carcinoma or multiple myeloma tumor cell lines. In Vivo. 2006;20:333–340.
28. Blanco B, Perez-Simon JA, Sanchez-Abarca LI, Carvajal-Vergara X, Mateos J, Vidriales B, Lopez-Holgado N, Maiso P, Alberca M, Villaron E, Schenkein D, Pandiella A, San Miguel J. Bortezomib induces selective depletion of alloreactive T lymphocytes and decreases the production of Th1 cytokines. Blood. 2006;107(9):3575–3582.
29. San Miguel J, Schlag R, Khuageva NK, Dimopouos MA, Shpilberg O, Kropff M, Spicka I, Petrucci MT, Palumbo A, Samoilova OS, Dmoszynska A, Abdulkadyrov KM, Schots R, Jiang B, Mateos M-V, Anderson KC, Esseltine DL, Liu K, Cakana A, van de Velde H, Richardson PG. Bortezomib plus melphalan and prednisone for initial treatment of multiple myeloma. N Engl J Med. 2008;359:906–917.
30. van Rhee F, Dhodapkar M, Shaughnessy JD, Anaissie E, Siegel D, Hoering A, Zeldis J, Jenkins B, Singhal S, Mehta J, Crowley J, Jagannath S, Barlogie B. First thalidomide clinical trial in multiple myeloma: a decade later. Blood. 2008;112:1035–1038.
31. Nair CKK, Parida DK, Nomura T. Radioprotectors in radiotherapy. J Radiat Res. 2001;42: 21–37.
32. Greenberger JS, et al. Radioprotective gene therapy. Curr Gene Ther. 2003;3:183–195.
33. Greenberger JS, Epperly MW. Radioprotective antioxidant gene therapy: potential mechanisms of action. Gene Ther Mol Biol. 2004;8:31–44.
34. van Kempen-Harteveld ML, Brand R, Kal HB, Verdonck LF, Hofman P, Schattenberg AV, Van Der Maazen RW, Cornelissen JJ, Eukenboom WMH, Van Der Lelie JP, Oldenburger F, Barge RM, Van Biezen A, Vossen JMJJ, Noorduk EM, Struikmans H. Results of hematopoietic stem cell transplantation after treatment with different high-dose total body irradiation regimens in five dutch centers. Int J Radiat Oncol Biol Phys. 2008;71(5):1444–1454.
35. Cheng JC, Schultheiss TE, Wong JYC. Impact of drug therapy, radiation dose, and dose rate on renal toxicity following bone marrow transplantation. Int J Radiat Oncol Biol Phys. 2008;71(5):1436–1443.
36. Greenberger JS. Toxic effects on the hematopoietic microenvironment. Exp Hematol. 1991;19:1101–1109.

37. Rajkumar SV, Rosinol L, Hussein M, Catalano J, Jedrzejczak W, Lucy L, Olesnyckyj M, Yu Z, Knight R, Zeldis JB, Blade J. Multicenter, randomized, double-blind, placebo-controlled study of thalidomide plus dexamethasone compared as initial therapy for newly diagnosed multiple myeloma. J Clin Oncol. 2008;26(13):2171–2177.
38. Hari P, Pasquini MC, Vesole DH. New questions about transplantation in multiple myeloma. Oncology. 2006;20(10):1230–1237.
39. Moreau P, Facon T, Attai M, Hulin C, Michallet M, Maloisel F, Sotto J-J, Guilhot F, Marit G, Doyen C, Jaubert J, Fuzibet J-G, Francois S, Benboubker L, Monconduit M, Voillat L, Macro M, Berthou C, Dorvaux V, Pignon B, Rio B, Matthes T, Casassus P, Caillot D, Najman N, Grosbois B, Bataille R, Harousseau J-L. Comparison of 200 mg/m^2 melphalan and 8 Gy total body irradiation plus 140 mg/m^2 melphalan as conditioning regimens for peripheral blood stem cell transplantation in patients with newly diagnosed multiple myeloma: final analysis of the Intergroupe Francophone du Myelome 9502 randomized trial. Blood. 2002;99(3): 731–742.
40. Jagannath S, Vesole DH, Glenn L, Crowley J, Barlogie B. Low-risk intensive therapy for multiple myeloma with combined autologous bone marrow and blood stem cell support. Blood. 1992;80(7):1666–1672.
41. Kyle RA, Rajkumar SV. Drug therapy multiple myeloma. N Engl J Med. 2004;351: 1860–1873.
42. Nera K-P, Kohonen P, Narvi E, Peippo A, Mustonen L, Terho P, Koskela K, Buerstedde J-M, Lassila O. Loss of Pax5 promotes plasma cell differentiation. Immunity. 2006;24:283–293.
43. Greenberger JS, FitzGerald TJ, Kleasen V, Anklesaria P, Bushnell D, Kase K, Sakakeeny MA. Alteration in hematopoietic stem cell seeding and proliferation by low-dose-rate irradiation of bone marrow stromal cells in vitro. Int J Radiat Oncol Biol Phys. 1988;14:85–94.
44. Oberley LW, Oberley TD. Free radicals, cancer, and aging. In: Johnson JE, Walford R, Harmon D, Miquel J, eds. Free Radicals, Aging, and Degenerative Diseases. New York: Alan R. Liss Inc.; 1986:325–381.

Chapter 5
Surgical Management of Bone Disease

Mohamad A. Hussein

Abstract Minimally invasive surgery plays an increasingly important role in the management of bone disease in patients with myeloma. The spine is the most common site of bone involvement in myeloma, and minimally invasive vertebral augmentation techniques have been developed which are safe and effective in relieving pain related to vertebral compression fractures in patients with myeloma. Vertebroplasty relieves pain and stabilizes the fractured vertebral body by injecting bone cement percutaneously into the cancellous area, however more recently its role in pain management has been questioned in two double blinded randomized clinical trials. Kyphoplasty is a similar technique, but uses an inflatable tamp to create a uniform cavity in which the bone cement is injected. Compared with vertebroplasty, kyphoplasty is associated with less cement leakage and has the added advantage of restoring vertebral height, which relieves stress on adjacent vertebral bodies and may reduce the risk of additional fractures. Continued improvements in myeloma therapy and the development of these minimally invasive techniques have increased the potential for more patients to be eligible for vertebral augmentation, which may have a favorable impact on pain, disability, quality of life, and even reduction in mortality. Vertebral augmentation is the procedure of choice for myeloma patients with severe pain related to vertebral compression fractures and may play a role in relieving pain and preventing impending fractures in patients with other conditions.

Keywords Surgery · Spine · Compression fracture · Vertebral augmentation · Vertebroplasty · Kyphoplasty

M.A. Hussein (✉)
Celgene Corporation, Summit, NJ 07901, USA
email: mhussein@celgene.com

G.D. Roodman (ed.), *Myeloma Bone Disease*, Current Clinical Oncology,
DOI 10.1007/978-1-60761-554-5_5, © Springer Science+Business Media, LLC 2010

5.1 Background

Recent advances in the treatment of multiple myeloma have extended the life expectancy of patients and are placing increased importance on their long-term supportive care and quality of life [1, 2]. Surgery remains a mainstay in the management of myeloma bone disease and bone-related pain, and recent breakthroughs in minimally invasive surgical techniques for spinal involvement have made surgery a viable treatment option for a greater number of patients.

Approximately 80% of patients with myeloma have evidence of lytic lesions, osteoporosis, or fractures at the time of diagnosis, which can limit mobility as well as increase morbidity and mortality [3]. The most commonly involved skeletal organ in plasma cell dyscrasias is the spine; other common sites include long bones (proximal portions of the humerus and femur), the skull, thoracic cage, and the pelvis.

Spinal involvement is associated with severe pain, disability, pulmonary dysfunction, and poor clinical outcomes [4]. Spinal involvement in patients with myeloma often manifests as vertebral compression fractures that shift the center of gravity forward (Figure 5.1) [5]. This creates a large bending moment, which places additional compressive stress on the anterior spine, particularly in areas adjacent to the fracture. Stress is also placed on surrounding muscles and ligaments, which can be a source of pain. As the center of gravity moves forward and compressive stress

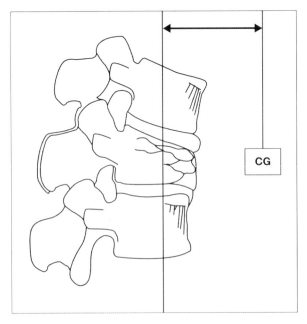

Fig. 5.1 Vertebral compression fractures shift the center of gravity forward. Reproduced with permission from Hussein et al. [5]

increases on adjacent vertebral bodies, the risk of further vertebral compressive fractures increases, creating a "domino effect" that manifests as progressive kyphosis. In patients with myeloma the consequences of kyphosis-related compression fractures can be severe and include compression of the abdominal contents and decreased lung capacity (Table 5.1) [5].

Table 5.1 Consequences of kyphosis [5]

Effect	Clinical consequences
Compression of abdominal contents	• Anorexia
	• Weight loss
Decreased lung capacity	• Limited exercise tolerance
	• Limited physical activity
Anterior loading of spine	• Subsequent fractures
	• Progressive kyphosis and deformity

The impact of vertebral compression fractures on outcomes in patients with myeloma has not been fully defined. However, in a study of nearly 10,000 women aged at least 65 years, in which 20% were found to have vertebral compression fractures related to osteoporosis, vertebral compression fractures were associated with increased morbidity and mortality [6]. Having multiple fractures was associated with a further increase in mortality from 19 per 1,000 woman-years in women without fractures to 44 per 1,000 woman-years in those with five or more fractures. The most common causes of death in women with vertebral fractures were pulmonary disease and cancer. These findings underscore the importance of rapid and effective correction of bone disease to prevent further morbidity and mortality, especially in patients with multiple myeloma where the humoral and cellular immune systems are compromised by the disease and/or its treatment.

5.2 Clinical Presentations of Skeletal Damage in Patients with Multiple Myeloma

Multiple myeloma could present as an unexpected pathologic fracture resulting in pain and diagnosis of the disease. Less often is the presentation of chest pain which could be related to rib lesions or fractures, but more importantly chest pains that are related to sternal pressure. The human straight posture is maintained by two structures: the spine and the sternum. In patients who are newly diagnosed with myeloma or those who have carried the diagnosis for some time, the development of significant spinal disease compromises the spinal structure from performing its physiologic function of supporting the body stature, resulting in increasing pressure on the sternum in order to support the normal posture. With the increasing pressure on the sternum and the sternal structure continuing to be compromised by progressive osteoporosis, the patient becomes at risk of fracturing the sternum. A fracture of the sternum, which is the last support posture structure, results in acute kyphosis and all of the resulting complications. Chest pain in patients with myeloma should alert physicians to the possibility of an impending sternal fracture, which in turn should trigger a thorough evaluation of the spine to stabilize and/or strengthen the vertebral bodies, thus avoiding a complex clinical situation with high morbidity and mortality.

5.3 The Role of Surgery in the Management of Myeloma Bone Disease

Although bisphosphonates have been shown to reduce the risk of skeletal-related events in patients with myeloma [7–14], many patients present with existing bone-related pain and evidence of bone abnormalities. With the exception of the spine, few studies have evaluated orthopedic surgery specifically in patients with myeloma [15–18]. In general, the surgical management of myeloma in weight-bearing bones is similar to the management of bony metastases of carcinomas. Traditional concepts of preventing a fracture apply to myeloma patients as well as to patients with other malignancies. Standard surgical techniques available for bony metastatic disease include internal fixation (e.g., plates and screws, intramedullary devices), reconstructive techniques involving endoprostheses, and augmentation with bone cement [19, 20]. The aim of orthopedic surgery is to restore skeletal function and maintain the ambulatory status of the patient. Compared with metastatic carcinoma, however, myeloma tends to produce more diffuse and extensive lesions in weight-bearing bones [18]. Massive osteolytic lesions, diffuse osteoporosis, and pathological fractures in the hip region are common in patients with myeloma due to infiltration of the acetabulum and proximal femur. Consequently, myeloma patients often require a more aggressive surgical approach in order to overcome the extensive disease adjacent to pathologic or impending fractures and the risk of disease progression. For example, in patients with pathological fractures of the head and neck of the femur, total hip replacement is preferred over internal fixation [18]. For fractures of the subtrochanteric region, intramedullary devices are preferred over plates and screws. Proximal femur replacement may be considered for select patients with extensive destruction of the proximal femur. Papagelopoulos et al. reported that total hip replacement is effective in myeloma patients with extensive lesions in the acetabulum and proximal femur that are not amenable to standard internal fixation techniques [18]. In a series of 50 patients who underwent 53 hip procedures, hip replacement relieved pain, restored bone integrity, preserved joint function, and resulted in satisfactory ambulation in most patients. Minimally invasive techniques, however, are also under investigation. Use of computed tomography (CT)-guided percutaneous acetabuloplasty resulted in pain relief and the ability to resume weight-bearing activities in one small study [21]. The acetabulum is a common site of metastasis, and standard surgical options for acetabular metastases include curettage of the lesion followed by bone cement packing and pin fixation, total hip replacement, and, rarely, hemipelvectomy [21]. Although the development of minimally invasive techniques might allow more patients with myeloma to become eligible for potentially beneficial orthopedic surgery, their efficacy relative to more invasive surgical techniques requires further investigation.

Treatment options for osteolytic lesions of the spine depend on a number of patient- and disease-related factors, such as the neurological and general condition of the patient, the number of disease sites, spinal level, location of lesions within the vertebra, extent of spinal canal involvement, and severity of pain [4]. Outdated traditional treatment options for vertebral collapse include bed rest, analgesics, and bracing [22]. For solitary spinal lesions, vertebrectomy with strut grafting or intra-operative use of bone cement may be considered. However, most patients with myeloma have multifocal disease and are, therefore, ineligible for surgical consolidation. In addition, many of these patients are poor candidates for open surgery due to advanced age and comorbidity factors, leading to longer recovery times and an increased risk of morbidity and mortality. Palliative radiation therapy is also an option and has been shown to relieve pain in up to 90% of patients [4, 23, 24]. However, these effects are delayed, usually occurring 10–14 days after initiating radiation and depending on the site and extent of radiation could compromise the bone marrow reserve for future or current therapy. The effects of radiation therapy on bone strength are also limited and are not evident until 2–4 months after the start of treatment, increasing the risk of vertebral collapse and neurological compression [4]. The limitations of these treatment options have led to the assessment of minimally invasive surgical techniques to relieve pain due to compression fractures and restore vertebral stability. These minimally invasive procedures could be used sequentially or simultaneously with chemotherapy and/or radiation, depending on the clinical status of the patient.

5.4 Minimally Invasive Vertebral Augmentation

5.4.1 Vertebroplasty

Vertebroplasty, a relatively new technique developed in France in the 1980s, involves the percutaneous injection of bone cement into the affected vertebral body using image guidance [25, 26]. Numerous reports have indicated that vertebroplasty reduces pain and strengthens bone in patients with vertebral compression fractures [27–34]. Although this minimally invasive technique offers several advantages over open surgery, it is associated with two inherent limitations: first, vertebroplasty does not restore vertebral height or correct spinal deformity and, second, it is associated with a high rate of leakage (30–60%) as the liquid bone cement is forced into the closed, collapsed space in the vertebral body. Leakage usually has no relevant clinical consequences; however, neurological compression is a rare but potentially devastating risk. Leakage can be largely avoided by injecting the bone cement during open surgery, but the benefits of this minimally invasive approach are then lost.

Few studies have specifically evaluated vertebroplasty in patients with multiple myeloma. In a study of vertebroplasty in patients with osteolytic metastases ($n = 29$) or myeloma ($n = 8$), partial or complete pain relief was achieved in 97% of patients [4, 35, 36]. However, asymptomatic cement leakage into epidural, intradiskal, and venous space occurred at 15, 8, and 2 levels, respectively. Two of eight foraminal leaks led to nerve root compression requiring decompression surgery, and 1 of 21 paravertebral leaks led to transient femoral neuropathy. More recently two randomized, one double blinded placebo controlled study, patients were assigned to vertebroplasty vs. a simulated procedure without cement (control group). In both studies there were no beneficial effect associated with osteoporotic compression fractures in patients treated with vertebroplasty vs. those patients in the control group [37, 38].

5.4.2 Kyphoplasty

Balloon kyphoplasty is a modified version of percutaneous vertebroplasty that was developed in the 1990s. Like vertebroplasty, kyphoplasty stabilizes the vertebral body, but it also restores vertebral body height, which reduces the risk of additional fractures in adjacent vertebrae and slows the progression of kyphosis. During kyphoplasty, the vertebral body is cannulated to allow the placement of an inflatable bone tamp at the site of compression (Fig. 5.2) [25]. The tamp is then inflated, restoring the height of the vertebral body, and the resulting cavity is filled with bone cement. Therefore, kyphoplasty overcomes some of the limitations of vertebroplasty by restoring vertebral body height, especially when performed within the first 6–12 months of the occurrence of the fracture, and reducing the rate of leakage by containing the bone cement within the tamp.

Several studies have evaluated kyphoplasty in patients with osteoporotic and osteolytic vertebral compression fractures [39–46]. The first prospective study [25] to evaluate kyphoplasty specifically in patients with myeloma was conducted at the Myeloma Program of the Cleveland Clinic Foundation (Table 5.2) [4, 25, 35, 36, 45–47]. Kyphoplasty was performed on 55 levels in 18 patients with osteolytic vertebral compression fractures due to myeloma. The average vertebral body height restoration after kyphoplasty was 34%. Significant improvements pre- and post-kyphoplasty were also seen in Short Form 36 Health Survey scores related to pain (23.2 vs. 55.4, respectively; $p = 0.0008$), physical functioning (21.3 vs. 50.6; $p = 0.001$), vitality (31.3 vs. 47.5; $p = 0.01$), and social functioning (40.6 vs. 64.8; $p = 0.014$). Leakage occurred in only 2 of the 55 procedures (4%) and was asymptomatic in both cases. No major complications related to the procedure were observed.

Pflugmacher et al. performed kyphoplasty on 48 vertebral bodies in 20 patients with myeloma [45]. After 1 year of follow-up, they found significant improvements in measures of pain (visual analog scale) and disability (Oswestry disability index). Vertebral height was restored and stabilized for up to 1 year. Kyphotic deformity, which was present in 14 of the 20 patients, was corrected in approximately 80% of

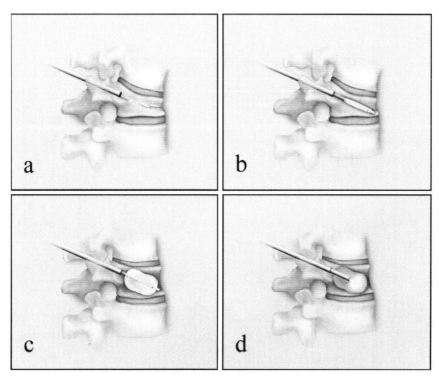

Fig. 5.2 Kyphoplasty. The collapsing vertebral body is cannulated (**a**) so that an inflatable bone tamp can be placed at the site of compression (**b**). The tamp is then inflated (**c**), which restores vertebral body height. Finally, the cavity created by the tamp is filled with bone cement (**d**). Reproduced with permission from Dudeney et al. [25]

cases; the mean correction was 6.3° with only minimal loss of correction (approximately 1.8°) seen 1 year after treatment. Clinically asymptomatic leakage occurred at five levels (10.4%).

In a retrospective study, Köse et al. analyzed quality-of-life outcomes after vertebral augmentation in 34 patients with myeloma and spinal compression fractures [46]. Kyphoplasty was performed on 22 levels in 18 patients, and vertebroplasty was performed on 28 levels in 16 patients. In patients who underwent kyphoplasty, improvement in mean overall pain score from baseline was seen 6 weeks, 6 months, and 12 months after treatment (36.0 vs. 12.1, 8.6, and 9.7, respectively; $p < 0.001$). A similar pattern was seen in those who underwent vertebroplasty (37.8 vs. 15.3, 12.2, and 13.5, respectively; $p < 0.001$). Notably, although mean pain scores were similar in both groups 6 weeks after treatment, the difference was significant after 6 and 12 months, favoring kyphoplasty.

Lane et al. reviewed outcomes after kyphoplasty in myeloma patients with vertebral compression fractures [47]. Kyphoplasty was performed on 46 levels in 19 patients. Overall, 16 of 19 patients had clinically meaningful improvements in

Table 5.2 Selected trials of percutaneous vertebroplasty or kyphoplasty in patients with myeloma [4, 25, 35, 36, 45–47]

Reference	No. of patients/ procedures	Relief of pain and disability	Vertebral height restoration	Cement leakage
Vertebroplasty				
References [4, 35, 36]	37 (8 had myeloma)/NR	97% of patient had partial or complete pain relief	NA	Paravertebral ($n = 21^a$), epidural ($n = 15$), intradiskal ($n = 8$), foraminal ($n = 8^b$), and venous ($n = 2$)
Kyphoplasty				
Dudeney et al. [25]	18/55	Postoperative improvement in SF-36 scores for bodily pain (23.2 vs. 55.4; $p = 0.0008$), physical functioning (21.3 vs. 50.6; $p = 0.001$), vitality (31.3 vs. 47.5; $p = 0.01$), and social functioning (40.6 vs. 64.8; $p = 0.014$)	Mean restoration: 34%	4% of procedures; asymptomatic
Pflugmacher et al. [45]	20/48	Postoperative improvement in pain (visual analog scale) and disability (Oswestry disability index)	Restored and stabilized for up to 1 year Kyphotic deformity ($n = 14$) was corrected in 80% of patients; mean correction: 6.3°; mean loss of correction after 1 year 1.8°	10.4% of procedures; asymptomatic

Table 5.2 (continued)

Reference	No. of patients/procedures	Relief of pain and disability	Vertebral height restoration	Cement leakage
Köse et al. [46]	34 patients: vertebroplasty 16/28 and kyphoplasty 18/22	Vertebroplasty: mean pain score was 37.8, 15.3, 12.2, and 13.5 at baseline, 6 weeks, 6 months, and 12 months, respectively ($p < 0.001$) Kyphoplasty: mean pain score was 36.0, 12.1, 8.6[c], and 9.7[c] at baseline, 6 weeks, 6 months, and 12 months, respectively ($p < 0.001$)	NR	None
Lane et al. [47]	19/46	84% had improvement in Oswestry disability index Mean score improvement: 16.5	Mean restoration: 37.9% (anterior 37.8% and mid-vertebral 53.4%) 76% of procedures resulted in height restoration (anterior 76% and mid-vertebral 91%)	26.3% of procedures

NA, not applicable; NR, not reported; SF-36, Short Form 36 Health Survey.

[a]One paravertebral leak led to transient femoral neuropathy.

[b]Two foraminal leaks led to nerve root compression requiring decompression surgery.

[c]Difference in mean pain scores at 6 and 12 months between vertebroplasty and kyphoplasty group was statistically significant, favoring kyphoplasty ($p = 0.024$ and $p = 0.027$, respectively).

Oswestry disability index scores (mean scores improved from 48.94 to 32.6 after treatment and the mean improvement in score was 16.5). Patients with pre-treatment scores lower than 28 had no significant improvement. Anterior vertebral height was restored in 35 of 46 levels (76%), and the average extent of defect restoration was 37.8%. Mid-vertebral height was restored in 42 of 46 levels (91%), and the average extent of defect restoration was 53.4%. In comparison with a historical control group that underwent kyphoplasty at the same institution for osteoporotic compression fractures, the study patients with myeloma compression fractures had similar outcomes with regard to pain and disability, despite the fact that they had a smaller extent of anterior height restoration (37.8 vs. 51.2%) and a slightly higher rate of cement extrusion (26.3 vs. 15.6%).

5.5 Practical Considerations

5.5.1 Indications

According to the International Myeloma Working Group, vertebral augmentation should be considered the procedure of choice to improve quality of life for painful vertebral compression fractures in patients with myeloma, rather than radiation therapy or intrathecal morphine pumps. Augmentation is indicated for patients with severe pain (>7/10 on visual analog scale) due to vertebral compression fractures and a high risk of further vertebral collapse based on evidence of osteolytic/osteopenic bone destruction [5]. In the absence of severe pain, vertebral augmentation may be considered for patients with significant loss of vertebral height and/or stability. Vertebral augmentation is also a viable option for patients with severe bone destruction and long life expectancy in order to maximize their quality of life by preventing possible compression fractures. Contraindications for vertebral augmentation are listed in Table 5.3 [5]. Myeloma patients with either acute or chronic fractures may be candidates for vertebral augmentation, although those with mechanical pain (e.g., pain that occurs mainly in an upright position, such as standing or walking, and is reduced while reclining) are most likely to benefit from vertebral augmentation.

In general, percutaneous vertebral augmentation should be considered for fractures in levels T_3-L_5. In experienced hands, augmentation to levels as high as the cervical area can be safe and effective. The effects of vertebral augmentation of the sacral or iliac region in patients with myeloma are currently unknown. Multiple augmentations at different levels are often necessary, particularly in patients with myeloma. However, the number of vertebrae treated in a single intervention should be limited to three or four, because the risk of pulmonary complications increases as the number of vertebrae treated increases. In some patients with myeloma, however, up to 16 levels have been successfully treated in separate sessions or stages [5]. Augmentation of unaffected vertebrae adjacent to compression fractures may

Table 5.3 Contraindications to vertebral augmentation

Absolute contraindications	Relative contraindications
• Contraindications to general or local anesthesia	• Lesions above T_3
• Pregnancy	• Osteoblastic metastases
• Bleeding disorder	• Aged <40 years
• Infection at site	• Technically not feasible (vertebra plana)
• Pain unrelated to vertebral collapse	• Fractures with obstructing plasmacytoma(ta)
• Cord compression	• Retropulsed bone
• Severe cardiopulmonary insufficiency	
• Allergy to procedure-related drugs or contrast media	

Reproduced with permission from Hussein et al. [5].

be necessary, particularly in cases of fracture with kyphosis in the thoracolumbar region, or for vertebra situated between two fractured vertebrae.

5.5.2 Methods

The decision between vertebroplasty and kyphoplasty is the treating physician's and should be based on the aims of the therapy [5]. However with the new data from two randomized studies vertebroplasty should be cautiously considered [37, 38]. The advantages of kyphoplasty are that it provides the possibility of vertebral height restoration and is associated with lower rates of cement leakage, compared with vertebroplasty [48]. However, vertebroplasty may be more appropriate than kypho-plasty for stabilizing an at-risk vertebral body with a subclinical metastasis, or vertebral bodies with minor, minimally displaced endplate fractures [49]. It has been suggested that vertebroplasty and kyphoplasty are not mutually exclusive proce-dures and should be considered as separate tools in the armamentarium for vertebral compression fractures [49]. Similarly, the type and amount of bone cement used [50–55] and the route of administration (i.e., unilateral or bilateral, transpedicular, or extrapedicular) are decisions left to the treating physician [5].

5.5.3 Diagnostic Workup

Before vertebral augmentation is performed, careful pain assessment is required to determine the severity of pain and confirm that the fracture is the actual source of pain [5]. Importantly, other types of pain, such as radicular, dysesthetic, discogenic, and degenerative pain, may coexist with compression fracture pain; these types of pain are unlikely to respond to vertebral augmentation. Magnetic resonance imag-ing (MRI), including short T1 inversion recovery (STIR) imaging, is essential in order to determine the presence or absence of spinal cord compression and edema. An assessment of other options for pain management, such as radiation therapy, bisphosphonates, and analgesics, should also be performed. In addition, the disease status should be evaluated to determine whether anti-myeloma treatment is needed.

5.5.4 Timing of Vertebral Augmentation

Immediate vertebral augmentation is indicated for patients with vertebral compression fractures and severe pain, or a high risk of progressive deformity especially in those with compromised spinal and sternal support [5]. Early initiation of treatment may provide rapid pain relief and restore vertebral height and stability, thereby proactively halting the cascade leading to additional fractures and progressive deformity. Trials comparing outcomes after early or delayed kyphoplasty are ongoing [5]. For patients with less severe pain and vertebral damage, a trial of analgesic therapy, bisphosphonates, systemic therapy, and other supportive measures may be considered, followed by surgery if necessary. One skeletal surgical rule of thumb is prevention; studies evaluating the susceptibility of a vertebral body to sustain a compression fracture and the impact of preventing such a fracture needs to be studied and evaluated especially in view of the advances in myeloma therapeutics allowing for longer overall survival.

5.5.5 Safety Considerations

The most common complication of vertebral augmentation is extravasation of bone cement, which is usually asymptomatic but can sometimes produce local and systemic effects, including pulmonary and neurological impairment [5]. Vertebroplasty is associated with a higher rate of leakage than kyphoplasty (Table 5.4) [44, 48]. The higher rate may be explained in part by the fact that vertebroplasty requires a less-viscous cement than kyphoplasty, so that the cement can pass through cortical defects to fill gaps between fracture fragments. During kyphoplasty, the cement is injected directly into the cavity in the vertebral body formed by the inflatable tamp; therefore, a higher viscosity is feasible, which reduces the rate of leakage.

Other less common complications of vertebral augmentation include spinal cord compression, radiculopathy, pneumothorax, retroperitoneal hematoma, and local or systemic infection [5, 48]. A meta-analysis indicated that the incidence of these events is similarly low after vertebroplasty and kyphoplasty, with the exception of myocardial infarction, which was significantly higher after kyphoplasty (0.5% with kyphoplasty vs. 0.005% with vertebroplasty; $p < 0.01$) [48]. Also, precautions should be taken to limit radiation exposure to the surgeon and patient during fluoroscopic

Table 5.4 Incidence of complications related to vertebroplasty and kyphoplasty [48]

Complication	Vertebroplasty (% of procedures)	Kyphoplasty (% of procedures)	p-Value
Cement leak	19.7	7.0	<0.001
Symptomatic leak	1.6	0.3	<0.01
New compression fracture	17.9	14.1	<0.01
Rib fracture	0.9	0.5	NS
Pulmonary embolism	0.9	0.4	NS
Myocardial infarction	0.05	0.5	<0.01
Pneumonia, hypoxia	0.1	0.5	NS
Hematoma	0.3	0.1	NS
Infection	0.1	0.3	NS
Change in blood pressure or heart rate	0.2	0.2	NS

NS, not significant.

navigation [56]. A physical rehabilitation program following vertebral augmentation is recommended. The program should be conducted under the supervision of a physiotherapist and include water aerobics and thoracolumbar stabilization with an extension directional focus.

5.6 Summary

In patients with multiple myeloma, the most commonly involved end organ is the skeletal system. Prevention of weight bearing bone fractures continues to be the main stay of therapy. Common bone disorders such as vertebral compression fractures are a considerable source of pain, disability, and increased morbidity and mortality. The development of minimally invasive vertebral augmentation techniques has made them a viable treatment option for many patients with vertebral compression fractures in order to relieve pain and stabilize the spine. Several technical aspects regarding the optimal timing and methods for vertebral augmentation require further study in myeloma. However, given the encouraging preliminary data on the efficacy and safety of vertebral augmentation, this procedure is already recommended for patients with myeloma and severe pain due to vertebral compression fractures. Kyphoplasty is associated with less cement leakage than vertebroplasty and has the added advantage of restoring vertebral height, which may relieve stress on adjacent vertebral bodies and reduce the risk of additional fractures. Additional studies are warranted to explore the ability of prophylactic vertebral augmentation to prevent fractures and progressive kyphosis.

References

1. Durie BG. New approaches to treatment for multiple myeloma: durable remission and quality of life as primary goals. Clin Lymphoma Myeloma. 2005;6:181–190.
2. Durie BG, Kyle RA, Belch A, et al. Myeloma management guidelines: a consensus report from the scientific advisors of the international myeloma foundation. Hematol J. 2003;4: 379–398.
3. Kyle RA. Multiple myeloma: review of 869 cases. Mayo Clin Proc. 1975;50:29–40.
4. Cotten A, Dewatre F, Cortet B, et al. Percutaneous vertebroplasty for osteolytic metastases and myeloma: effects of the percentage of lesion filling and the leakage of methyl methacrylate at clinical follow-up. Radiology. 1996;200:525–530.
5. Hussein MA, Vrionis FD, Allison R, et al. The role of vertebral augmentation in multiple myeloma: international myeloma working group consensus statement. Leukemia. 2008;22:1479–1484.
6. Kado DM, Browner WS, Palermo L, Nevitt MC, Genant HK, Cummings SR. Vertebral fractures and mortality in older women: a prospective study. Study of Osteoporotic Fractures Research Group. Arch Intern Med. 1999;159:1215–1220.
7. Djulbegovic B, Wheatley K, Ross J, et al. Cochrane Database Syst Rev. 2002;2: CD003188.
8. Berenson JR, Hillner BE, Kyle RA, et al. American Society of Clinical Oncology bisphosphonates expert panel. American Society of Clinical Oncology clinical practice guidelines: the role of bisphosphonates in multiple myeloma. J Clin Oncol. 2002;20: 3719–3736.
9. Berenson JR, Lichtenstein A, Porter L, et al. Long-term pamidronate treatment of advanced multiple myeloma patients reduces skeletal events. Myeloma Aredia Study Group. J Clin Oncol. 1998;16:593–602.
10. Berenson JR, Lichtenstein A, Porter L, et al. Efficacy of pamidronate in reducing skeletal events in patients with advanced multiple myeloma. Myeloma Aredia Study Group. N Engl J Med. 1996;334:488–493.
11. McCloskey EV, MacLennan IC, Drayson MT, Chapman C, Dunn J, Kanis JA. A randomized trial of the effect of clodronate on skeletal morbidity in multiple myeloma. MRC working party of leukaemia in adults. Br J Haematol. 1998;100:317–325.
12. McCloskey EV, Dunn JA, Kanis JA, MacLennan IC, Drayson MT. Long-term follow-up of a prospective, double-blind, placebo-controlled randomized trial of clodronate in multiple myeloma. Br J Haematol. 2001;113:1035–1043.
13. Gertz BJ, Holland SD, Kline WF, et al. Studies of the oral bioavailability of alendronate. Clin Pharmacol Ther. 1995;58:288–298.
14. Rosen LS, Gordon D, Kaminski M, et al. Zoledronic acid versus pamidronate in the treatment of skeletal metastases in patients with breast cancer or osteolytic lesions of multiple myeloma: a phase III, double-blind, comparative trial. Cancer J. 2001;7:377–387.
15. Zeifang F, Zahlten-Hinguranage A, Goldschmidt H, Cremer F, Bernd L, Sabo D. Long-term survival after surgical intervention for bone disease in multiple myeloma. Ann Oncol. 2005;16:222–227.
16. Chang SA, Lee SS, Ueng SW, Yuan LJ, Shih CH. Surgical treatment for pathological long bone fracture in patients with multiple myeloma: a retrospective analysis of 22 cases. Chang Gung Med J. 2001;24:300–306.
17. Harrington KD. Orthopedic surgical management of skeletal complications of malignancy. Cancer. 1997;80(8 Suppl):1614–1627.
18. Papagelopoulos PJ, Galanis EC, Greipp PR, Sim FH. Prosthetic hip replacement for pathologic or impending pathologic fractures in myeloma. Clin Orthop Relat Res. 1997;341: 192–205.
19. Colyer RA. Surgical stabilization of pathological neoplastic fractures. Curr Probl Cancer. 1986;10:117–168.

20. Jacofsky DJ, Haidukewych GJ. Management of pathologic fractures of the proximal femur: state of the art. J Orthop Trauma. 2004;18:459–469.

21. Sapkota BH, Hirsch AE, Yoo AJ, et al. Treatment of metastatic carcinoma to the hip with CT-guided percutaneous acetabuloplasty: report of four cases. J Vasc Interv Radiol. 2009;20:548–552.

22. Lieberman I, Reinhardt MK. Vertebroplasty and kyphoplasty for osteolytic vertebral collapse. Clin Orthop Relat Res. 2003;415(Suppl):S176–S186.

23. Shepherd S. Radiotherapy and the management of metastatic bone pain. Clin Radiol. 1988;39:547–550.

24. Yeh HS, Berenson JR. Treatment for myeloma bone disease. Clin Cancer Res. 2006;12(20 Part 2):6279s–6284s.

25. Dudeney S, Lieberman IH, Reinhardt MK, Hussein M. Kyphoplasty in the treatment of osteolytic vertebral compression fractures as a result of multiple myeloma. J Clin Oncol. 2002;20:2382–2387.

26. Galibert P, Deramond H, Rosat P, Le Gars D. [Preliminary note on the treatment of vertebral angioma by percutaneous acrylic vertebroplasty]. Neurochirurgie. 1987;33:166–168 (French).

27. Deramond H, Depriester C, Galibert P, Le Gars D. Percutaneous vertebroplasty with polymethylmethacrylate. Technique, indications, and results. Radiol Clin North Am. 1998;36:533–546.

28. Deramond H, Wright NT, Belkoff SM. Temperature elevation caused by bone cement polymerization during vertebroplasty. Bone. 1999;25(2 Suppl):17S–21S.

29. Jensen ME, Evans AJ, Mathis JM, Kallmes DF, Cloft HJ, Dion JE. Percutaneous polymethyl-methacrylate vertebroplasty in the treatment of osteoporotic vertebral body compression fractures: technical aspects. AJNR Am J Neuroradiol. 1997;18:1897–1904.

30. Kayanja M, Evans K, Milks R, Lieberman IH. The mechanics of polymethylmethacrylate augmentation. Clin Orthop Relat Res. 2006;443:124–130.

31. Kayanja MM, Schlenk R, Togawa D, Ferrara L, Lieberman I. The biomechanics of 1, 2, and 3 levels of vertebral augmentation with polymethylmethacrylate in multilevel spinal segments. Spine. 2006;31:769–774.

32. Pateder DB, Khanna AJ, Lieberman IH. Vertebroplasty and kyphoplasty for the management of osteoporotic vertebral compression fractures. Orthop Clin North Am. 2007;38: 409–418.

33. Barr JD, Barr MS, Lemley TJ, McCann RM. Percutaneous vertebroplasty for pain relief and spinal stabilization. Spine. 2000;25:923–928.

34. Keller TS, Kosmopoulos V, Lieberman IH. Vertebroplasty and kyphoplasty affect vertebral motion segment stiffness and stress distributions: a microstructural finite-element study. Spine. 2005;30:1258–1265.

35. Cortet B, Cotten A, Boutry N, et al. Percutaneous vertebroplasty in patients with osteolytic metastases or multiple myeloma. Rev Rhum Engl Ed. 1997;64:177–183.

36. Cotten A, Boutry N, Cortet B, et al. Percutaneous vertebroplasty: state of the art. Radiographics. 1998;18:311–320.

37. Buchbinder R, Osborne RH, Ebeling PR, Wark JD, Mitchell P, Wriedt C, Graves S, Staples MP, Murphy B. A randomized trial of vertebroplasty for painful osteoporotic vertebral fractures. N Engl J Med. 2009;361:557–568.

38. Kallmes DF, Comstock BA, Heagerty PJ, Turner JA, Wilson DJ, Diamond TH, Edwards R, Gray LA, Stout L, Owen S, Hollingworth W, Ghdoke B, Annesley-Williams DJ, Ralston SH, Jarvik JG. A randomized trial of vertebroplasty for osteoporotic spinal fractures. N Engl J Med. 2009;361:569–579.

39. Wardlaw D, Cummings SR, Van Meirhaeghe J, et al. Efficacy and safety of balloon kyphoplasty compared with non-surgical care for vertebral compression fracture (FREE): a randomised controlled trial. Lancet. 2009;373:1016–1024.

40. Vrionis FD, Hamm A, Stanton N, Sullivan M, Obadia M, Miguel RV. Kyphoplasty for tumor-associated spinal fractures. Tech Reg Anesth Pain Manag. 2005;9:35–39.

41. Khanna AJ, Reinhardt MK, Togawa D, Lieberman IH. Functional outcomes of kyphoplasty for the treatment of osteoporotic and osteolytic vertebral compression fractures. Osteoporos Int. 2006;17:817–826.

42. Shedid D, Togawa D, Lieberman IH. Kyphoplasty: vertebral augmentation for compression fractures. Clin Geriatr Med. 2006;22:535–544.

43. Harrop JS, Prpa B, Reinhardt MK, Lieberman I. Primary and secondary osteoporosis' incidence of subsequent vertebral compression fractures after kyphoplasty. Spine. 2004;29: 2120–2125.

44. Lieberman IH, Dudeney S, Reinhardt MK, Bell G. Initial outcome and efficacy of "kyphoplasty" in the treatment of painful osteoporotic vertebral compression fractures. Spine. 2001;26:1631–1638.

45. Pflugmacher R, Agarwal A, Kandziora F, K-Klostermann C. Balloon kyphoplasty combined with posterior instrumentation for the treatment of burst fractures of the spine – 1-year results. J Orthop Trauma. 2009;23:126–131.

46. Phillips FM, Wetzel FT, Lieberman I, Campbell-Hupp M. An in vivo comparison of the potential for extravertebral cement leak after vertebroplasty and kyphoplasty. Spine. 2002;27:2173–2179.

47. Pflugmacher R, Kandziora F, Schoeder RJ, Melcher I, Haas NP, Klostermann CK. Percutaneous balloon kyphoplasty in the treatment of pathological vertebral body fracture and deformity in multiple myeloma: a one-year follow-up. Acta Radiol. 2006;47:369–376.

48. Köse KC, Cebesoy O, Akan B, Altinel L, Dinçer D, Yazar T. Functional results of vertebral augmentation techniques in pathological vertebral fractures of myelomatous patients. J Natl Med Assoc. 2006;98:1654–1658.

49. Lane JM, Hong R, Koob J, et al. Kyphoplasty enhances function and structural alignment in multiple myeloma. Clin Orthop Relat Res. 2004;426:49–53.

50. Eck JC, Nachtigall D, Humphreys SC, Hodges SD. Comparison of vertebroplasty and balloon kyphoplasty for treatment of vertebral compression fractures: a meta-analysis of the literature. Spine J. 2008;8:488–497.

51. Khanna AJ, Neubauer P, Togawa D, Kay Reinhardt M, Lieberman IH. Kyphoplasty and vertebroplasty for the treatment of spinal metastases. Support Cancer Ther. 2005;3:21–25.

52. Lieberman I, Goins M, An H, Phillips F. Summary statement: kyphoplasty and nucleus pulposus prosthesis. Spine J. 2005;5(6 Suppl):325S.

53. Lieberman IH, Togawa D, Kayanja MM. Vertebroplasty and kyphoplasty: filler materials. Spin J. 2005;5(6 Suppl):305S–316S.

54. Bostrom MP, Lane JM.. Future directions. Augmentation of osteoporotic vertebral bodies. Spine. 1997;22(24 Suppl):38S–42S.

55. Togawa D, Bauer TW, Lieberman IH, Takikawa S. Histologic evaluation of human vertebral bodies after vertebral augmentation with polymethyl methacrylate. Spine. 2003;28: 1521–1527.

56. Togawa D, Lieberman IH, Bauer TW, Reinhardt MK, Kayanja MM. Histological evaluation of biopsies obtained from vertebral compression fractures: unsuspected myeloma and osteomalacia. Spine. 2005;30:781–786.

57. Togawa D, Kovacic JJ, Bauer TW, Reinhardt MK, Brodke DS, Lieberman IH. Radiographic and histologic findings of vertebral augmentation using polymethylacrylate in the primate spine: percutaneous vertebroplasty versus kyphoplasty. Spine. 2006;31:E4–E10.

58. Mroz TE, Yamashita T, Davros WJ, Lieberman IH. Radiation exposure to the surgeon and the patient during kyphoplasty. J Spinal Disord Tech. 2008;21:96–100.

Chapter 6
Bisphosphonates in the Treatment of Myeloma Bone Disease

James R. Berenson

Abstract Multiple myeloma (MM) is a B-cell malignancy characterized by enhanced bone loss commonly associated with diffuse osteopenia, focal lytic lesions, pathological fractures, hypercalcemia, and bony pain. As a result, these patients often require radiotherapy and surgical procedures to relieve pain and to treat actual and impending fractures and spinal cord compression or collapse. Bisphosphonates have been shown to be potent inhibitors of bone loss through their inhibitory effects on bone-resorbing osteoclasts. In laboratory studies, nitrogen-containing bisphosphonates through their inhibition of farnesyl diphosphate synthase have shown more potent inhibitory effects on osteoclasts than non-nitrogen-containing compounds. In large randomized clinical trials, monthly intravenous infusion of the nitrogen-containing bisphosphonates pamidronate or zoledronic acid has been shown to reduce skeletal complications in MM patients and are now a mainstay of myeloma therapy. Orally administered and weaker non-nitrogen-containing bisphosphonates, in contrast, have shown little ability to slow the development of skeletal complications in these patients. Complications including osteonecrosis of the jaw and worsening of renal function have been reported with these drugs but these side effects can be minimized with proper clinical management. Preclinical studies also show that nitrogen-containing bisphosphonates especially zoledronic acid have potent antitumor effects, and enhance the anti-MM effects of other agents shown to be active for the treatment of myeloma. Although case reports and subsets of patients have shown an improvement in survival with the use of these agents in MM, more clinical studies are needed to confirm this effect.

Keywords Bisphosphonates · Myeloma bone disease · MGUS · Myeloma treatment · Pamidronate · Zolendronate

J.R. Berenson (✉)
Medical and Scientific Director, Institute for Myeloma & Bone Cancer Research, West Hollywood, CA, 90069, USA
e-mail: jberenson@imbcr.org

G.D. Roodman (ed.), *Myeloma Bone Disease*, Current Clinical Oncology, DOI 10.1007/978-1-60761-554-5_6, © Springer Science+Business Media, LLC 2010

6.1 Introduction

Multiple myeloma (MM) is a B-cell malignancy that substantially causes skeletal dysfunction during the course of the disease. MM induces osteolysis and shifts the normal balance of bone formation toward bone resorption [1]. As a result, diffuse osteopenia, focal lytic lesions, pathological fractures, hypercalcemia, and bony pain are common clinical manifestations in MM patients. These prominent clinical features are major causes of morbidity and mortality [2]. The lytic process observed in MM is very different from other cancers that metastasize to bone in which bone destruction is followed by new bone formation. Even when MM patients respond to anti-MM therapies, they may still have progression of skeletal events [3, 4] without repair of osteolytic lesions. Prior to use of intravenous bisphosphonates, these patients frequently developed bone pain, hypercalcemia, and fractures that often required treatment with radiation, surgery, and use of analgesics. The monthly infusions of intravenous pamidronate or zoledronic acid have reduced these complications; and, as a result, dramatically improved the quality of lives of myeloma patients. Preclinical studies suggest that these agents also possess antitumor effects; and, thus, these drugs also may prolong the survival of MM patients. Although some clinical data suggest this effect in MM and other tumor types, clinical trials clearly demonstrating this have not been completed in MM patients.

6.2 Fracture Risk in MM

Although older studies suggested that a minority of myeloma patients presented with at least one fracture, more recent studies with the addition of MRI assessment show a much higher proportion of patients actually have fractures at presentation [5]. Notably, the use of MRI increases the proportion of patients found to develop fractures during the course of their disease as shown in two studies [6, 7]. In one of the placebo-controlled bisphosphonate trials, approximately one-third of myeloma patients with lytic bone disease not receiving bisphosphonate treatment (placebo arm) developed new fractures as assessed by plain x-rays after just 9 months of follow-up [8]. These fractures may result from direct myelomatous involvement of the bone that shows the fracture but also may simply result from the generalized bone loss that is a hallmark of myeloma. The most common site of fracture is in the spine (55–70% of patients) especially in the lower thoracic or lumbar vertebral bodies [9]. Other common sites of fracture include the femur, pelvis, ribs, and humerus.

Melton et al. also has reported an increased fracture risk among patients with monoclonal gammopathy of undetermined significance (MGUS) in a retrospective cohort study [10]. There was nearly a threefold increase in risk of vertebral compression fractures compared to a control group from Olmsted County, Minnesota. Furthermore, Melton et al. revealed fracture risk in MM significantly increases around the time of diagnosis of myeloma [11]. The majority of these fractures were pathological. This is consistent with the notion that these patients have a higher prevalence of osteopenia and osteoporosis than the normal population and generally have a higher risk of fracture particularly in the weight-bearing areas of the spine [12].

6.3 Bisphosphonates for the Treatment of Myeloma Bone Disease

Bisphosphonates are specific inhibitors of osteoclastic activity and are effective in the treatment of hypercalcemia associated with malignancy. They are nonhydrolyzable analogs of inorganic pyrophosphate that bind avidly to hydroxyapatite crystals and are subsequently released during the process of bone resorption. The released bisphosphonate is taken up by osteoclasts leading to the inhibition of that cell's activity and survival. Once internalized, bisphosphonates are cytotoxic to osteoclasts and the more potent bisphosphonates interfere with intracellular signaling pathways required for osteoclast activity and survival. Newer nitrogen-containing bisphosphonates, such as zoledronic acid, pamidronate and ibandronate, have a unique mechanism of action and greater clinical activity than first-generation bisphosphonates that lack nitrogen such as etidronate and clodronate (see Table 6.1) [13]. Non-nitrogen-containing drugs become incorporated into adenosine triphosphate and its analogs whereas nitrogen-containing compounds have been shown to block enzymes (specifically farnesyl diphosphate synthase) involved in synthesis of fatty acids including geranylgeranylated derivatives [14]. In fact, drugs such as simvastatin used in the treatment of hypercholesterolemia block earlier steps in this pathway. These statins have been shown to produce similar effects in laboratory studies but their lack of affinity to bone makes these agents inactive in inhibiting osteoclast function. Many proteins including GTPases such as Ras, Rho, Rac, Cdc42, and Rab family members require geranylgeranylation in order to function properly. Notably, the anti-bone-resorptive actions of these specific bisphosphonates can be overcome with the addition of these fatty acid derivatives in preclinical studies. The lack of geranylgeranylated derivatives in cells prevents proper functioning of many proteins. Osteoclasts and their precursors are especially sensitive to this effect and undergo apoptosis; and, as a result, the loss of these bone-resorbing cells prevents bone loss. Clinically, both oral and intravenously administered bisphosphonates with or without nitrogen have been evaluated to determine whether these anti-bone-resorptive agents can reduce skeletal problems in large randomized trials over the past two decades. The following are the summaries of the impact of bisphosphonates on skeletal disease as well as its clinical manifestations in MM patients.

6.3.1 Etidronate

In the Canadian study involving etidronate [3], 173 newly diagnosed patients all received intermittent oral melphalan and prednisone as primary chemotherapy, and

Table 6.1 Types of bisphosphonates

	Relative potency[a]	Dose (mg)	Mode of administration	Adverse effects
Non-nitrogen				
Clodronate	1	1,600	Oral	Hypersensitivity, renal insufficiency, hypocalcemia, hyperkalemia, hyperpara thyroidism, hypocalcemia, abdominal pain, arthralgia
Single nitrogen				
Pamidronate	20	90	2 h i.v.	Fever in 20% hypophosphatemia, hypocalcemia, hypomagnesemia, loss of appetite, nausea, vomiting, renal impairment, ONJ
Ibandronate	857	6 50	1 h i.v. oral	Rash, abdominal pain, constipation, diarrhea, dyspepsia, nausea, arthralgia, back pain, dizziness, headache
Two nitrogens				
Zoledronic acid	16,700	4	15 min i.v.	Minor; fever, rarely hypocalcemia, hypophosphatemia, loss of appetite, nausea, vomiting, renal impairment, ONJ

[a] Green and Rogers (2002).

166 were then randomized to receive either daily oral etidronate (5 mg/kg) or placebo until death or stopping the treatment due to side effects. The primary objective of this study was to evaluate whether etidronate would retard skeletal progression of multiple myeloma, based on patient's height, vertebral height and deformity, hypercalcemia, development of pathological fractures, and bone pain. Although significant height loss occurred in both placebo- and etidronate-treated patients, no difference was found between the two arms. Similarly, the other outcome measures (new fractures, hypercalcemic episodes, and bone pain) showed no

differences between the two arms. Lack of improvement with etidronate may be due to low absorption and potency and incorrect selection of regular daily therapy.

6.3.2 Clodronate

Three large randomized trials have been published using oral clodronate in myeloma patients and the clinical results are variable. In the Finnish trial [15], 350 previously untreated patients were entered and 336 randomized to receive either clodronate (2.4 g) or placebo daily for 2 years. All patients were also treated with intermittent oral melphalan and prednisolone. The proportion of patients with progression of lytic lesions was less in the clodronate-treated group (12%) than in the placebo group (24%). However, the progression of overall pathological fractures, as well as both vertebral and nonvertebral fractures, was not different between the arms. In addition, the number of patients developing hypercalcemia was similar in the two arms. Changes in pain index and use of analgesics were similar in both arms.

Clodronate has also been evaluated in an open-label randomized German trial [16]. In this study, 170 previously untreated patients were randomized to receive either no bisphosphonate or oral clodronate (1.6 g) daily for 1 year. All patients were also treated with intermittent intravenous melphalan and oral prednisone. Unfortunately, premature termination occurred in more than half of the patients despite the short length of the study (1 year). The results showed no difference in progression of bone disease as assessed by plain radiographs in the two arms.

Third, a clinical trial conducted by the Medical Research Council has evaluated 536 recently diagnosed myeloma patients randomized to receive either oral clodronate 1.6 g or placebo daily in addition to alkylator-based chemotherapy [17]. After combining the proportion of patients developing either nonvertebral fractures or severe hypercalcemia including those leaving the trial due to severe hypercalcemia, there were less clodronate-treated patients experiencing these combined events than placebo patients. The number of patients experiencing nonvertebral fractures was lower in the clodronate group. Back pain and poor performance status were not significantly different between the two groups except at one time point (24 months). There was no difference in the time to the first skeletal event, the proportion of patients requiring radiotherapy or overall survival between the arms.

6.3.3 Oral Pamidronate

Daily oral pamidronate (300 mg/day) was evaluated in a double-blind randomized trial by a Danish–Swedish cooperative group compared to placebo in 300 newly diagnosed myeloma patients [18]. After a median duration of 18 months, there was no significant reduction in the primary endpoint defined as skeletal-related morbidity (bone fracture, surgery for impending fracture, vertebral collapse, or increase in number and/or size of lytic lesions), hypercalcemic episodes, or survival between the arms. Fewer episodes of severe pain and less height loss were observed in the oral pamidronate-treated patients, however. Poor bioavailability of oral pamidronate may be the reason for the lack of efficacy shown in this trial.

6.3.4 Intravenous Pamidronate

Results of small open-label trials lasting up to 24 months suggested that pamidronate disodium might be effective in reducing skeletal complications for MM patients [19, 20]. Thus, a large randomized, double-blind study was conducted to determine whether monthly 90 mg infusions of pamidronate compared to placebo for 21 months reduced skeletal events in patients with multiple myeloma who were receiving chemotherapy [21]. This study included patients with Durie–Salmon Stage III multiple myeloma and at least one osteolytic lesion. Unlike the etidronate and clodronate trials, which involved untreated patients, patients were required to receive an unchanged chemotherapy regimen for at least 2 months prior to enrollment. The patients were stratified according to whether they were receiving first-line (stra-tum 1) or second-line (stratum 2) antimyeloma chemotherapy at entry into the study.

At the preplanned primary endpoint after nine cycles of therapy [22], the proportions of myeloma patients having any skeletal event was 41% in patients receiving placebo but only 24% in pamidronate-treated patients. The proportion of pamidronate-treated patients with skeletal events was lower in both stratum 1 (first-line therapy) and stratum 2 ($\geq$ second-line therapy). The patients who received pamidronate also had significant decreases in bone pain, no increase in analgesic usage, and showed no deterioration in performance status and quality of life at the end of 9 months. The proportion of patients developing any skeletal event and the skeletal morbidity rate continued to remain significantly lower in the pamidronate group than the placebo group during the additional 12 cycles of treatment [21]. Notably, those myeloma patients with failed front-line therapy lived significantly longer when treated with pamidronate (stratum II patients with adjusted survival based on the levels of β2-microglobulin and Eastern Cooperative Oncology Group performance scores), whereas myeloma patients responding to front-line therapy (stratum I) had no significant survival benefit from the pamidronate treatment. The lack of a difference in survival in stratum I patients may have been due to the heterogeneity of the chemotherapeutic regimens the patients were receiving, the short period of follow-up (median, 17 months), or the fact that pamidronate does not have direct anti-MM effects.

6.3.5 Ibandronate

Ibandronate is a nitrogen-containing bisphosphonate that, in preclinical models, shows more anti-bone-resorptive potency than pamidronate and the other non-nitrogen-containing bisphosphonates. The results of a Phase III placebo-controlled trial of 214 stage II or III myeloma patients with osteolytic bone disease were recently published [23]. Patients either received monthly injections of 2 mg of ibandronate or placebo in addition to their antineoplastic therapy. Ninety-nine patients were evaluable in each arm for efficacy. The mean number of events per patient year on treatment was similar in both groups (ibandronate 2.13 vs. placebo 2.05). In addition, there was no difference in pain, analgesic usage, or quality of life between the arms. However, among patients treated with ibandronate who showed a sustained and marked reduction in bone-resorption markers, fewer skeletal complications occurred. There was no difference in overall survival. Thus, this monthly dose of intravenous ibandronate did not show significant benefits in reducing skeletal complications in myeloma patients with lytic bone disease. These disappointing data in myeloma patients may be attributed to an insufficiently low ibandronate dose, as a study of breast cancer patients showed that a higher dose of ibandronate at 6 mg i.v. once every 4 weeks was effective in reducing the incidence of skeletal-related events [24]. Moreover, the study outcome may have been biased favorably to placebo because of an unbalanced dropout behavior after the first skeletal-related event.

6.3.6 Zoledronic Acid

Zoledronic acid is an imidazole-containing bisphosphonate that shows more potency in preclinical studies than any other bisphosphonate currently available [25].

6.3.6.1 Phase I and II Trials

Two small Phase I trials established the safety and marked sustained reduction in bone-resorption markers for patients with myeloma and other cancers associated with metastatic bone disease with monthly infusions of small doses given over several minutes [26, 27]. A large randomized Phase II study compared this newer bisphosphonate to pamidronate in 280 patients with lytic bone metastases from either multiple myeloma ($n = 108$) or breast cancer ($n = 172$) [28]. Patients were randomized to nine monthly infusions of 0.4 mg, 2.0 mg, or 4.0 mg of zoledronic acid, or to 90 mg of pamidronate as a 2-h infusion. The primary endpoint was to determine a dose of zoledronic acid that reduced the need for radiation therapy to less than 30% of treated patients, although all skeletal events were also analyzed similar to those determined in the Phase III pamidronate trials outlined above. Radiation therapy was required in a similar proportion of patients receiving pamidronate and zoledronic acid at 2.0 and 4.0 mg (18–21%), whereas more patients receiving the lowest dose of zoledronic acid underwent radiotherapy (24%). Similarly, the proportion of patients with any skeletal event was lower in these same groups compared to patients receiving 0.4 mg of zoledronic acid. Interestingly, significant increases in bone density (>6% in the lumbar spine) and inhibition of bone-resorption markers were observed in this latter cohort but this failed to translate to any clinical benefit. Although the results of this study suggested that 0.4 mg was an inadequate monthly dose of zoledronic acid to be of clinical use in the prevention of skeletal complications for patients with myeloma or breast cancer metastatic to bone, the small size of this Phase II trial did not allow for a complete assessment of the efficacy of higher doses (2 mg or 4 mg) of zoledronic acid compared to pamidronate.

6.3.6.2 Phase III Trial: Zoledronic Acid vs. Pamidronate

A large Phase III trial that evaluated two doses of zoledronic acid (4 and 8 mg) compared to pamidronate (90 mg) infused every 3–4 weeks for treatment of myeloma or breast cancer patients with metastatic bone disease was conducted [29]. The doses and infusion time (5 min) of zoledronic acid were selected based on the safety and superiority of these doses in reversing hypercalcemia of malignancy compared to pamidronate (90 mg) [30]. Importantly, the primary efficacy endpoint of this trial was to show the noninferiority of zoledronic acid compared to pamidronate in reducing skeletal complications for patients with myeloma or breast cancer metastatic to bone. The trial involved 1,643 patients who were stratified among individuals with myeloma ($n = 513$) or breast cancer on either hormonal therapy or chemotherapy ($n = 1130$). The results of the study showed that the proportion of patients with any skeletal event did not differ among the three treatment arms. In addition, the time to first skeletal event and analgesic use was similar in the three groups (12–13 months). Moreover, after 25 months of follow-up, the overall proportions of patients developing skeletal events remained similar between the zoledronic acid (4 mg) and pamidronate-treated patients [31]. However, using an additional preplanned analysis, the multiple events analysis, zoledronic acid-treated patients showed a 16% reduced risk of developing skeletal complications compared to those patients who received pamidronate. These long-term results show the efficacy and convenience of this more potent bisphosphonate for treating myeloma patients with skeletal involvement.

Importantly, during the clinical trial, rises in creatinine were more frequently observed in the zoledronic acid arms when administered over 5 min. Because of the renal toxicity, infusion time of zoledronic acid was increased to 15 min. Because of ongoing kidney problems (rises in creatinine) in the 8 mg zoledronic acid group, these patients subsequently had their dosage reduced to 4 mg. Long-term follow-up data are now available and show no difference in the renal profile between patients receiving 4 mg zoledronic acid infused over 15 min compared to 90 mg pamidronate infused over 120 min [31].

6.4 Bisphosphonates for MGUS Patients

A recent open-label study of 54 patients with MGUS and either osteoporosis or osteopenia demonstrated that zoledronic acid 4 mg significantly improved bone density when administered at 0, 6, and 12 months [32]. After 13 months of treatment, BMD of the posteroanterior lumbar spine and nondominant proximal femur increased by 22 and 8%, respectively. Another study showed that 18 months of treatment with oral alendronate 70 mg/week for MGUS patients also increased BMD [33]. Specifically, individuals with evidence of either osteoporosis or VCF were included in the trial, and bone density increased 6.1% in the lumbar spine and 1.5% in the hip, although this effect was less than observed with zoledronic acid. No randomized studies comparing these two bisphosphonates to placebo or each other have been completed to date. However, since these patients, unlike cancer patients, were not on other treatments that may have improved their bone density, these two studies suggest the benefits of bisphosphonates for treatment of MGUS-associated osteopenia/osteoporosis.

6.5 Bisphosphonates: Side Effects

Although monthly administration of intravenous bisphosphonates is generally well-tolerated, patients may experience several side effects. Flu-like symptoms may occur for several hours in 10–15% of patients usually 24–48 h after dosing [22, 31]. This side effect is self-limiting and rarely occurs by the time of the third infusion. More serious complications may involve renal impairment with ongoing treatment and osteonecrosis of the jaw (see below).

6.5.1 Renal Issues

Recent concern by the FDA regarding the potential risk of rises in creatinine from chronic administration of zoledronic acid [34] has prompted a risk-adapted approach to dosing this bisphosphonate based on the patient's calculated creatinine clearance. Patients with a calculated creatinine clearance >60 mL/min as determined using the Cockcroft–Gault formula should receive 4 mg, whereas patients with lower levels (between 30 and <60) are to receive lower doses depending upon the calculated number. This adjustment in dose is made only at the time of determining the initial dose and all subsequent doses are to be given at the same dose. Whether these adjustments in dose are either necessary or will reduce the already low risk of renal toxicity from this bisphosphonate is unknown. Renal safety of long-term administration of both pamidronate (90 mg) and zoledronic acid (4 mg) has been suggested in two recent studies [35, 36]. In fact, the development of renal risk in preclinical models is felt to be related to the $C_{\max}$ (maximal concentration of the drug in the blood) which is related to rate of infusion rather than the dose per se.

Monthly monitoring of serum creatinine is critical in identifying patients who may be experiencing renal issues although most of the time these changes in kidney function result from worsening of the myeloma, other co-morbid conditions, or other nephrotoxic medications. It is recommended that the dose be held if the creatinine increases more than 0.5 and 1.0 mg/dL from its baseline value for those with a normal or elevated baseline creatinine, respectively, and the treating physician believes that the bisphosphonate is the cause of the increase in creatinine. Treatment can be resumed when the creatinine returns to within 10% of baseline and increasing the infusion time may reduce the risk of recurrence of this problem.

6.5.2 Osteonecrosis of the Jaw

Another complication that may result from bisphosphonate therapy is osteonecrosis of the jaw (ONJ). Recent reports suggest this potential complication develops among cancer patients receiving either chronic zoledronic acid or pamidronate treatment [37–40]. The frequency with which this complication occurs in cancer patients receiving bisphosphonate therapy is unknown. However, it appears that there is a higher risk of this complication among patients particularly among those with myeloma who receive these drugs. Risk factors include trauma and prior dental procedures especially dental extraction and implants [40, 41]. Lesser dental procedures including root canal procedures are felt not to increase the risk of ONJ. A recent report identified polymorphisms of P450 *CYP2C8* with this complication in a large study of MM patients also treated with polychemotherapy and autologous transplantation [42]. Most cases are associated with exposed jaw bone with minimal symptoms but patients may require more extensive intervention including surgical procedures to treat this problem. Approximately two-thirds of cases occur in the mandibular bone and the remainder in the maxillary bone. Because of this dental complication, a number of recommendations have come from panels of dental medical experts [43–45]. It is now recommended that patients receiving bisphosphonates, including the vast majority of myeloma patients, should be evaluated early on in their treatment for dental problems. Any dental problems requiring extraction of teeth and directly involving jaw bones should be done prior to initiation of these drugs, and treatment with these drugs should not start for several months after these procedures are done. These types of surgeries should also be avoided while patients are receiving these drugs. If patients undergo these types of procedures, it has been suggested that patients may want to refrain from receiving these drugs for several months before and after these surgeries are done although there is no evidence to support this recommendation. While receiving bisphosphonates, patients should also be encouraged to maintain excellent dental hygiene and undergo regular dental exams. It should be noted that there is no evidence that discontinuation of the bisphosphonate or replacement with other bisphosphonates changes the course of this complication. Interestingly, a recent large multicenter retrospective study suggests that patients experiencing ONJ may have less skeletal events and show an improved survival [46].

6.6 Guidelines for the Use of Bisphosphonates in Multiple Myeloma

Several guidelines have been developed for the use of bisphosphonates to treat myeloma bone disease during the past several years [47–49]. The first guideline from an American Society of Clinical Oncology (ASCO) Panel recommended that, for multiple myeloma patients who have, on plain radiographs, evidence of lytic bone disease, receive either intravenous zoledronic acid 4 mg infused over 15 min or pamidronate 90 mg delivered over 120 min every 3–4 weeks [47]. The panel also believed it was reasonable to start these agents for patients with osteopenia but without evidence of lytic bone disease. Although this panel recommended that the intravenous bisphosphonate be continued until there was a substantial decline in the patient's performance status, a recent update of this guideline from ASCO suggested that the drugs be continued for only 2 years among patients with stable or responsive disease [48]. This panel only recommended that the drug be restarted among patients developing new skeletal events. A similar recommendation has been made in a recent Mayo Consensus Statement [49]. However, studies have recently shown that the development of skeletal events is associated with a shortened survival for myeloma patients [46, 50] so waiting for these events to occur to reinitiate therapy may actually put patients at high risk not only for new untoward skeletal problems but also for a shortened survival as well. Unfortunately, because the large randomized trials were only carried out for 2 years during which continued benefit was seen with monthly intravenous bisphosphonate treatment, no data exist beyond this time point on which to base firm recommendations for duration of therapy. In addition, the Mayo Clinic suggested that for patients requiring active treatment, the time between these infusions should be lengthened to every 3 months after 2 years. However, there are no data on which to base this recommendation although current ongoing studies are being conducted to evaluate alternative schedules after initial monthly treatment. Moreover, both the recent ASCO and Mayo Clinic statements suggested that MM patients should be treated with pamidronate rather than zoledronic acid because of the potential higher risk of ONJ with the more potent zoledronic acid. However, a recently completed prospective trial started in the last few years shows a very high risk of ONJ among MM patients treated with 90 mg of pamidronate monthly [51]. Thus, the perception of a difference in risk may have resulted from the difference in survival as well as the use of antimyeloma medications that were not available during the widespread use of pamidronate in the 1990s. Because the survival was shorter during the pamidronate era, the time at risk for this complication was much shorter for patients treated with this bisphosphonate compared to those treated with zoledronic acid more recently during a time in which MM patients are living much longer. Moreover, many of the drugs recently used to treat myeloma may be additional risk factors for ONJ and were not available during the time in which pamidronate was used widely. In fact, several recent studies suggest that some of these newer drugs such as thalidomide that were not in widespread use in the pamidronate era increase the risk of ONJ in MM patients [41].

The guidelines also recommended intermittent monitoring of renal function as well as urinary protein evaluation to assess possible renal dysfunction that may occur from these agents. Monitoring of renal function with evaluation of serum creatinine prior to each dose of drug should be standard procedure for MM patients receiving these agents (see above). The guidelines have recommended adjustment of doses of both drugs based on renal function although no data exist to support that these changes will reduce the risk of these patients developing impaired renal function.

For patients with either solitary plasmacytoma or indolent myeloma, the guidelines suggested that patients do not receive either drug because of the lack of data from clinical studies. However, a recent study suggests that monthly zoledronic acid reduces skeletal events and progression of bone disease among patients with asymptomatic MM not requiring additional anti-MM treatments [52]. In addition, although patients with MGUS show significant amounts of bone loss and a higher risk of fracture especially of vertebral bodies, the panel did not recommend treatment of these patients with bisphosphonates. However, two recent studies [32, 33] suggest that use of bisphosphonates improves bone density in these patients; and, thus, is likely to reduce the high risk of fracture in these individuals.

6.7 Antimyeloma Effects of Bisphosphonates

The role of bisphosphonates for myeloma patients may go beyond simply inhibiting bone resorption and the resulting skeletal complications. Radl et al. suggested that pamidronate might reduce myeloma tumor burden in treated mice [53]. Treating bone marrow mononucleated cells of patients with MM with increasing concentrations of zoledronic acid in vitro, investigators found modified patterns of expression of adhesion molecules in plasma cell binding and an increase in apoptosis of myeloma bone marrow stromal cells [54]. In vitro studies also suggest that pamidronate may possess antimyeloma properties as demonstrated by its ability to induce apoptosis of myeloma cells [55] and suppression of IL-6 production [56]. Several studies indicate that bisphosphonates may be markedly antiangiogenic [57–59]. Interestingly, the antitumor effects of bisphosphonates appear to be synergistic with glucocorticoids, an investigational farnesyl transferase inhibitor, a recently FDA-approved histone deacetylase inhibitor, and thalidomide in preclinical and early clinical studies [60–63]. The potent antitumor effects of bisphosphonates observed in the laboratory suggest that higher doses of bisphosphonates given at slower rate may establish possible antitumor effects clinically in MM patients. Subset analysis of large clinical trials [21] and case reports [64] suggest that these agents may possess anti-MM effects that improve survival and that zoledronic acid provides additional benefits compared to pamidronate in this regard [65] but confirmation of these impacts on survival will depend on large prospective studies. Support of the potential antitumor effect of intravenous bisphosphonate treatment clinically comes from recently published results from a large randomized study involving premenopausal women with estrogen-receptor-positive early breast cancer administered zoledronic acid 4 mg every 6 months in conjunction with endocrine therapy [66]. This treatment led to a 36% relative reduction in the risk of disease progression and a 3.2% absolute reduction in disease recurrence with a strong trend in this early analysis toward an improvement in overall survival among the zoledronic acid-treated patients.

6.8 Conclusions

The major clinical problems that arise in myeloma patients relate to the enhanced bone loss that commonly occurs in these patients. The results of two large Phase III clinical trials have shown the efficacy of monthly administration of intravenously administered pamidronate and zoledronic acid in reducing bone complications in myeloma patients. In fact, a recent retrospective study [46] showed that patients treated with monthly zoledronic acid in conjunction with other antimyeloma therapies had a skeletal morbidity rate (# of skeletal events/year) of only 0.112 (1 event every 9 years) which is markedly lower than in previous studies [22, 29]. This dramatic reduction in skeletal morbidity has had a major positive impact on the quality of lives for patients with myeloma. As a result, monthly treatment with intravenous bisphosphonates should now be considered for all myeloma patients with evidence of bone loss. The optimal duration of monthly therapy still has not been clearly established. The risk of ONJ associated with administration of these drugs can be minimized with proper dental care and avoidance of dental procedures involving the jaw bones. Renal impairment may occur from use of these agents but this risk can be reduced with recommended infusion times and monitoring of renal function prior to each dose of drug. Although preclinical studies suggest nitrogen-containing bisphosphonates have potent antitumor effects, clinical trials will be required to clearly establish their antitumor effects clinically. Overall, treatment of myeloma patients with long-term monthly intravenous bisphosphonates has had a major positive impact on the lives of patients with myeloma over the past two decades, and remains a mainstay of the therapeutic armamentarium for this B-cell malignancy.

References

1. Mundy GR, Bertoline DR. Bone destruction and hypercalcemia in plasma cell myeloma. Semin Oncol. 1986;13:291–299.
2. Kyle RA. Multiple myeloma, review of 869 cases. Mayo Clin Proc. 1975;50: 29–40.
3. Belch AR, Bergsagel DE, Wilson K, et al. Effect of daily etidronate on the osteolysis of multiple myeloma. J Clin Oncol. 1991;9:1397–1402.
4. Kyle RA, Jowsey J, Kelly PJ, et al. Multiple myeloma bone disease. The comparative effect of sodium fluoride and calcium carbonate or placebo. N Engl J Med. 1975;293:1334–1338.
5. Angtuaco EJ, Justus M, Sethi R, et al. Analysis of compression fractures in patients with newly diagnosed multiple myeloma on comprehensive therapy (abstr). Radiology. 2001;221(P):138.
6. Moulopoulos LA, Dimopoulos MA, Alexanian R, et al. Multiple myeloma: MR patterns of response to treatment. Radiology. 1994;193:441–446.
7. Lecouvet FE, Malghem J, Michaux L, et al. Vertebral compression fractures in multiple myeloma. II. Assessment of fracture risk with MR imaging of spinal bone marrow. Radiology. 1997;204:201–205.
8. Berenson JR, Lichtenstein A, Porter L, et al. Efficacy of pamidronate in reducing the skeletal events in patients with advanced multiple myeloma. N Engl J Med. 1996;334: 488–493.
9. Lecouvet FE, Vande Berg BC, Maldague BE, et al. Vertebral compression fractures in multiple myeloma. I. Distribution and appearance at MR imaging. Radiology. 1997;204:195–199.

10. Melton LJ 3rd, Rajkumar SV, Khosla S, Achenbach SJ, Oberg AL, Kyle RA. Fracture risk in monoclonal gammopathy of undetermined significance. J Bone Miner Res. January 2004;19(1):25–30.
11. Melton LJ 3rd, Kyle RA, Achenbach SJ, Oberg AL, Rajkumar SV. Fracture risk with multiple myeloma: a population-based study. J Bone Miner Res. March 2005;20(3):487–493; Epub November 29, 2004.
12. Bataille R, Chappard D, Basle MF. Quantifiable excess of bone resorption in monoclonal gammopathy is an early symptom of malignancy: a prospective study of 87 bone biopsies. Blood. 1996;87:4762–4769.
13. Green JR, Rogers MJ. Pharmacologic profile of zoledronic acid: a highly potent inhibitor of bone resorption. Drug Dev Res. 2002;55:210–224.
14. Rogers MJ. From molds and macrophages to mevalonate: a decade of progress in understanding the molecular mode of action of bisphosphonates. Calcif Tissue Int. 2004;75: 451–461.
15. Lahtinen R, Laakso M, Palva I, et al. Randomised, placebo-controlled multicentre trial of clodronate in multiple myeloma. Lancet. 1992;340:1049–1052.
16. Heim ME, Clemens MR, Queisser W, et al. Prospective randomized trial of dichloromethylene bisphosphonate (clodronate) in patients with multiple myeloma requiring treatment: a multicenter study. Onkologie. 1995;18:439–448.
17. McCloskey EV, MacLennan CM, Drayson MT, et al. A randomized trial on the effect of clodronate on skeletal morbidity in multiple myeloma. Br J Haematol. 1998;101:317–325.
18. Brincker H, Westin J, Abildgaard N, et al. Failure of oral pamidronate to reduce skeletal morbidity in multiple myeloma: a double-blind placebo-controlled trial. Br J Haematol. 1998;101:280–286.
19. Man Z, Otero AB, Rendo P, et al. Use of pamidronate for multiple myeloma osteolytic lesions. Lancet. 1990;335:663.
20. Purohit OP, Anthony C, Radstone CR, et al. High-dose pamidronate for metastatic bone pain. Br J Cancer. 1994;70:554–558.
21. Berenson J, Lichtenstein A, Porter L, et al. Long-term pamidronate treatment of advanced multiple myeloma patients reduces skeletal events. J Clin Oncol. 1998;16:593–602.
22. Berenson JR, Lichtenstein A, Porter L, et al. Efficacy of pamidronate in reducing the skeletal events in patients with advanced multiple myeloma. N Engl J Med. 1996;334: 488–493.
23. Menssen HD, Saklova A, Fontana A, et al. Effects of long-term intravenous ibandronate therapy on skeletal-related events, survival, and bone resorption markers in patients with advanced multiple myeloma. J Clin Oncol. 2002;20:2353–2359.
24. Body JJ, Lichinitser MR, Diehl I, et al. Double blind-placebo controlled trial of intravenous ibandronate in breast cancer metastatic to bone. Proc Am Soc Clin Oncol. 1999;35:575a (abstr 2222)
25. Green JR, Muller K, Jaeggi KA. Preclinical pharmacology of CGP 42'446, a new, potent, heterocyclic bisphosphonate compound. J Bone Miner Res. 1994;9:745–751.
26. Berenson JR, Vescio R, Henick K, et al. A phase I open label, dose ranging trial of intravenous bolus zolderonic acid, a novel bisphosphonate, in cancer patients with metastatic bone disease. Cancer. 2001;91:144–154.
27. Berenson J, Vescio R, Rosen LS, et al. A phase I dose-ranging trial of monthly infusions of zoledronic acid for the treatment of metastatic bone disease. Clin Cancer Res. 2001;7: 478–485.
28. Berenson J, Rosen LS, Howell A, et al. Zoledronic acid reduces skeletal-related events in patients with osteolytic metastases. Cancer. 2001;91:1191–1200.
29. Rosen LS, Gordon D, Antonio BS, et al. Zoledronic acid versus pamidronate in the treatment of skeletal metastases in patients with breast cancer or osteolytic lesions of multiple myeloma: A phase III, double-blind, comparative trial. Cancer J. 2001;7:377–387.
30. Major P, Lortholary A, Hon J, et al. Zoledronic acid is superior to pamidronate in the treatment of hypercalcemia of malignancy: a pooled analysis of two randomized, controlled clinical trials. J Clin Oncol. 2001;19:558–567.

31. Rosen LS, Gordon D, Kaminski M, et al. Long-term efficacy and safety of zoledronic acid compared with pamidronate disodium in the treatment of skeletal complications in patients with advanced multiple myeloma or breast carcinoma: a randomized, double-blind, multicenter, comparative trial. Cancer. 2003;98:1735–1744.

32. Berenson J, Yellin O, Boccia RV, et al. Zoledronic acid markedly improves bone mineral density for patients with monoclonal gammopathy of undetermined significance and bone loss. Clin Cancer Res. 2008;14:6289–6295.

33. Pepe J, Petrucci MT, Mascia ML, et al. The effects of alendronate treatment in osteoporotic patients affected by monoclonal gammopathy of undetermined significance. Calcif Tissue Int. 2008;82:418–426.

34. Chang JT, Green L, Beitz J., Tarassoff P, Hei Y-J, Maladorno D. Letters to the editor: renal failure with the use of zoledronic acid. N Engl J Med. 2003;349:1676–1679.

35. Guarneri V, Donati S, Nicolini M, et al. Renal safety and efficacy of iv bisphosphonates in patients with skeletal metastases treated for up to 10 years. Oncologist. 2005;10:842–848.

36. Ali SM, Esteva FJ, Hortobagyi G, et al. Safety and efficacy of bisphosphonates beyond 24 months in cancer patients. J Clin Oncol. 2001;19:3434–3437.

37. Ruggiero SL, Mehrotra B, Rosenberg TJ, Engroff SL. Osteonecrosis of the jaws associated with the use of bisphosphonates: a review of 63 cases. J Oral Maxillofac Surg. 2004;62:527–534.

38. Woo S-B, Hellstein JW and Kalamr JR. Systematic review: bisphosphonates and osteonecrosis of the jaws. Ann Intern Med. 2006;144:753–761.

39. Van Poznak C, Estilo C. Osteonecrosis of the jaw in cancer patients receiving IV bisphosphonates. Oncology. 2006;20:1053–1062.

40. Bamias A, Kastritis E, Bamia C, et al. Osteonecrosis of the jaw in cancer after treatment with bisphosphonates: incidence and risk factors. J Clin Oncol. 2005;23:8580–8587.

41. Badros A, Weikel D, Salama A, et al. Osteonecrosis of the jaw in multiple myeloma patients: clinical features and risk factors. J Clin Oncol. 2006;24:945–952.

42. Sarasquete ME, Garcia-Sanz R, Marin L, et al. Bisphosphonate-related osteonecrosis of the jaw is associated with polymorphisms of the cytochrome P450 CYP2C8 in multiple myeloma: a genome-wide single nucleotide polymorphism analysis. Blood. 2008;112:2709–2712.

43. American Dental Association Council on Scientific Affairs. Dental management of patients receiving oral bisphosphonate therapy – Expert panel recommendations. JADA. 2006;137:1144–1150.

44. Ruggerio S, Gralow J, Marx RE, et al. Practical guidelines for the prevention, diagnosis, and treatment of osteonecrosis of the jaw in patients with cancer. J Oncol Pract. 2006;2:7–13.

45. Migliorati CA, Casiglia J, Epstein J, et al. Managing the care of patients with bisphosphonate-associated osteonecrosis – an American Academy of Oral Medicine position paper. JADA. 2005;136:1658–1681.

46. Berenson JR, Yellin O, Crowley J, et al. Overall survival among patients with multiple myeloma (MM) treated with zoledronic acid. Clin Lymphoma Myeloma. 2009;9:Abstract 101:E30.

47. Berenson JR, Hillner BE, Kyle RA, et al. American Society of Clinical Oncology bisphosphonates expert panel. American Society of Clinical Oncology clinical practice guidelines: the role of bisphosphonates in multiple myeloma. J Clin Oncol. 2002;20:3719–3736.

48. Kyle RA, Yee GC, Somerfield MR, et al. American Society of Clinical Oncology 2007 clinical practice guideline update on the role of bisphosphonates in multiple myleoma. J Clin Oncol. 2007;25:2462–2472.

49. Lacy MQ, Dispenzieri A, Gertz MA, et al. Mayo Clinic consensus statement for the use of bisphosphonates in multiple myeloma. Mayo Clin Proc. 2006;81:1047–1053.

50. Berenson J, Cook R, Lipton A, et al. Increased levels of N-telopeptide of Type I collagen correlate with reduced survival in patients with advanced multiple myeloma. Blood. 2007;110:449a.

51. Gimsing P, Carlson K, Fayers P, et al. Randomised study on prophylactic pamidronate 30 mg vs. 90 mg in multiple myeloma (Nordic Myeloma Study Group). Blood. 2007;110:164a.

52. Musto P, Petrucci MT, Bringhen S, et al. Final analysis of a multicenter, randomised study comparing zoledronate vs. observation in patients with asymptomatic myeloma. Blood. 2007;110:164a.
53. Radl J, Croese JW, Zircher C, et al. Influence of treatment with APD-bisphosphonate on the bone lesions in the mouse 5T2 multiple myeloma. Cancer. 1985;55:1030–1040.
54. Corso A, Ferretti E, Lunghi M, Zappasodi P, Mangiacavalli S, De Amici M, Rusconi C, Varettoni M, Lazzarino M. Zoledronic acid down-regulates adhesion molecules of bone marrow stromal cells in multiple myeloma: a possible mechanism for its antitumor effect. Cancer. 2005;104:118–125.
55. Aparicio A, Gardner A, Tu Y, Savage A, Berenson J, et al. In vitro cytoreductive effects on multiple myeloma cells induced by bisphosphonates. Leukemia. 1998;12:220–229.
56. Savage AD, Belson DJ, Vescio RA, et al. Pamidronate reduces IL-6 production by bone marrow stroma from multiple myeloma patients. Blood. 1996;88:105a.
57. Wood J, Bonjean K, Ruetsz S, et al. Novel antiangiogenic effects of the bisphosphonate compound zoledronic acid. J Pharmacol Exp Ther. 2002;302:1055–1061.
58. Fournier P, Boissier S, Filleur S, et al. Bisphosphonates inhibit angiogenesis in vitro and testosterone-stimulated vascular regrowth in the ventral prostate in castrated rats. Cancer Res. 2002;62:6538–6544.
59. Chen H, Wang CS, Li M, et al. A novel screening method for screening anti-angiogenic compounds: the chorioallantoic membrane (CAM)/feather bud (FB) assay. Blood. 2008;112:663.
60. Tassone P, Forciniti S, Galea E, et al. Growth inhibition and synergistic induction of apoptosis by zoledronate and dexamethasone in human myeloma cell lines. Leukemia. 2000;14:841–844.
61. Ochiai N, Yamada N, Uchida R, Fuchida S, Okano A, Okamoto M, Ashihara E, Inaba T, Shimazaki C. Nitrogen-containing bisphosphonate incadronate augments the inhibitory effect of farnesyl transferase inhibitor tipifarnib on the growth of fresh and cloned myeloma cells in vitro. Leuk Lymphoma. 2005;46:1619–1625.
62. Sonnemann J, Bumbul B, Beck JF. Synergistic activity of the histone deacetylase inhibitor suberoylanilide hydroxamic acid and the bisphosphonate zoledronic acid against prostate cancer cells in vitro. Mol Cancer Ther. 2007;6:2976–2984.
63. Ochiai N, Yamada N, Uchida R, Fuchida S, Okano A, Hatsuse M, Okamoto M, Ashihara E, Shimazaki C. Combination therapy with thalidomide, incadronate, and dexamethasone for relapsed or refractory multiple myeloma. Int J Hematol. 2005;82:243–247.
64. Dhodapkar MV, Singh J, Mehta J, et al. Anti-myeloma activity of pamidronate in vivo. Br J Haematol. 1998;103:530–532.
65. Berenson J, Shirina N, Chen YM, et al. Survival in patients with multiple myeloma receiving zoledronic acid: stratification by baseline bone alkaline phosphatase levels. J Clin Oncol. 2006;24:Abstract # 7505;4235.
66. Gnant M, Mlineritsch B, Schippinger W, et al. Endocrine therapy plus zoledronic acid in premenopausal breast cancer. N Engl J Med. 2009;360:679–691.

Chapter 7
Osteonecrosis of the Jaw

Ashraf Badros

Abstract Osteonecrosis of the jaw (ONJ), defined as an oral soft tissue defect with superficial necrosis of the underlying exposed bone, is a severe but uncommon side effect of bisphosphonates (BP). ONJ typically follows a mucosal injury, such as a dental extraction. The exact incidence is unknown but seems to range between 3 and 4%. ONJ occurs after a median of 4 years of "continuous" BP use. There is no specific therapy and 60% of the patients will heal spontaneously in 6–9 months. It seems reasonable to stop BP once ONJ develops until the mucosal lesions heal and then restart BP if clinically indicated; stopping BP before dental procedures is recommended. The use of pamidronate rather than zoledronic acid and less frequent infusions 3-monthly after the first 2 years of monthly infusions may decrease the risk of ONJ, although definitive data are absent. Implementation of preventative measures such as good dental hygiene and limiting the invasiveness of dental procedures seems to decrease the risk of ONJ. Pathogenesis of BP-induced ONJ is unknown. In this chapter, the incidence and risks of ONJ, the clinical presentation, diagnostic workup will be reviewed followed by a summary of the current hypotheses of pathogenesis.

Keywords Osteonecrosis · Bisphosphonates · Pathogenesis · Clinical presentation · Myeloma

7.1 Introduction

Bisphosphonates (BP) are effective in the prevention of skeletal-related events and treatment of lytic bone disease in multiple myeloma (MM) and cancer patients with bone metastases. Their use in many benign conditions such as osteoporosis

A. Badros (✉)
Associate Professor of Medicine, Greenebaum Cancer Center, University of Maryland, Baltimore, MD 21201, USA
e-mail: abadros@umm.edu

G.D. Roodman (ed.), *Myeloma Bone Disease*, Current Clinical Oncology,
DOI 10.1007/978-1-60761-554-5_7, © Springer Science+Business Media, LLC 2010

is increasing [1]. BP accumulate at sites of active bone formation and inhibits osteoclast function by altering cell attachment and differentiation inducing apoptosis and
leading to reduction in bone resorption [2].

The toxicity profile of these drugs has been favorable supporting their long-
term/indefinite use. In 2002, less than 1 year after the most potent intravenous
BP, zoledronic acid, received regulatory approval for marketing, the FDA received
reports of nine patients with cancer, all treated with zoledronic acid, who unexpect-
edly developed oral mucosal lesions [3]. This was followed by reports from three
oral surgeons describing 104 cancer patients with what they called osteonecrosis
of the jaw (ONJ) as a complication of BP administration [4–6]. In the last 5 years,
hundreds of cases have been published, mostly as case reports and retrospective case
series. The reports focused on cancer patients, with MM compromising the majority of the cases. ONJ has also been described in the none-cancer setting and with
oral BP.

ONJ is defined as an oral soft tissue defect with superficial necrosis of the
underlying exposed bone. ONJ typically follows a mucosal injury, such as a dental extraction. There is no effective therapy for established cases; approximately
half the cases heal spontaneously. Implementation of preventative measures such
as good dental hygiene and limiting the invasiveness of dental procedures seems
to decrease the risk of ONJ. Pathogenesis of BP-induced ONJ is unknown. Several
hypotheses have been proposed to explain the condition that include: suppression of
bone turnover, inhibition of angiogenesis, infection and damage to the soft tissues
that lead to impaired healing following minor trauma.

In this chapter, the incidence and risks of ONJ, the clinical presentation, diagnostic workup will be reviewed followed by a summary of the current hypotheses
of pathogenesis. It is very important to emphasize that ONJ is an infrequent event;
in few patients it can have a significant impact on quality of life. Consequently,
because BP therapy has a relatively low risk and considerable benefit, the clinician
and the patient should not avoid or delay using BP therapy when indicated.

7.2 Clinical Presentation of ONJ

The criteria used to diagnose ONJ in the published cases have been inconsistent.
Several associations and expert panels provided consensus statements for criteria
to diagnose ONJ, the details have been recently reviewed [7]. BP-related ONJ is
defined as "an area of exposed bone in the maxillofacial region that has not healed
within 8 weeks after identification by a healthcare provider in a patient who is
receiving or has been exposed to a BP without local evidence of malignancy and
no prior radiotherapy to the affected region," Fig. 7.1 [8]. ONJ may occur spontaneously, though most cases follow a tooth extraction or a dental procedure. Patients
may present with pain, feelings of numbness or heaviness of the jaw. Other symptoms include soft tissue swelling, loosening of teeth, and infection. In many cases,
ONJ is asymptomatic and is detected by the examining physician who finds an

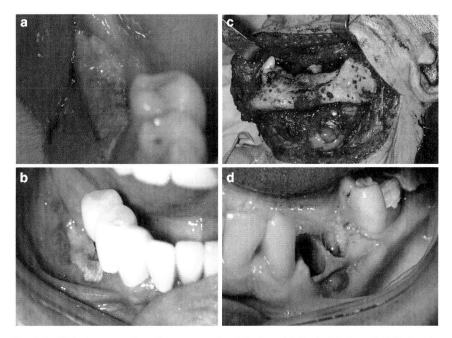

Fig. 7.1 Clinical presentation of osteonecrosis of the jaw. (**a**) Typical lesion of ONJ showing exposed infected bone involving the mylohyoid ridge. (**b**) ONJ bone below dental implant. (**c**) Spontaneous exfoliated teeth with underlying exposed dead bone. (**d**) Operative picture showing well-demarcated dead bone involving the whole alveolus

exposed bone in the jaw. The mandible is the main affected site, and most lesions occur posterior to the cuspid teeth. Staging of ONJ has been suggested as a standard tool to compare the results of the published cases (Table 7.1). Its clinical use and widespread utility have been limited [9].

Before a diagnosis of ONJ is established, a dental professional who is familiar with ONJ needs to evaluate the patient mostly to rule out other causes of exposed bone in the oral cavity in cancer patients that include: infectious osteomyelitis, gingivitis or mucositis, periodontal disease, sinusitis, temporo-mandibular joint disease, periapical pathology due to a carious infection, osteoradionecrosis, neuralgia-inducing cavitational osteonecrosis, and bone tumors or metastases. The differential diagnosis should also exclude other conditions that may present as exposed bone

Table 7.1 American Academy of oral and facial surgeons staging of bisphosphonate-related osteonecrosis of the jaw

Stage 1: Patients asymptomatic with no evidence of infection, but with exposed or necrotic bone

Stage 2: Patients have exposed or necrotic bone, along with pain and clinical evidence of infection

Stage 3: Includes all the elements of stages 1 and 2, and one or more of the following: pathological fracture, extraoral fistula, or osteolysis extending to the inferior border without a history of malignancy or BP use, including benign sequestration of the lingual plate, odontogenic infections leading to osteomyelitis, trauma, and human immunodeficiency virus-associated necrotizing ulcerative periodontitis [10]. The diagnosis of ONJ is a clinical one but can be supported pathologically. ONJ lesions are characterized by necrotic and acellular bone usually with quiescent bone surface and absence of osteoblastic and osteoclastic activity, Fig. 7.2 [11]. In many cases foci of mixed inflammatory cellular infiltration are seen, suggesting that infection may play a role in ONJ and justifying the empiric use of systemic and oral antimicrobials for prevention and therapy [12].

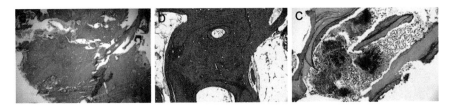

Fig. 7.2 Pathology of surgically removed bone from patients with osteonecrosis of the jaw. (**a**) Acellular bone with osteoclastic activity at irregular bone surfaces (hematoxylin–eosin stain, 100×). (**b**) A quiescent bone surface, complete absence of osteoblastic and osteoclastic cells (hematoxylin–eosin, 200×). (**c**) Foci of filamentous organisms *Actinomycetes* (*arrow*) in the vicinity of acellular bone surrounded by mixed inflammatory cellular infiltration (PAS stain, 200×)

7.3 Incidence and Risk Factors of Osteonecrosis of the Jaw

Current estimates on the incidence of ONJ in BP-treated MM patients are unknown. Manufacturer-sponsored epidemiological studies reported an ONJ estimate ranging from 0.1 to 1.8%. By contrast, independent epidemiological reports from clinicians and the International Myeloma Foundation the incidence estimates are higher, between 5 and 10%. The results of selected trails that focus on homogenous MM patients had an incidence range between 3.2 and 10%, Table 7.2. At the University of Maryland, we reported a 3% incidence of ONJ (11 of 340 patients) and the incidence remains stable in our prospective follow-up. Using matched case–controls, we found that the risk factors predictive of developing ONJ were dental extraction ($p = 0.009$), sequential treatment with pamidronate followed by zoledronic acid ($p = 0.009$), longer follow-up time based on longer survival ($p = 0.03$), and older age at diagnosis of MM ($p = 0.006$) [11]. A retrospective chart review from Boston identified similar incidence of ONJ (11 of 292 MM patients 3.8%; 95% CI: 1.6–6.0%) [13]. Large Canadian retrospective study of 655 MM patients reported an incidence of 3.2%. Risk factors reported were: longer duration of pamidronate therapy ($p < 0.001$), dental extractions ($p < 0.001$), cyclophosphamide therapy ($p < 0.014$), prednisone therapy ($p < 0.014$), erythropoietin therapy ($p = 0.006$), low hemoglobin levels ($p < 0.001$), renal dialysis ($p < 0.016$), and advanced age ($p < 0.001$) [14].

Table 7.2 Representative studies reporting the incidence of osteonecrosis of the jaw in multiple myeloma patients

Author	Study design	Pts, ONJ No.	Incidence
Bamias et al. [16]	Prospective	111, 11	10%
Durie et al. [18]	Web survey	904, 62	6.9
Wilkinson et al. [18]	SEER/Medicare	14,349	5.4
Badros et al. [11]	Retrospective	340, 11	3.2
Hoff, 2006 [15]	Retrospective	548, 13	2.4
Jadu, 2007 [14]	Retrospective	655, 21	3.2
Wang et al. [13]	Retrospective	292, 11	3.8

In the Greek Multiple Myeloma Study Group, the incidence of ONJ was 9.9% (11 of 111 patients) in a prospective follow-up study [16]. The risk increased with the duration of exposure to BP from 1.5% among patients treated for 4–12 months to 7.7% in those treated for 37–48 months. The cumulative hazard was significantly higher with zoledronic acid compared with pamidronate alone or pamidronate and zoledronic acid sequentially ($p < 0.001$). Another study from Greece reported an incidence of 11% (28 of 254 patients) [16]. Again zoledronic acid was associated with a 9.5-fold greater risk for developing ONJ than pamidronate alone ($p = 0.042$) and a 4.5-fold greater risk than sequential use of pamidronate and zoledronic acid ($p = 0.018$). The use of thalidomide was reported to increase the risk for ONJ 2.4-fold ($p = 0.043$).

A web-based survey of 1,203 MM patients identified 152 ONJ patients. ONJ was reported in 10% of 211 patients receiving zoledronic acid and in 4% of 413 patients receiving pamidronate. The data are hampered by selection bias, unreliability of self-reported data, and lack of health-care confirmation of the diagnosis [17]. Two large studies investigated dental toxicities as a surrogate diagnosis for ONJ. One by linking data from the Surveillance, Epidemiology, and End Results (SEER) program to Medicare claims ($n = 14,349$) and one by review of medical claims alone (714,217 patients on oral or intravenous BP) reported an absolute risk at 6 years for any jaw toxicity of 5.48 events per 100 patients using intravenous BP. Oral BP carries a lower risk of "jaw complications," $p = 0.05$ [18, 19].

7.4 Natural History of ONJ in MM Patients

All published reports describing ONJ focused on the outcome of severe cases and ignored or misdiagnosed the mild cases, giving a frightening picture of ONJ both to patients and physicians. We have performed a prospective, observational study of 97 patients with MM who had been diagnosed with ONJ to report on the natural history of ONJ [20]. A unique feature of this study was that it compared patients from two geographic locations: the United States (US) ($n = 37$) and Greece ($n = 60$). The median age at MM diagnosis was 60 years old, the median time from diagnosis of MM to ONJ was 4 years and the median follow-up time was 3.9 years. All parameters were similar in both groups. Primary therapy of MM included autologous stem cell transplant in 73% of the US patients, but only 28% of the Greek group ($p < 0.0001$). More US patients had relapsed disease at the time of their first ONJ episode, compared to the Greek patients (51% vs. 23%, $p = 0.008$) and more were receiving MM salvage therapy with novel agents (70% vs. 23%, $p = 0.0001$). Additionally, US patients more frequently had diabetes mellitus (24% vs. 8%, $p = 0.0002$) and renal insufficiency ($p = 0.002$) at diagnosis of ONJ. Dental extraction preceded ONJ in 46 of 97 patients (47%), with similar frequencies in both groups. Surgical interventions for ONJ were performed more often in the US patients than in Greece, 17 of 37 (45%) vs. 19 of 60 (32%).

ONJ resolved in 62% of cases, recurred after healing in 12% in the same site and/or in a new location, and did not resolve in 26% during a follow-up of 9 months. The recurrence rate was highest among US patients than Greek patients (22% vs. 7%, respectively). Dental extractions preceded diagnosis of ONJ in 47% of cases and these procedures were more common in patients with a single episode of ONJ than in those with recurrent and nonhealing disease (58% vs. 30%).

7.5 Imaging Studies of ONJ

Radiographic studies have a limited role in confirming the diagnosis, but they may help in the differential diagnosis of ONJ, Fig. 7.3. Regular X-rays "panoramic views" show bone sclerosis and fragmentation [21]. The use of CT scan can clearly define the areas of cortical bone loss and fragmented sequestra in the mandible and can also detect soft tissue fullness around the mandible [22]. The use of F-18 fluoride and F-18 fluorodeoxyglucose (FDG) positron-emission tomography (PET) was recently assessed in a cohort of nine patients with ONJ [23]. Although fairly sensitive the uptake "SUV" did not correlate with the severity of ONJ [24]. MRI was helpful in the assessment of bone lesions caused by ONJ as well as in detection of subclinical lesions [25]. Of 14 patients undergoing MRI 26 focal lesions were detected clinically and 36 lesions detected radiologically. The significance of focal lesions detectable on radiological examination but without clinical ONJ and their possible progression over time to clinical ONJ remain to be determined. This may need to be fully evaluated in a prospective study especially if a decision is to be made to stop or continue BP therapy.

Two studies using 99Tc(m)-MDP 3-phase bone scans were carried out in patients with ONJ and compared to conventional radiography, CT, and MRI. Both showed that 99Tc(m)-MDP three-phase bone scans were the most sensitive tool to detect early stages of ONJ [26, 27]. However, the changes were none specific and should be differentiated from other causes of increased uptake such as infection [28].

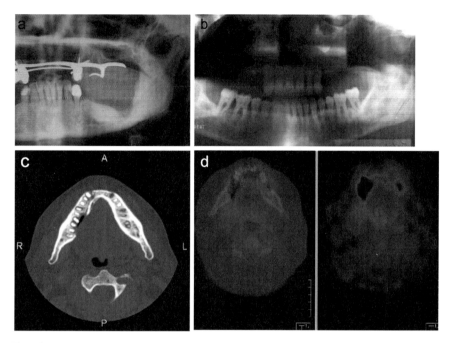

Fig. 7.3 Radiological imaging of osteonecrosis of the jaw. (**a**) Dense sclerotic bone adjacent to an osteonecrosis site. (**b**) Bilateral condensing osteitis and widened periodontal ligaments. (**c**) CT scan showing cortical bone loss on the *right side* of the mandible. (**d**) A fusion PET/CT scan showing metabolic activity at the site of ONJ

7.6 Pathogenesis of Bisphosphonate-Related Osteonecrosis of the Jaw

Although the pathogenesis of ONJ is not understood, indirect evidence suggests that it is multifactorial and is clearly linked to long-term BP use. Based on the biological activity of BP, ONJ was linked to adynamic bone, inhibition of angiogenesis and microbial infections. A possible hypothesis is summarized in Fig. 7.4. Briefly, after years of BP therapy, the skeleton is saturated and BP pharmacokinetics is altered favoring higher concentrations in the saliva following intravenous infusions; these levels may significantly increase following dental procedures such as extractions or even minor trauma. BP inhibits soft tissue healing, in vitro studies showed that a brief exposure to low levels of BP inhibits proliferation and induces apoptosis of human gingival fibroblasts and oral epidermal mucosal cells (see below). The loss of mucosal integrity leads to the formation of a microbial biofilm from oral pathogens on the exposed bone. This chronic infection leads to release of inflammatory cytokines that further free bone-bound BP that sustains the soft tissue defect. The disruption of the periosteum interrupts the blood supply to the cortical bone and the direct inhibition of endothelial progenitor cells by BP impairs angiogenesis and bone healing.

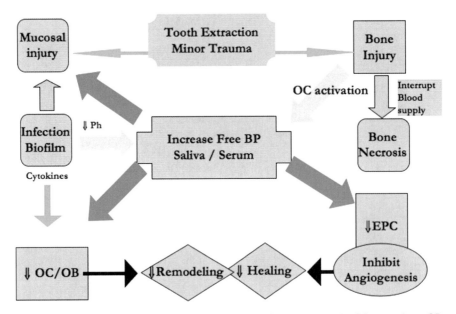

Fig. 7.4 A hypothesis for pathogenesis of osteonecrosis of the jaw. Legends: OC, osteoclasts; OB, osteoblasts, EPC, endothelial progenitor cells; BP, bisphosphonates

One of the first propositions to explain ONJ was related to BP effects on the bone. BP inhibits osteoclast activity and reduce bone turnover, impairing its ability to repair bone micro-fractures thus leaving the bone susceptible to necrosis [29]. In our initial series, among 22 ONJ patients, 8 (36%) had other bone pathology while on long-term BP therapy [11]. Four patients had avascular necrosis of the hip, 1 before and 3 after the diagnosis of ONJ. Three patients had no pathological long-bone fractures. We suspected that ONJ might be the tip of the iceberg with other bone pathology to follow, but this has not been confirmed in other studies. As bone is resorbed by osteoclast activity, the collagen remnants of the matrix degradation products, amino-terminal (NTX-I) and carboxy-terminal (CTX-I) cross-linked telopeptide, can be detected in the urine and serum, respectively [30]. Although initially used in clinical trials to assess the effect of BP therapy on bone turnover, its use has been abandoned. The use of serum CTX-I has recently been proposed to predict the risk for ONJ after an invasive dental procedure in patients receiving oral BP therapy. Patients who had a morning fasting serum CTX-I levels >150 pg/mL were considered to have adequate residual bone remodeling capacity and subsequently at minimal risk of developing ONJ [31]. We have assessed over 100 MM patients for CTX and other bone turnover markers including NTX, bone-specific alkaline phosphatase, serum 25-hydroxyvitamin D, parathyroid hormone, calcium, and phosphorus levels and did not find a difference between patients with ONJ ($n = 12$) and those without or between those receiving monthly versus 3-monthly BP infusions [32]. Several published reports cast doubt on the reliability of CTX-I for predicting ONJ since they failed to demonstrate a significant relationship between the marker and the severity of ONJ. In fact, many patients with active ONJ have bone markers that are within the normal range [33, 34].

Although bone necrosis is the cardinal sign of ONJ, one issue that is recently debated is whether BP may lead to mucosal damage and whether the ONJ lesions start in the soft tissue rather than in the underlying bone. The first study to address this question was recently published by Landesberg et al., where exposure of mucosal cells (murine oral keratinocytes) to pamidronate at a range of clinically relevant concentrations inhibited proliferation of oral keratinocytes and consequently wound healing [35]. We investigated the effects of zoledronic acid on soft tissues using human oral mucosal cells in vitro, Fig. 7.5 [36]. In this study, human gingival fibroblast and keratinocyte cell lines were exposed to different concentrations of zoledronic acid (0.25–3 μmol/L). A dose–response effect on apoptosis and cell proliferation was observed with increasing zoledronic acid concentrations. Western

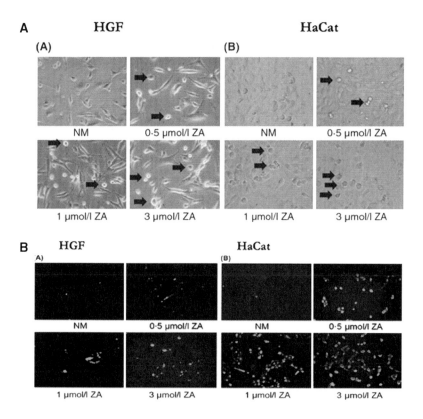

Fig. 7.5 Bisphosphonate induces apoptosis and inhibits proliferation of mucosal cells. Apoptosis in human gingival fibroblasts (HGF) and mucosal cells (HaCat) was seen at different concentrations of zoledronic acid microscopically (**a**) and by TUNEL assays (**b**). Inhibition of proliferation is also dose dependent (**c**). Caspase-3 upregulation and survivin downregulation detected by western blot analysis may play a critical in BP-induced mucosal damage (**d**)

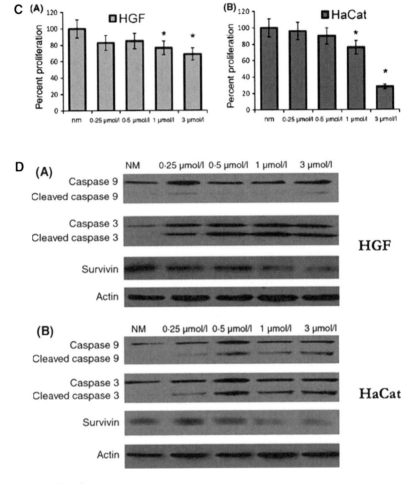

Fig. 7.5 (continued)

blot analysis confirmed the presence of activated forms of caspase-3 and caspase-9 and underexpression of survivin protein expression. These preliminary findings support the potential role of soft tissue injury as an initiating/potentiating event in ONJ following BP infusions.

It is well established that BP as a class inhibit angiogenesis [37]. Zoledronic acid inhibits the proliferation of human umbilical vein endothelial cell in vitro and blocks in vivo angiogenesis in CAM and Matrigel assays at high concentrations [38–40]. How BP suppress angiogenesis within the osseous tissue is not clear BP has been shown to decrease endothelial cell numbers and inhibit proliferation in vitro and in vivo [41–43]. Endothelial progenitor cells (EPC) are produced within the bone marrow and released into the circulation upon tissue injury promoting angiogenesis [44, 45]. Allegra et al., recently reported that the number of EPC was reduced in

BP-treated patients as compared to control subjects [46]. This reduction of EPC may impair bone and soft tissue repair/regeneration following BP infusions contributing to ONJ.

One of the main differences between the jaw and other bones in the body is the microbial flora in close proximity to the oral bones. There are 200 species that colonize the oral cavity so super-infection of an exposed surface is common. In fact, all ONJ lesions become infected, however, no specific organism has been identified. Infection seems to be a secondary event, rather than a causative factor. In most cases it is rather chronic/subclinical [47]. In our initial experience with ONJ, several organisms were frequently isolated from tissues cultured from ONJ lesions, including *Actinomyces*, *Streptococcus*, *Peptostreptococcus*, *Eikenella*, *Prevotella*, *Porphyromonas*, and *Fusobacterium* species [11, 48]. Whether microbial infections can modify the oral environment and directly cause bone destruction or indirectly modify cytokine secretion leading to release of bone-bound BP that further affect tissue healing, remains unknown [49, 50]. Furthermore, studying the microbial signature is a challenge in ONJ patients that needs to be addressed in a prospective fashion to establish a relationship between BP, alterations in the nature and magnitude of the oral microflora, and ONJ [51].

A study was recently published using 500, 568 single-nucleotide polymorphisms in two cohorts of MM patients, one with ONJ ($n = 22$) and another without ONJ ($n = 65$, matched controls) [52]. All patients received BP therapy, either pamidronate (16 ONJ cases and 57 controls) or zoledronic acid (6 ONJ cases and 8 controls) for 2 years. The rs1934951 polymorphism mapped within the cytochrome P450-2C polypeptide 8 genes (CYP2C8) was associated with increased risk for the development of ONJ in MM patients who receive intravenous BP. An accompanying editorial questioned a biological link between the rs1934951 polymorphism of the CYP2C8 and the development of ONJ in MM patients who receive BP, as CYP2C8 is not involved in the metabolism of BP and the rs1934951 polymorphism is placed in an intrinsic region, which theoretically should not imply alterations at the protein level. A gene transcriptional profiling study of 10 MM patients with ONJ showed that genes and proteins involved in osteoblast and osteoclast signaling cascades were significantly downregulated in patients with ONJ suggesting that altered bone remodeling, evidenced by suppression of both bone resorption and formation may be a factor in ONJ [24]. Both studies are not conclusive and lead to more questions than answers, but they open a new area of research linking genetic variables with the development of ONJ.

The measurement of free zoledronic acid in the saliva and blood of patients on long-term BP therapy needs to be investigated to understand the pathogenesis of the soft tissue and bone components of ONJ. Few PK studies of zoledronic acid have been performed in BP-naïve patients, mostly in patients with bone metastasis. These studies demonstrated a wide range of serum and urinary levels, from 1 to 10 μM/L, following a 15-min i.v. infusion and no data were provided for the concentrations of zoledronic acid in the saliva. In one study, zoledronic acid levels in the plasma and urine were determined by radioimmunoassay after three consecutive infusions, every 28 days, 4 mg infused over 5 min ($n = 5$), 4 mg infused over 15 min ($n = 7$),

8 mg infused over 15 min ($n = 12$), or 16 mg infused over 15 min ($n = 12$) [53]. Zoledronic acid plasma disposition was multiphasic, with an early, rapid decline of concentrations from the end-of-infusion to <1% at 24 h postdose and half-lives of 39 and 4526 h. AUC 0–24 h and C_{max} were dose proportional and no accumulation, AUC 0–24 h ratio between the third and first dose was 1.28. Prolonging the infusion from 5 to 15 min lowered C_{max} by 34%, with no effect on AUC 0–24 h. The notion that the skeleton has an infinite ability to retain BP is inaccurate. Within 6 weeks of initiation of BP treatment for osteoporosis and within days of first dose of BP in cancer therapy bone remodeling and resorption rates are suppressed by 70–80% [54, 55]. This suppression is most profound at the trabecular and endocortical surfaces, where BP is most predominantly distributed [56]. Once the patients receive BP, most bone surfaces are quiet and resting and as therapy progresses and continues the resorbing surface and formation surface decrease in comparison to BP-naïve patients. So, deposition of bisphosphonates in bones decreases and secretion in kidney and possibly saliva increases. This shift in favor of elimination of the drug leads to both renal damage and possibly contributing to ONJ soft tissue damage as mentioned above. Thus, the skeleton of a patient on active BP therapy, with lower turnover rate, collect and retain less BP than that of a BP-naïve patient [57].

To better understand the pathophysiology of ONJ several investigators attempted to supplement the ongoing clinical research with animal studies. Efforts to develop an animal model had been difficult; remodeling suppression, disrupted angiogenesis, and infection have all been tried with no clear success. A recent report studying the dog as a potential model of ONJ was published [58]. Another group developed a rat model, which replicated many of the clinical, radiographic, and histological features described in ONJ [59]. After treatment with a sequence of zoledronic acid and dexamethasone over a 1–3 week period rats developed ONJ-like changes in bony and soft tissue changes following extraction of mandibular or maxillary molars. The application of these models is in preliminary stages.

7.7 Therapeutic and Prevention Strategies

Currently, there is no effective therapy for ONJ. A conservative "supportive" non-surgical approach has been recommended. This conservative treatment includes: chlorhexidine 0.12% oral rinses, intermittent systemic antibiotics, and careful sequestrectomy. One study showed that this conservative treatment of ONJ leads to mucosal closure in 53% of patients [60]. It is worth emphasizing that standard osseous sequestrectomy and other surgical interventions have been associated with worsening lesions and should be avoided. The size of the lesion predicted healing in few studies, which may be simply a reflection of early detection and implantation of corrective measures such as stopping BP [61]. Ozone therapy, hyperbaric oxygen, and VSP Er: YAG lasers have been used in several cases of ONJ with mixed results [62–65]. The data are preliminary and further analysis of the chemical, physical, and pharmacological aspects of these therapies are necessary to establish reliable treatment protocols for ONJ patients.

Discontinuation of BP is recommended until the ONJ lesions heal. Restarting BP therapy is a controversial issue with no available data. The risk of ONJ recurrence seems low especially in patients who had the first episode of ONJ after a dental procedure. However, patients with no predisposing cause for the first ONJ episode are at an increased risk of recurrence on restarting BP. In this setting, the benefit of therapy and the risk should be discussed with the patient and the decision made after consultation with an oral surgeon experienced in ONJ [20].

The American Society of Clinical Oncology (ASCO) provided guidelines, suggesting a limit to the duration of BP therapy of 2 years in MM patients who respond to myeloma therapy or have stable disease, instead of continued use until there is evidence of a substantial decline in a patient's general performance status [66]. This is currently being studied in LOTUZ (LOng-Term Use of Zometa), a multicenter, prospective, pharmaco-epidemiological trial evaluating the safety and efficacy of the long-term use of zoledronic acid beyond 2 years in patients. It is worth mentioning that there are no data that show that less-frequent BP infusions decrease the risk of ONJ. An even more controversial topic is the preferred BP to use in MM patients. No clear data favor pamidronate over zoledronic acid with regard to overall toxicity profile, but many authors recommend that pamidronate be the first choice for patients [67], mostly due to a higher risk for ONJ in patients treated with zoledronic acid.

Although prevention is effective in reducing the incidence of ONJ in MM patients [51], in the absence of a clear initiating event for ONJ, development of prevention strategies is difficult. Patients on BP should be informed of the benefits and risks of treatment [68]. Dental assessment should include a panoramic radiograph to diagnosis caries and periodontal disease and identify other bony pathology. If BP therapy can be delayed, preventive surgery to eliminate potential sites of infection should be performed. Also, optimal dental health during treatment is essential, and all patients should be informed of the importance of good oral hygiene and the use of chlorhexidine rinses. In addition, regular visual inspections by the treating physician and routine assessments (at least annually) by a dental specialist are warranted. Whenever dental interventions are necessary, the less invasive techniques with preservation of the dental root are preferred. Only when teeth have a mobility score ≥ 3 should extraction be considered, and it should be performed as atraumatically as possible. Some authors suggest the withdrawal of BP therapy for 1–3 months before performing invasive dental procedures. Considering the long half-life of BP in bone, it is doubtful that a short drug holiday can restore adequate osteoclast function.

7.8 Summary

ONJ is a severe but uncommon side effect that occurs in MM patients receiving BP. The incidence is unknown but seems to range between 3 and 4%. It occurs at a median of 4 years of "continuous" BP use. There is no specific therapy and 60% of the patients will heal spontaneously in <9 months of follow-up. Prevention and close attention to dental care in patients receiving BP may decrease the risk. It seems reasonable to stop BP once ONJ develops until the mucosal lesions heal and then restart BP if clinically indicated. Stopping BP before dental procedures is recommended but again with no data. Whether pamidronate is safer than zoledronic acid is unclear. Similarly there are no data that less frequent infusions will decrease the risk of ONJ. The pathogenesis is unknown, but seems to be multifactorial. There is an urgent need to understand the patho-physiological mechanisms underlying ONJ and the exact risk factors to optimize strategies for prevention and treatment.

References

1. Dunstan CR, Felsenberg D, Seibel MJ. Therapy insight: the risks and benefits of bisphosphonates for the treatment of tumor-induced bone disease. Nat Clin Pract Oncol. 2007;4:42–55.
2. Yuasa T, Kimura S, Ashihara E, Habuchi T, Maekawa T. Zoledronic acid – a multiplicity of anti-cancer action. Curr Med Chem. 2007;14:2126–2135.
3. Edwards BJ, Gounder M, McKoy JM, et al. Pharmacovigilance and reporting oversight in US FDA fast-track process: bisphosphonates and osteonecrosis of the jaw. Lancet Oncol. 2008;9:1166–1172.
4. Carter GD, Goss AN. Bisphosphonates and avascular necrosis of the jaws. Aust Dent J. 2003;48:268.
5. Marx RE. Pamidronate (Aredia) and zoledronate (Zometa) induced avascular necrosis of the jaws: a growing epidemic. J Oral Maxillofac Surg. 2003;61:1115–1117.
6. Ruggiero SL, Mehrotra B, Rosenberg TJ, Engroff SL. Osteonecrosis of the jaws associated with the use of bisphosphonates: a review of 63 cases. J Oral Maxillofac Surg. 2004;62: 527–534.
7. Silverman SL, Landesberg R. Osteonecrosis of the jaw and the role of bisphosphonates: a critical review. Am J Med. 2009;122:S33–S45.
8. American Association of Oral and Maxillofacial Surgeons position paper on bisphosphonate-related osteonecrosis of the jaws. J Oral Maxillofac Surg. 2007;65:369–376.
9. Boonyapakorn T, Schirmer I, Reichart PA, Sturm I, Massenkeil G. Bisphosphonate-induced osteonecrosis of the jaws: prospective study of 80 patients with multiple myeloma and other malignancies. Oral Oncol. 2008;44:857–869.
10. Khosla S, Burr D, Cauley J, et al. Bisphosphonate-associated osteonecrosis of the jaw: report of a task force of the American Society for Bone and Mineral Research. J Bone Miner Res. 2007;22:1479–1491.
11. Badros A, Weikel D, Salama A, et al. Osteonecrosis of the jaw in multiple myeloma patients: clinical features and risk factors. J Clin Oncol. 2006;24:945–952.
12. Dental management of patients receiving oral bisphosphonate therapy: expert panel recommendations. J Am Dent Assoc. 2006;137:1144–1150.
13. Wang EP, Kaban LB, Strewler GJ, Raje N, Troulis MJ. Incidence of osteonecrosis of the jaw in patients with multiple myeloma and breast or prostate cancer on intravenous bisphosphonate therapy. J Oral Maxillofac Surg. 2007;65:1328–1331.
14. Jadu F, Lee L, Pharoah M, Reece D, Wang L. A retrospective study assessing the incidence, risk factors and comorbidities of pamidronate-related necrosis of the jaws in multiple myeloma patients. Ann Oncol. 2007;18:2015–2019.
15. Hoff AO, Toth BB, Altundag K, et al. Frequency and risk factors associated with osteonecrosis of the jaw in cancer patients treated with intravenous bisphosphonates. J Bone Miner Res. 2008;23:826–836.
16. Bamias A, Kastritis E, Bamia C, et al. Osteonecrosis of the jaw in cancer after treatment with bisphosphonates: incidence and risk factors. J Clin Oncol. 2005;23:8580–8587.

17. Zervas K, Verrou E, Teleioudis Z, et al. Incidence, risk factors and management of osteonecrosis of the jaw in patients with multiple myeloma: a single-centre experience in 303 patients. Br J Haematol. 2006;134:620–623.
18. Durie BG, Katz M, Crowley J. Osteonecrosis of the jaw and bisphosphonates. N Engl J Med. 2005;353:99–102; discussion 199–102.
19. Wilkinson GS, Kuo YF, Freeman JL, Goodwin JS. Intravenous bisphosphonate therapy and inflammatory conditions or surgery of the jaw: a population-based analysis. J Natl Cancer Inst. 2007;99:1016–1024.
20. Cartsos VM, Zhu S, Zavras AI. Bisphosphonate use and the risk of adverse jaw outcomes: a medical claims study of 714,217 people. J Am Dent Assoc. 2008;139:23–30.
21. Badros A, Terpos E, Katodritou E, et al. Natural history of osteonecrosis of the jaw in patients with multiple myeloma. J Clin Oncol. 2008;26:5904–5909.
22. Phal PM, Myall RW, Assael LA, Weissman JL. Imaging findings of bisphosphonate-associated osteonecrosis of the jaws. Am J Neuroradiol. 2007;28:1139–1145.
23. Carneiro E, Vibhute P, Montazem A, Som PM. Bisphosphonate-associated mandibular osteonecrosis. Am J Neuroradiol. 2006;27:1096–1097.
24. Wilde F, Steinhoff K, Frerich B, et al. Positron-emission tomography imaging in the diagnosis of bisphosphonate-related osteonecrosis of the jaw. Oral Surg Oral Med Oral Pathol Oral Radiol Endod. 2009;107(3):412–419.
25. Raje N, Woo SB, Hande K, et al. Clinical, radiographic, and biochemical characterization of multiple myeloma patients with osteonecrosis of the jaw. Clin Cancer Res. 2008;14: 2387–2395.
26. Garcia-Ferrer L, Bagan JV, Martinez-Sanjuan V, et al. MRI of mandibular osteonecrosis secondary to bisphosphonates. AJR Am J Roentgenol. 2008;190:949–955.
27. Chiandussi S, Biasotto M, Dore F, Cavalli F, Cova MA, Di Lenarda R. Clinical and diagnostic imaging of bisphosphonate-associated osteonecrosis of the jaws. Dentomaxillofac Radiol. 2006;35:236–243.
28. Dore F, Filippi L, Biasotto M, Chiandussi S, Cavalli F, Di Lenarda R. Bone scintigraphy and SPECT/CT of bisphosphonate-induced osteonecrosis of the jaw. J Nucl Med. 2009;50: 30–35.
29. Zanglis A, Andreopoulos D, Dima M, Baltas G, Baziotis N. Jaw uptake of technetium-99 methylene diphosphonate in patients on biphosphonates: a word of caution. Hell J Nucl Med. 2007;10:177–180.
30. Yang KH, Won JH, Yoon HK, Ryu JH, Choo KS, Kim JS. High concentrations of pamidronate in bone weaken the mechanical properties of intact femora in a rat model. Yonsei Med J. 2007;48:653–658.
31. Meier C, Seibel MJ, Kraenzlin ME. Use of bone turnover markers in the real world: are we there yet? J Bone Miner Res. 2009;24:386–388.
32. Marx RE, Cillo JE Jr, Ulloa JJ. Oral bisphosphonate-induced osteonecrosis: risk factors, prediction of risk using serum CTX testing, prevention, and treatment. J Oral Maxillofac Surg. 2007;65:2397–2410.
33. Badros A, Goloubeva O, Terpos E, Milliron T, Baer MR, Streeten E. Prevalence and significance of vitamin D deficiency in multiple myeloma patients. Br J Haematol. 2008;142(3): 492–494.
34. Lehrer S, Montazem A, Ramanathan L, et al. Bisphosphonate-induced osteonecrosis of the jaws, bone markers, and a hypothesized candidate gene. J Oral Maxillofac Surg. 2009;67: 159–161.
35. Bagan JV, Jimenez Y, Gomez D, Sirera R, Poveda R, Scully C. Collagen telopeptide (serum CTX) and its relationship with the size and number of lesions in osteonecrosis of the jaws in cancer patients on intravenous bisphosphonates. Oral Oncol. 2008;44:1088–1089.
36. Landesberg R, Cozin M, Cremers S, et al. Inhibition of oral mucosal cell wound healing by bisphosphonates. J Oral Maxillofac Surg. 2008;66:839–847.
37. Scheper MA, Badros A, Chaisuparat R, Cullen KJ, Meiller TF. Effect of zoledronic acid on oral fibroblasts and epithelial cells: a potential mechanism of bisphosphonate-associated osteonecrosis. Br J Haematol. 2009;144:667–676.

38. Yamada J, Tsuno NH, Kitayama J, et al. Anti-angiogenic property of zoledronic acid by inhibition of endothelial progenitor cell differentiation. J Surg Res. 2009;151:115–120.

39. Wood J, Bonjean K, Ruetz S, et al. Novel antiangiogenic effects of the bisphosphonate compound zoledronic acid. J Pharmacol Exp Ther. 2002;302:1055–1061.

40. Hasmim M, Bieler G, Ruegg C. Zoledronate inhibits endothelial cell adhesion, migration and survival through the suppression of multiple, prenylation-dependent signaling pathways. J Thromb Haemost. 2007;5:166–173.

41. Bezzi M, Hasmim M, Bieler G, Dormond O, Ruegg C. Zoledronate sensitizes endothelial cells to tumor necrosis factor-induced programmed cell death: evidence for the suppression of sustained activation of focal adhesion kinase and protein kinase B/Akt. J Biol Chem. 2003;278:43603–43614.

42. Santini D, Vincenzi B, Galluzzo S, et al. Repeated intermittent low-dose therapy with zoledronic acid induces an early, sustained, and long-lasting decrease of peripheral vascular endothelial growth factor levels in cancer patients. Clin Cancer Res. 2007;13:4482–4486.

43. Santini D, Vincenzi B, Dicuonzo G, et al. Zoledronic acid induces significant and long-lasting modifications of circulating angiogenic factors in cancer patients. Clin Cancer Res. 2003;9:2893–2897.

44. Scavelli C, Di Pietro G, Cirulli T, et al. Zoledronic acid affects over-angiogenic phenotype of endothelial cells in patients with multiple myeloma. Mol Cancer Ther. 2007;6:3256–3262.

45. Bellahcene A, Chaplet M, Bonjean K, Castronovo V. Zoledronate inhibits alphavbeta3 and alphavbeta5 integrin cell surface expression in endothelial cells. Endothelium. 2007;14: 123–130.

46. Koto K, Horie N, Kimura S, et al. Clinically relevant dose of zoledronic acid inhibits spontaneous lung metastasis in a murine osteosarcoma model. Cancer Lett. 2009;274:271–278.

47. Allegra A, Oteri G, Nastro E, et al. Patients with bisphosphonates-associated osteonecrosis of the jaw have reduced circulating endothelial cells. Hematol Oncol. 2007;25:164–169.

48. Napenas JJ, Brennan MT, Bahrani-Mougeot FK, Fox PC, Lockhart PB. Relationship between mucositis and changes in oral microflora during cancer chemotherapy. Oral Surg Oral Med Oral Pathol Oral Radiol Endod. 2007;103:48–59.

49. Hansen T, Kunkel M, Springer E, et al. Actinomycosis of the jaws – histopathological study of 45 patients shows significant involvement in bisphosphonate-associated osteonecrosis and infected osteoradionecrosis. Virchows Arch. 2007;451:1009–1017.

50. Sedghizadeh PP, Kumar SK, Gorur A, Schaudinn C, Shuler CF, Costerton JW. Identification of microbial biofilms in osteonecrosis of the jaws secondary to bisphosphonate therapy. J Oral Maxillofac Surg. 2008;66:767–775.

51. Bahrani-Mougeot FK, Paster BJ, Coleman S, Ashar J, Barbuto S, Lockhart PB. Diverse and novel oral bacterial species in blood following dental procedures. J Clin Microbiol. 2008;46:2129–2132.

52. Dimopoulos MA, Kastritis E, Bamia C, et al. Reduction of osteonecrosis of the jaw (ONJ) after implementation of preventive measures in patients with multiple myeloma treated with zoledronic acid. Ann Oncol. 2009;20:117–120.

53. Sarasquete ME, Garcia-Sanz R, Marin L, et al. Bisphosphonate-related osteonecrosis of the jaw is associated with polymorphisms of the cytochrome P450 CYP2C8 in multiple myeloma: a genome-wide single nucleotide polymorphism analysis. Blood. 2008;112: 2709–2712.

54. Chen T, Berenson J, Vescio R, et al. Pharmacokinetics and pharmacodynamics of zoledronic acid in cancer patients with bone metastases. J Clin Pharmacol. 2002;42:1228–1236.

55. Cremers S, Sparidans R. den HJ, Hamdy N, Vermeij P, Papapoulos S. A pharmacokinetic and pharmacodynamic model for intravenous bisphosphonate (pamidronate) in osteoporosis. Eur J Clin Pharmacol. 2002;57:883–890.

56. Khan SA, Kanis JA, Vasikaran S, et al. Elimination and biochemical responses to intravenous alendronate in postmenopausal osteoporosis. J Bone Miner Res. 1997;12:1700–1707.

57. Bone HG, Downs RW Jr, Tucci JR, et al. Dose–response relationships for alendronate treatment in osteoporotic elderly women. Alendronate Elderly Osteoporosis Study Centers. J Clin Endocrinol Metab. 1997;82:265–274.
58. Fogelman I, Bessent RG, Turner JG, Citrin DL, Boyle IT, Greig WR. The use of whole-body retention of Tc-99m diphosphonate in the diagnosis of metabolic bone disease. J Nucl Med. 1978;19:270–275.
59. Allen MR. Bisphosphonates and osteonecrosis of the jaw: moving from the bedside to the bench. Cells Tissues Organs. 2009;189:289–294.
60. Sonis ST, Watkins BA, Lyng GD, Lerman MA, Anderson KC. Bony changes in the jaws of rats treated with zoledronic acid and dexamethasone before dental extractions mimic bisphosphonate-related osteonecrosis in cancer patients. Oral Oncol. 2009;45:164–172.
61. Van den Wyngaert T, Claeys T, Huizing MT, Vermorken JB, Fossion E. Initial experience with conservative treatment in cancer patients with osteonecrosis of the jaw (ONJ) and predictors of outcome. Ann Oncol. 2009;20:331–336.
62. Saussez S, Javadian R, Hupin C, et al. Bisphosphonate-related osteonecrosis of the jaw and its associated risk factors: a Belgian case series. Laryngoscope. 2009;119:323–329.
63. Freiberger JJ, Padilla-Burgos R, Chhoeu AH, et al. Hyperbaric oxygen treatment and bisphosphonate-induced osteonecrosis of the jaw: a case series. J Oral Maxillofac Surg. 2007;65:1321–1327.
64. Shimura K, Shimazaki C, Taniguchi K, et al. Hyperbaric oxygen in addition to antibiotic therapy is effective for bisphosphonate-induced osteonecrosis of the jaw in a patient with multiple myeloma. Int J Hematol. 2006;84:343–345.
65. Petrucci MT, Gallucci C, Agrillo A, Mustazza MC, Foa R. Role of ozone therapy in the treatment of osteonecrosis of the jaws in multiple myeloma patients. Haematologica. 2007;92:1289–1290.
66. Stubinger S, Dissmann JP, Pinho NC, Saldamli B, Seitz O, Sader R. A preliminary report about treatment of bisphosphonate related osteonecrosis of the jaw with Er:YAG laser ablation. Lasers Surg Med. 2009;41:26–30.
67. Kyle RA, Yee GC, Somerfield MR, et al. American Society of Clinical Oncology 2007 clinical practice guideline update on the role of bisphosphonates in multiple myeloma. J Clin Oncol. 2007;25:2464–2472.
68. Lacy MQ, Dispenzieri A, Gertz MA, et al. Mayo clinic consensus statement for the use of bisphosphonates in multiple myeloma. Mayo Clin Proc. 2006;81:1047–1053.
69. Migliorati CA, Schubert MM, Peterson DE, Seneda LM. Bisphosphonate-associated osteonecrosis of mandibular and maxillary bone: an emerging oral complication of supportive cancer therapy. Cancer. 2005;104:83–93.

Chapter 8
Murine Models of Myeloma Bone Disease: The Importance of Choice

Peter I. Croucher, Karin Vanderkerken, Joshua Epstein, and Babatunde Oyajobi

Abstract Murine models of human disease have contributed significantly to our understanding of the pathophysiology of disease and played a key role in development of new treatments. The study of myeloma bone disease is no exception. In recent decades we have seen the development of a number of different models of myeloma bone disease. These include the syngeneic models, such as the 5TMM series, and the SCID models, including the SCID-hu model and those based upon engraftment of human cell lines. They have contributed directly to the identification of key molecules such as MIP-1α, facilitated establishing a critical role for the RANKL pathway, and been used to identify new agents for treatment including RANKL inhibition therapies and the bisphosphonates. More recently, they have been used to establish the role for osteoblast inhibition in the development of myeloma bone disease and contributed to the study of molecular pathways that regulate osteoblast suppression. In addition, these models have played a key role in understanding the importance of the bone microenvironment in supporting myeloma cell growth and survival in bone. It is likely that further refinements to our understanding of these models will lead to further insights into the mechanisms of myeloma bone disease. Murine models of myeloma bone disease will remain central to the development of new therapeutic approaches to treating this important clinical feature of myeloma.

Keywords Myeloma · RANKL · Bone disease · Mouse models · OPG

8.1 Introduction

Murine models of human disease have provided fundamental information about the etiology, pathophysiology, and development of disease processes. They have provided new insights into the mechanisms responsible for the clinical manifestation

P.I. Croucher (✉)
Department of Human Metabolism, Faculty of Medicine, Dentistry and Health, University of Sheffield, Sheffield S10 2RX, UK
e-mail: p.croucher@sheffield.ac.uk

G.D. Roodman (ed.), *Myeloma Bone Disease*, Current Clinical Oncology,   151
DOI 10.1007/978-1-60761-554-5_8, © Springer Science+Business Media, LLC 2010

of disease and allowed us to critically evaluate new approaches to treating a broad range of disorders, including cancer. Importantly, they provide a means to study complex interactions in a controlled setting. The study of multiple myeloma has also benefited from murine models.

Over recent years the myeloma research community has recognized the value of murine models of myeloma bone disease and considerable effort has been put into their development and characterization. This has facilitated the study of a range of biological processes including myeloma-induced osteoclastogenesis, the suppression of bone formation, and the interdependence between myeloma and the bone microenvironment. These models have also allowed us to evaluate new approaches to targeting the disease. This has involved determining the efficacy of a known, or novel, agent, evaluating new approaches to managing myeloma development in bone and/or the clinical manifestations of myeloma. However, for a model to be of real value it is critical that it accurately reflects the human disease or specific features of the disease under investigation. In myeloma, a good model, ideally, would be characterized by the clonal growth of myeloma cells in the bone marrow and not in other sites, akin to its growth in patients. Myeloma growth would be associated with the development of a serum paraprotein of the M-protein isotype that reflects tumor burden. Finally, the development of myeloma should be associated with appropriate clinical manifestations including the presence of osteolytic bone disease, increased angiogenesis, neutropenia, and anemia. These are ambitious requirements; however, over recent years significant progress has been made in the development of such murine models of myeloma.

The purpose of this chapter is to describe the murine models of myeloma bone disease that have been established over recent years. We will focus on those models that develop in the bone marrow and give rise to the characteristic bone disease and discuss the advantages and disadvantages of these different systems. We will also use specific examples to illustrate the importance of selecting appropriate models to address specific hypotheses and demonstrate that choice of model can determine experimental outcome.

8.2 Models of Multiple Myeloma Bone Disease

The last decade has seen the development of a number of different murine models of myeloma bone disease, which can loosely be divided into two groups. The first, are the syngeneic models, which involves implanting primary murine myeloma cells or murine myeloma cell lines into young recipient mice of the same donor strain. The second are SCID mouse-based models. These typically involve xenografting primary human myeloma cells or human myeloma cell lines into the bones of SCID mice or bone explants engrafted onto the flanks of SCID mice.

8.2.1 The 5TMM Syngeneic Models of Multiple Myeloma

The 5TMM series of syngeneic murine models were originally developed by Radl et al. [1]. Multiple myeloma was shown to develop spontaneously, at a frequency of 0.5%, in inbred C57BL/KaLwRij mice that were older than 2 years. Myeloma cells were localized in the bone marrow, and the serum paraprotein concentration correlated with disease development. This rise in paraprotein was associated with a decrease in polyclonal immunoglobulins. When diseased bone marrow was transplanted, intravenously, into young syngeneic animals all animals developed myeloma. Subsequently, the repeated *in vivo* transfer of bone marrow has resulted in the development of several *in vivo* growing 5TMM lines. Each of these lines was derived from a different mouse with myeloma and has its own characteristics. The 5TMM models have all arisen spontaneously in mice and have many features in common with the human disease [2]. These include the localization of tumor cells in the bone marrow, the presence of a serum paraprotein that reflects tumor burden, increased neovascularization in areas of tumor involvement, and in some lines the development of osteolytic bone disease [2, 3]. 5TMM myeloma cells can also be found in the spleen, a hemopoietic organ in the mouse, but are not typically found in other organs. All of the original 5TMM lines are maintained and propagated by in vivo transfer into recipient C57BL/KaLwRij mice [2, 4]. The cells will not grow in other intact strains of mouse, which make access to this particular strain of mouse of critical importance. These cells will grow in immunocompromised mice; however, there is a concern that some of the defining characteristics of this model may be lost in the SCID background, for example, the cells dependence upon the bone marrow microenvironment for their survival. The original cell lines will not grow *in vitro*, in common with primary myeloma cells, making propagation of the models more difficult. Although a number of lines were established originally, only two systems have been studied extensively, the 5T2MM and the 5T33MM models, and lines derived from them.

8.2.1.1 The 5T2MM Model

The 5T2MM model is the best characterized model. It is associated with a moderate rate of growth (12 weeks to signs of morbidity) and a disease that is confined to the bone marrow and spleen. Cytogenetic analysis has confirmed that chromosomal abnormalities are similar to those observed in humans [5]. Monoclonal antibodies have been raised against the 5T2MM idiotype allowing the detection of the serum paraprotein by ELISA, the specific identification of tumor cells by flow cytometric analysis and immunohistochemical detection in tissue sections [6]. Mice bearing 5T2MM cells develop increased angiogenesis [3], an osteolytic bone disease characterized by the presence of osteolytic bone lesions, a decrease in cancellous bone volume, a decrease in bone mineral density, increased osteoclast number, and decreased osteoblast number, all features seen in patients with myeloma [6–9].

The 5T2MM model has been used in studies aimed at unraveling key cellular and molecular mechanisms within the bone marrow microenvironment that contribute to the development of multiple myeloma and the associated bone disease. For example, studies investigating the mechanisms responsible for the "homing" of myeloma cell to the bone marrow have shown that a number of molecules play a role. These include the demonstration that MCP-1, secreted by bone marrow endothelial cells, is chemotactic for 5T2MM cell [10], and CD44v10 is involved in their adhesion to bone marrow endothelial cells [11]. Laminin-1, a component of the basement membrane, by binding the 67 kDa receptor, attracts 5T2MM cells [12], and IGF-1, secreted by the bone marrow fibroblasts, is also chemotactic for 5T2MM cells [13]. Bone marrow endothelial cells were also shown to participate in this homing process by upregulating the expression of the IGF-1R [14] and MMP9 [15], and the interactions between the MM cells and the endothelial cells resulted in an induction of angiogenesis [3]. Studies have shown that once in bone, 5T2MM cell promotes osteoclastogenesis and suppresses bone formation. This has led to studies examining the effects of bisphosphonates, including pamidronate and zoledronic acid, on the development of myeloma bone disease. Both of these agents have been shown to inhibit bone resorption and stop the development of lytic bone lesions [16, 17]. Zoledronic acid has also been shown to decrease serum paraprotein and increase survival in this model [17]. 5T2MM cells have also been reported to express the critical osteoclastogenic factor, the ligand for receptor activator of NF-kB (RANKL) [8]. Targeting the interaction between RANKL and its receptor RANK, with recombinant osteoprotegerin (OPG), or OPG peptidomimetic, prevents the development of myeloma bone disease and decreases serum paraprotein concentrations [8, 18]. Furthermore, inhibition of p38MAPK prevents development of bone lesions in this model [19].

Recent studies have shown that 5T2MM cells may express the soluble Wnt antagonist dickkopf-1 (dkk1). Inhibiting dkk1 with an anti-dkk1 antibody was shown to prevent suppression of osteoblastogenesis and stop development of osteolytic bone disease [9]. Furthermore, other approaches believed to promote bone formation, such as the proteosome inhibitor bortezomib, have also been shown to prevent myeloma bone disease in this model [20].

8.2.1.2 The 5T33MM Model

The 5T33MM myeloma model also arose spontaneously in an aged C57BL/KaLwRij mouse [1]. The 5T33MM model develops more quickly than the 5T2MM model with signs of morbidity being observed after 4 weeks. 5T33MM cells are found in the bone marrow, but can also be seen in the liver [6]. As with the 5T2MM model, the presence of a serum paraprotein can be used to assess tumor burden. 5T33MM cells induce angiogenesis [3] and 5T33MM-bearing mice are also reported to develop osteolytic bone disease although this is diffuse rather than the more pronounced, focal lesions see in 5T2MM-bearing mice [21]. However, not all reports have been able to confirm this, suggesting that different sublines have been selected in different laboratories over time. This may also reflect the fact that it is the *in vitro* growing variants (see below) that were used rather than the parental cells. As a consequence the 5T33MM model has not been used to study bone disease in a systematic manner and the subline 5TGM1 is preferred for such studies (see below). The 5T33MM model has been used in studies investigating mechanisms of myeloma cell "homing" and growth. Furthermore, this system has also been used to investigate the efficacy of novel approaches to treating myeloma and the associated clinical manifestations. These include the demonstration that immunization of 5T33MM-bearing mice with DNA vaccines may be effective in protecting against myeloma growth and that recombinant OPG treatment can decrease tumor burden and increase survival [22, 23].

In vitro, stroma-independent growing variants of the 5T33MM line, which are clonally identical to the in vivo growing line, have also been developed [21, 24, 25]. This includes the 5TGM1 line which is discussed below. These lines have proved valuable in confirming and extending many of the in vivo-based studies reported with 5T2MM and 5T33MM cells. The expression profile of the 5T33MM in vitro and in vivo growing cells differs. Inoculation of these 5T33MM in vitro cells into the bone marrow microenvironment induces the expression of a number of molecules including IGF-1 receptor, CD44v6, and MMP9 [14, 15], demonstrating the key role of this in vivo syngeneic environment. The use of these cells in studies looking at interactions between myeloma cells and osteoclast and osteoblasts is less widespread.

8.2.1.3 The 5TGM1 Model

5TGM1 murine myeloma cells were derived from the IgG2b-secreting 5T33MM cells. The 5TGM1 variant of 5T33MM grows more avidly and causes more bone destruction in vivo. In contrast to 5T33MM this variant grows well in vitro, without the requirement for supplementation with IL-6 or stromal cell-conditioned media. Like the other 5TMM Radl myeloma models, the 5TGM1 development is largely confined to bone marrow and the spleen. However, in contrast to the 5T2MM model, the course of the disease in the 5TGM1 tumor-bearing mice is more rapid with development of paraparesis/paraplegia in 4–5 weeks. Characterization of 5TGM1 cells in vitro and in vivo has been described in detail previously [26]. In addition to the parental 5TGM1 cell line, a green fluorescent protein (GFP)-expressing 5TGM1 subclone has also been generated, which has facilitated in vivo whole-body fluorescence imaging of mice, thereby enabling temporal monitoring of tumor burden in bone which has hitherto not been feasible [27].

In common with the 5T2MM model, the 5TGM1 model has proved invaluable in studies aimed at gaining fundamental insights into the pathogenesis of myeloma and the associated bone disease. For example, early studies with 5TGM1 cells demonstrated that cell–cell interactions between marrow stromal cells and myeloma cells, mediated via VCAM-1 and $\alpha 4\beta 1$ integrin, enhanced osteoclast activity [28]. Subsequently, this led to studies showing that neutralizing anti-α_4 antibodies reduce osteolysis and myeloma tumor burden in vivo [29, 30]. More recently, studies showed that increasing Wnt signaling in the bone marrow microenvironment, with LiCl treatment of 5TGM1-bearing mice, inhibits the development of myeloma bone disease and reduces tumor load [31]. Similarly, the 5TGM1 model has been instrumental in a variety of settings requiring evaluation of myeloma survival and growth in bone in vivo in the context of an intact immune system. For example, in studies investigating mechanisms by which myeloma evades the immune system, the 5TGM1 model was used to show that inhibition of p38 MAPK restores the function of dendritic cells in myeloma in vivo [32]. Similarly, Th1 cells were shown to be tumoricidal, whereas Th2 cells were shown to promote 5TGM1 tumor growth in vivo thus contributing valuable insight into the role of idiotype-specific T cells in myeloma cell growth and survival [33].

In addition, because 5TGM1 cells can be maintained continuously as a cell line in vitro, a precise number of cells can be injected into mice thereby facilitating the preclinical evaluation of efficacy of potential anti-osteolytic and anti-myeloma agents as have been shown for the bisphosphonate ibandronate, anti-MIP-1alpha-neutralizing antibodies, and bortezomib [26, 34, 35]. Other examples include the use of the 5TGM1 model to demonstrate the feasibility of novel skeletally targeted radiovirotherapy in reducing myeloma tumor burden in vivo [36, 37] and anti-myeloma efficacy of potential immunotherapeutic agents such as anti-CD 137 [38].

8.2.2 The SCID Mouse Models of Multiple Myeloma

The SCID mouse has provided a unique opportunity for developing models of multiple myeloma that fulfills many of the criteria outlined above. These now include those based upon the engraftment of human myeloma cell lines or primary human myeloma cells into SCID mice or the injection of human myeloma cells into human fetal bone explants xenografted into SCID mice.

8.2.2.1 The SCID/Human Cell Line Models

A number of human myeloma cell lines, and Epstein–Barr virus-transformed lymphoblastoid cell lines, have now been xenografted into SCID mice. These models have proved valuable in examining direct anti-myeloma activity of agents when implanted subcutaneously or intraperitoneally, where they grow largely as solitary plasmacytomas. However, there are only a limited number of examples in which cells are injected intravenously, migrate to bone, and give rise to bone disease. In all cases cells also grow in other organs, although the patterns of growth differ between models.

The best studied of the human cell lines grafted in this way is the ARH-77 cell line. This is not a true myeloma cell line, having been established from cells taken from the peripheral blood of a patient with a plasma cell leukemia and shown to be EBV-transformed and B-lymphoblastoid in nature. However, injection of ARH-77 cells into irradiated SCID mice leads to the development of tumors in the bone marrow, brain, lung, and less frequently in the liver and kidney [39]. Human immunoglobulin, derived from the ARH-77 cells, can be detected in the serum and is of value in monitoring disease [39]. SCID mice-bearing ARH-77 cells develop a bone disease characterized by the presence of hypercalcemia, osteolytic bone lesions on X-ray, a decrease in cancellous bone area, and increased osteoclast formation [40]. ARH-77 cells were the first shown to produce macrophage inflammatory protein 1alpha (MIP-1α), an osteoclast-stimulating factor; inhibition with antibodies to MIP-1α or MIP-1α anti-sense constructs prevented the development of lytic bone disease [41, 42]. Subsequently, the role of this molecule has been examined in some of the syngeneic models. Due to the relative ease of manipulation this system has also been used to study the effect of overexpression of OPG on bone disease. Lentiviral delivery of OPG was shown to reduce the development of bone lesions [43]. Agents that target osteoclasts, including the bisphosphonate ibandronate have also been shown to inhibit the development of lytic bone disease in this model [44].

A number of the accepted myeloma cell lines have also been shown to engraft in SCID mice and promote bone disease. They include the JJN-3 line and a subline JJN-3T1. Although these cells grow in the skeleton they can also be found in other sites including liver, brain, and brown adipose tissue [45]. Once in bone, the JJN-3T1 cells were shown to suppress osteoblast numbers and bone formation. These cells express hepatocyte growth factor and this system has been used to explore its role in myeloma and the associated bone disease. The KMS-12-BM cell line, injected via the tail vein, has also been shown to successfully engraft into the bone of beta2M-NOD/SCID mice [46]. Engraftment was associated with increased osteoclastic bone resorption, suppression of bone formation, and a decrease in bone volume. Injection of mesenchymal stem cells (MSC), lentivirally transduced to express OPG, prevented KMS-12-BM-induced bone loss [46].

Although other lines have been shown to engraft in bone and give rise to bone disease, they are often evaluated to illustrate that the model accurately reflects the human disease rather than as a system to study the bone disease per se. Examples of such lines include the KPPM2 line [47] and a number of GFP-labeled lines including RPMI8226-GFP cells [48] and INA-6-GFP cells [49]. As such, these models are not widely used to study myeloma bone disease.

8.2.2.2 The SCID/Primary Human Cell Models

Primary human myeloma cells have also been engrafted into SCID or NOD/SCID mice. Early studies demonstrated that intraperitoneal injection of bone marrow mononuclear cells resulted in the appearance of light chain in the serum and growth of myeloma, particularly in the fat tissue surrounding the pancreas and spleen [50, 51]. More recently, Pilarski et al. have reported that intracardiac injection of peripheral blood mononuclear cells, or CD34 selected cells, isolated from patients with myeloma, results in the development of myeloma in the bone marrow [52]. These animals develop characteristic lytic bone lesions. Intraosseous injection results in the development of myeloma in the primary site and subsequent development of lytic bone lesions at distant sites. It is unclear how reproducible this system is and as a result this has not been widely adopted.

8.2.2.3 The SCID-hu Model

The introduction of human myeloma cells into SCID mice allows for the study of the interaction between human myeloma cells and the murine bone marrow. However, the development of the SCID-hu system has allowed primary human myeloma cells/human bone marrow microenvironment interactions to be studied. This model involves implanting human fetal bone grafts into the flanks of SCID mice [53]. Human myeloma cell lines [48, 54, 49], patient bone marrow cells, or purified primary myeloma cells [55, 56] are then injected directly into the bone marrow cavity of the fetal bone grafts.

The most informative of these studies have been with primary myeloma cells. Growth of injected myeloma cells is restricted to the human bones and induces changes in the human bone marrow microenvironment, most notably increases in microvessel density, increased osteoclast activity, and decreases in osteoblast numbers. Growth of myeloma cells is also associated with typical myeloma manifestations, the most dramatic of which is osteolysis of the human bone [55]. By supporting the growth of primary human myeloma cells in a human bone marrow microenvironment, the SCID-hu model has provided a platform for studying important aspects of myeloma biology and therapy, among them whether myeloma plasma cells are proliferative and the role of the bone marrow microenvironment in the development of the disease process.

Injection of myeloma plasma cells, purified from bone marrow aspirates of patients with myeloma, demonstrated unequivocally that such cells, with recognizable plasma cell morphology and phenotype, produce myeloma in the SCID-hu model with all its manifestations. Moreover, myeloma cells could be sequentially transferred from one SCID-hu mouse to another, demonstrating that myeloma plasma cells have the capacity of sustained proliferation. In contrast, the myeloma plasma cell-depleted bone marrow and blood specimens or purified B cells from patients with myeloma did not produce myeloma in SCID-hu mice [56]. When myeloma cells were injected only into one human bone in mice implanted with two contralaterally placed bones, the myeloma developed plasma cells disseminated, presumably through the circulation, to the second bone. However, no myeloma cells were detected in any of the murine tissues, demonstrating the total dependence of the cells on the human bone marrow. In this model in most cases, myeloma cells grow only within the bone marrow of the human bone. The only exception is when cells from patients with extramedullary disease are injected and in this case cells grow also along the outer surface of the human bone. This growth pattern indicates that extramedullary disease, while still dependent on a human microenvironment, no longer requires elements present only in the bone marrow, highlighting a biological difference between these and classical myeloma cells [57].

The absolute dependence of the myeloma cells on the human microenvironment has offered an opportunity to study the effects of myeloma cells on the bone microenvironment and also whether the changes in the microenvironment associated with their growth are merely consequences of, or are important for, disease development. To examine this, anti-angiogenic and anti-osteoclastic agents have been used to inhibit myeloma-induced angiogenesis and osteoclastogenesis. Thalidomide treatment demonstrated anti-myeloma activity only in SCID-hu mice that contained human liver implants, demonstrating that metabolism is important for the drug's anti-myeloma efficacy. While anti-myeloma activity was associated with reduced microvessel density, cause and effect could not be determined [58]. Endostatin, another inhibitor of angiogenesis, elicited a response in 50% of cases, suggesting that in some cases, angiogenesis may have a key role in the disease process [59]. Treatment with the bisphosphonates, pamidronate and zoledronic acid, or the antagonist of RANKL, RANK-Fc, prevented the destruction of the human bones. Zoledronic acid and RANK-Fc treatments both reduced the number of osteoclasts, whereas pamidronate had no effect on osteoclast number. However, each of these agents also decreased paraprotein concentration and tumor burden demonstrating profound anti-myeloma effects and indicating that myeloma may depend on osteoclast activity. In contrast to classical myeloma, while myeloma cells from patients with extramedullary disease were sensitive to thalidomide, they were completely resistant to the activities of anti-osteoclastic agents, highlighting their independence on a bone marrow-specific microenvironment [57].

In addition to stimulating osteoclast activity, development of myeloma in the SCID-hu model, as in patients, is associated with a reduction in osteoblast number and activity [55], via a mechanism likely involving inhibition of Wnt signaling by the myeloma cell-secreted inhibitor dickkopf (Dkk-1) [60]. Reversing the loss of osteoblasts by injection of mesenchymal stem cells [61], blocking Dkk-1 activity [62], or by stimulating Wnt3a signaling [63] has been shown to increase bone formation, to prevent bone destruction, and is associated with an inhibition of myeloma growth in the SCID-hu system.

In an effort to widen use of this system rabbit rather than human bone explants have also been used [64]. As in the 5T2MM and 5TGM1 model, the proteosome inhibitor bortezomib stimulates bone formation and suppresses myeloma growth in this model [65]. Although this system overcomes some of the regulatory and ethical difficulties in gaining access to human fetal bone explants, this introduces an additional species, which may result in false positives or false negatives. Unlike mouse and rat, there is very little published on the differences and/or commonalities between rabbit and human bone.

8.3 The Importance of the Bone Marrow Microenvironment

The bone marrow clearly provides an important microenvironment for the growth and survival of myeloma cells. The fact that myeloma cells do not grow in other organs demonstrates that this environment is critical for their growth and survival. Consequently, an essential feature of any model of myeloma should be its ability to support the growth of myeloma cells in the bone marrow and preferably not in other organs. The exception to this is that in the later stages of myeloma the tumor cells lose their dependence on the bone marrow microenvironment, enter the circulation, and can be found at extramedullary sites. Models based upon cells derived from extramedullary disease may therefore be modeling a different aspect of myeloma to those originally derived from bone marrow-confined disease. This can be seen in the studies performed in the SCID-hu system.

Of the models that are currently available, a number have bone marrow-confined disease, do not grow in vitro, and can be described as *bone marrow-dependent* models (5T2MM, 5T33MM, and SCID-hu) (Fig. 8.1). In contrast, the majority of the cell lines engrafted in SCID or syngeneic mice also grow in vitro without the requirement for exogenous stimuli for their survival. By definition they are not dependent upon the bone microenvironment for key survival signals. They may well respond to changes in this environment but are not necessarily dependent upon it for their survival. Indeed, when these cells are injected into recipient mice, although they grow in bone, they can often be found in other sites outside of the skeleton. As a direct consequence, they may not necessarily respond to changes in the bone microenvironment. These models could be described as being *bone marrow-independent* models (5TGM1, human cell line models). This should not necessarily be seen as a weakness and is not a contraindication for their use, but should be considered when selecting models for experimentation.

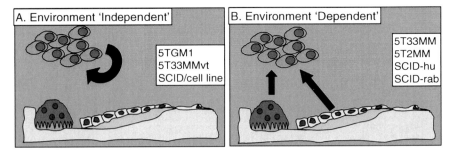

Fig. 8.1 The relationship between myeloma cells and the cells of bone. (**a**) Myeloma cells may grow in bone but are not necessarily dependent upon bone for key survival signals. The cells used in these models grow in vitro. These may be called "microenvironment-independent" models. (**b**) Myeloma cells grow largely only in bone and will not grow in vitro. These can be called "microenvironment-dependent" models

The importance of this distinction between bone marrow microenvironment dependent versus independent models is evident from studies using bisphosphonates. Bisphosphonates are potent inhibitors of osteoclastic bone resorption and have been investigated for their ability to prevent the development of myeloma bone disease. The bisphosphonates pamidronate and zoledronic acid have both been studied in the 5T2MM and SCID-hu models [16, 17, 57]. In these studies, the bisphosphonates were reported to be effective at preventing the development of myeloma bone disease. The bisphosphonate ibandronate has been studied in the 5TGM1 syngeneic model and the ARH77 system [26, 44]. In both ibandronate was also shown to be effective in preventing the development of osteolytic bone disease. However, a distinction can be made between these studies when examining the effect of inhibiting osteoclasts on myeloma growth itself. Both pamidronate and zoledronic acid treatment have been reported to be associated with decreases in tumor burden. In the case of zoledronic acid this is accompanied with an increase in time to morbidity [17]. In contrast, studies with ibandronate were unable to show any effect on indices of myeloma activity. Since these are all nitrogen-containing bisphosphonates it is unlikely that this difference is the result of differences in mechanism of action or potency. A more likely explanation is that this is a consequence of the different models being used. The studies with pamidronate and zoledronic acid were performed in the 5T2MM and SCID-hu systems, models in which the myeloma cells are dependent upon the bone marrow microenvironment for their growth. In contrast, the ibandronate studies were undertaken in the ARH-77/SCID model and the 5TGM1 model. These both involve the injection of cell lines that grow independently in vitro into either SCID or syngeneic mice. Although these cells grow in the bone marrow and cause lytic bone disease, by their nature they are not necessarily dependent upon this environment for their growth and survival. That is not to say that they cannot be influenced by the situation in which they find themselves. This is supported further by the observation that injection of myeloma cells, isolated from patients with extramedullary disease or plasma cell leukemia, in fetal bone explants grown in SCID mice, will grow on the outer surface of the bone explant and do not respond to bisphosphonates [57]. Although there are often additional mechanisms that could account for these observations, and no systematic studies have been undertaken comparing more than one bisphosphonates in the different models, this highlights the potential importance of microenvironment dependence when selecting models for experimentation.

Indeed, this concept is supported further by other strategies designed to inhibit osteoclastic bone resorption. RANKL has been strongly implicated in the development of myeloma bone disease and been inhibited in a number of these mouse models. These include the use of recombinant osteoprotegerin (Fc.OPG) [8], a recombinant soluble form of receptor activator of NF-kB (RANK-Fc) [57, 66, 67], and the OPG peptidomimetics, OP3-4 [18]. All are effective in preventing the development of myeloma bone disease in all of the models examined. However, the effect of inhibiting bone resorption with these agents on tumor burden in bone is less clear. Treatment of 5T2MM or 5T33MM-bearing mice with Fc.OPG was associated with a decrease in paraprotein and in the 5T33MM model an increase in time to morbidity [8, 23]. RANK-Fc treatment was also associated with a decrease in serum paraprotein in the SCID-hu system (except when cells from patients with extramedullary disease were used) [57, 67]. Both of these models are "microenvironment-dependent" models. However, when RANK-Fc was examined in the ARH77/SCID mouse model, a microenvironment-independent model, treatment had no effect on serum paraprotein concentration, an effect that is consistent with those observed with bisphosphonates [67]. The exception to this appears to be studies of RANK-Fc in the 5TGM1 model. Treatment was associated with a decrease in osteolytic bone disease and tumor burden [66, 68]. This may reveal important differences in the relative dependence of cells on osteoclastic resorption or the stage of osteoclast differentiation.

Although it is recognized that it will not always be possible to use microenvironment-dependent models for studies investigating the interdependence between myeloma cells and bone, it would be desirable to use these models. At the very least there should be recognition of the issues associated with the use of the different models.

8.4 The Importance of Selecting Appropriate Models

The models that are currently available have certain advantages and disadvantages (Table 8.1). Since they all offer something different it is critical that appropriate models are chosen to best test the hypothesis under examination. A good example of how different models can result in different conclusions can be seen in the studies investigating the effect of bisphosphonates. All of the bisphosphonates have been shown to prevent bone disease in each of the models selected. Typically, this was the primary endpoint to each of these studies. As such these studies can be considered to have been successful. However, in these studies myeloma burden, and in some cases survival, was also examined; however, this was often as a secondary endpoint. When "microenvironment-dependent" models were used evidence was presented that bisphosphonate treatment was associated with a reduction in myeloma burden. In contrast, when "microenvironment-independent" models were used no effect was observed. Although in some studies the reduction in myeloma burden was modest, these data show that a limited understanding of the models could lead to false positives/negatives and inappropriate conclusions.

Thus, when considering appropriate models consideration needs to be given to the specific hypothesis under examination. We also need to be aware that for the majority of models we are only investigating the effects of a single cell line/strain derived from a single patient/mouse. This amounts to studying the equivalent of one person's myeloma in what is a heterogenous disease. This is not the case with the SCID-hu models in which many patient samples can be studied. Some of the issues that need to be considered include:

- The importance of studying true myeloma cells versus cells that are lymphoblastoid in nature, but still give rise to bone disease.
- Whether the study of human or murine cells is required.
- Whether the models give rise to classical myeloma bone disease with increased resorption, decreased formation, and the development of osteolytic bone lesions or not.
- The need for microenvironment-dependent or microenvironment-independent models.
- The importance of the immune status of the host. Clearly an intact immune system is critical if studying mechanisms/molecules that are likely to impact on the immune system.

Table 8.1 Characteristics of some of the commonly used models of myeloma bone disease

Variables	Murine model of myeloma bone disease						
	5T2MM	5T33MM[a]	5TGM1	SCID-hu	ARH77	JJN-3	KMS-12-BM[b]
Cell type	Myeloma	Myeloma	Myeloma	Myeloma	Lymphoblastoid	Myeloma	Myeloma
Route of injection	Intravenous	Intravenous	Intravenous	Intraosseous	Intravenous	Intravenous	Intravenous
Develops lytic bone disease	Yes	?[c]	Yes	Yes	Yes	Yes	Yes
Increased osteoclastic resorption	Yes	?[c]	Yes	Yes	Yes	No	Yes
Suppressed bone formation	Yes	?[c]	Yes	Yes	?[c]	Yes	Yes
Syngeneic versus xenograft	Syngeneic	Syngeneic	Syngeneic	Xenograft	Xenograft	Xenograft	Xenograft
Immune competent	Yes	Yes	Yes	No	No	No	No
Environment dependent	Yes	Yes	No	Yes	No	No	No
Suitability for preclinical evaluation	Yes	Yes	Yes	No	Yes	Yes	Yes
Ability to manipulate cells	Difficult	Difficult	Simple	Difficult	Simple	Simple	Simple

[a]Evidence that 5T33MM cells develop osteolytic disease is limited and based upon all lines.
[b]KMS-12-BM is used as an example of human myeloma cell lines only.
[c]Currently unclear whether osteoblastic bone formation and/or osteoclastic activity are altered.
[d]This has not been studied systematically in parental cell. If pre

- The need to manipulate cells in order to study molecular mechanisms. This is challenging for the 5T2MM and SCID-hu system but more practical with cell lines.
- The requirement to perform classical preclinical studies. This is more practical with cell lines than with primary myeloma cells.
- Whether early events, such as colonization of the skeleton, are being studied. Such studies require cells to enter the bone marrow via the vasculature rather than via direct injection into the bone.

Considering these issues not only are important in experimental design but will also generate insights into the biology of myeloma and the associated bone disease.

8.5 Conclusions

Murine models have been used to identify, successfully, some of the key molecular mechanisms responsible for myeloma bone disease provided functional data to support a causal role, and been used to develop new approaches to treating myeloma bone disease. In this regard these models have provided fundamentally important information. For example, they have contributed directly to the identification of key molecules such as MIP-1α, facilitated establishing a critical role for the RANKL pathway and been used to identify new agents for treatment, for example, RANKL inhibition therapies and the bisphosphonates. However, as we move forward they will now be used to investigate other aspects of myeloma bone disease. This will include establishing the role of osteoblast suppression in the development of bone disease and determined whether promoting bone formation can prevent bone disease and/or facilitate repair of bone lesions. Equally, new models, based upon introduction of key transgenes, for example, MYC [69], are likely to give new insights into the pathogenesis of myeloma bone disease and may prove of value in developing new treatments. Furthermore, one area in which these models will undoubtedly play a key role will be in understanding the role of the bone microenvironment in supporting myeloma cell growth and survival in bone. This will require further refinements to our understanding and our use of these models. In this regard a more detailed understanding of their development is necessary. Given the key role that these models have played to date this is worthy objective and they are likely to provide further critical insights in the future.

Acknowledgements Peter Croucher is supported by the Leukaemia Research Fund and Karin Vanderkerken is supported by the VUB, Fonds voor Wetenschappelijk (FWO) – Vlaanderen and Stichting tegen Kanker. Joshua Epstein is supported by grants CA-55819 and CA-113992 from the National Cancer Institute and Babatunde Oyajobi is supported by grants KO1 CA104180 and PO1 CA000435 from the National Cancer Institute.

References

1. Radl J, et al. Transplantation of the paraprotein-producing clone from old to young C57BL/KaLwRij mice. J Immunol. 1979;122:609–613.
2. Radl J, et al. Animal model of human disease: multiple myeloma. Am J Pathol. 1988;132: 177–181.
3. Van Valckenborgh E, et al. Murine 5T multiple myeloma cells induce angiogenesis in vitro and in vivo. Br J Cancer. 2002;86:796–802.
4. Radl J. Age-related monoclonal gammopathies: clinical lessons from the aging C57BL mouse. Immunol Today. 1990;11:234–236.
5. van den Akker TW, et al. Cytogenetic findings in mouse multiple myeloma and Waldenstrom's Macroglobulinemia. Cancer Genet Cytogenet. 1996;86:156–161.
6. Vanderkerken K, et al. Organ involvement and phenotypic adhesion profile of 5T2 and 5T33MM cells in the C57BL/KaLwRij mouse. Br J Cancer. 1997;76:451–460.
7. Vanderkerken K, et al. Follow-up of bone lesions in an experimental multiple myeloma mouse model: description of an in vivo technique using radiography dedicated for mammography. Br J Cancer. 1996;73:1463–1465.
8. Croucher PI, et al. Osteoprotegerin inhibits the development of osteolytic bone disease in multiple myeloma. Blood. 2001;98:3534–3540.
9. Heath DJ, et al. Inhibiting Dickkopf1 (Dkk1) removes suppression of bone formation and prevents the development of osteolytic bone disease in multiple myeloma. J Bone Miner Res. 2009;24:425–436.
10. Vanderkerken K, et al. Monocyte chemoattractant protein-1 (MCP-1), secreted by bone marrow endothelial cells, induces chemoattraction of 5T multiple myeloma cells. Clin Exp Metast. 2002;19:87–90.
11. Asosingh K, et al. A unique pathway in the homing of murine multiple myeloma cells: CD44v10 mediates binding to bone marrow endothelium. Cancer Res. 2001;61:2862–2865.
12. Vande Broek I, et al. Laminin-1-induced migration of multiple myeloma cells involves the high-affinity 67kD laminin receptor. Br J Cancer. 2001;85:1387–1395.
13. Vanderkerken K, et al. Insulin like growth factor-1 acts as a chemoattractant for 5T2 multiple myeloma cells. Blood. 1999;93:235–241.
14. Asosingh K, et al. In vivo induction of insulin-like growth factor-I receptor and CD44v6 confers homing and adhesion to murine multiple myeloma cells. Cancer Res. 2000;60: 3096–3104.
15. Van Valckenborgh E, et al. Upregulation of matrix metalloproteinase-9 in murine 5T33 multiple myeloma cells by interaction with bone marrow endothelial cells. Int J Cancer. 2002;101:512–518.
16. Radl J, et al. Influence of treatment with APD-bisphosphonate on the bone lesions in the mouse 5T2 multiple myeloma. Cancer. 1985;55:1030–1040.
17. Croucher PI, et al. Zoledronic acid treatment of 5T2MM-bearing mice inhibits the development of myeloma bone disease: evidence for decreased osteolysis, tumor burden and angiogenesis, and increased survival. J Bone Miner Res. 2003;18(3):482–492.
18. Heath DJ, et al. An osteoprotegerin-like peptidomimetic inhibits osteoclastic bone resorption and osteolytic bone disease in myeloma. Cancer Res. 2007;67:202–208.
19. Vanderkerken K, et al. Inhibition of p38alpha mitogen-activated protein kinase prevents the development of osteolytic bone disease, reduces tumor burden, and increases survival in murine models of multiple myeloma. Cancer Res. 2007;67:4572–4577.
20. Deleu S, et al. Bortezomib alone or in combination with the histone deacetylase inhibitor JNJ-26481585: effect on myeloma bone disease in the 5T2MM murine model of myeloma. Cancer Res. 2009;69:5307–5311.
21. Garrett IR, et al. A murine model of human myeloma bone disease. Bone. 1997;20:515–520.
22. King CA, et al. DNA vaccines with single-chain Fv fused to fragment C of tetanus toxin induce protective immunity against lymphoma and myeloma. Nat Med. 1998;4:1281–1286.

23. Vanderkerken K, et al. Recombinant osteoprotegerin decreases tumor burden and increases survival in a murine model of multiple myeloma. Cancer Res. 2003;63: 287–289.
24. Manning LS, et al. A model of multiple myeloma: culture of 5T33 murine myeloma cells and evaluation of tumorigenicity in the C57BL/KaLwRij mouse. Br J Cancer. 1992;66: 1088–1093.
25. Asosingh K, et al. The 5TMM series: a useful in vivo mouse model of human multiple myeloma. Hematol J. 2000;1:351–356.
26. Dallas SL, et al. Ibandronate reduces osteolytic lesions but not tumor burden in a murine model of myeloma bone disease. Blood. 1999;93:1697–1706.
27. Oyajobi BO, et al. Detection of myeloma in skeleton of mice by whole-body optical fluorescence imaging. Mol Cancer Ther. 2007;6:1701–1708.
28. Michigami T, et al. Cell-cell contact between marrow stromal cells and myeloma cells via VCAM-1 and alpha(4)beta(1)-integrin enhances production of osteoclast-stimulating activity. Blood. 2000;96:1953–1960.
29. Mori Y, et al. Anti-alpha4 integrin antibody suppresses the development of multiple myeloma and associated osteoclastic osteolysis. Blood. 2004;104:2149–2154.
30. Olson DL, et al. Anti-alpha4 integrin monoclonal antibody inhibits multiple myeloma growth in a murine model. Mol Cancer Ther. 2005;4:91–99.
31. Edwards CM, et al. Increasing Wnt signaling in the bone marrow microenvironment inhibits the development of myeloma bone disease and reduces tumor burden in bone in vivo. Blood. 2008;111:2833–2842.
32. Wang S, et al. Tumor evasion of the immune system: inhibiting p38 MAPK signaling restores the function of dendritic cells in multiple myeloma. Blood. 2006;107:2432–2439.
33. Hong S, et al. Roles of idiotype-specific T cells in myeloma cell growth and survival: Th1 and CTL cells are tumoricidal while Th2 cells promote tumor growth. Cancer Res. 2008;68:8456–8464.
34. Oyajobi BO, et al. Dual effects of macrophage inflammatory protein-1alpha on osteolysis and tumor burden in the murine 5TGM1 model of myeloma bone disease. Blood. 2003;102: 311–319.
35. Oyajobi BO, et al. Stimulation of new bone formation by the proteasome inhibitor, bortezomib: implications for myeloma bone disease. Br J Haematol. 2007;139:434–438.
36. Goel A, et al. Synergistic activity of the proteasome inhibitor PS-341 with non-myeloablative 153-Sm-EDTMP skeletally targeted radiotherapy in an orthotopic model of multiple myeloma. Blood. 2006;107:4063–4070.
37. Goel A, et al. Radioiodide imaging and radiovirotherapy of multiple myeloma using VSV(Delta51)-NIS, an attenuated vesicular stomatitis virus encoding the sodium iodide symporter gene. Blood. 2007;110:2342–2350.
38. Murillo O, et al. Therapeutic antitumor efficacy of anti-CD137 agonistic monoclonal antibody in mouse models of myeloma. Clin Cancer Res. 2008;14:6895–6906.
39. Huang YW, et al. Disseminated growth of a human multiple myeloma cell line in mice with severe combined immunodeficiency disease. Cancer Res. 1993;53:1392–1396.
40. Alsina M, et al. Development of an in vivo model of human multiple myeloma bone disease. Blood. 1996;87:1495–1501.
41. Choi SJ, et al. Macrophage inflammatory protein 1-alpha is a potential osteoclast stimulatory factor in multiple myeloma. Blood. 2000;96:671–675.
42. Choi SJ, et al. Antisense inhibition of macrophage inflammatory protein 1-a blocks bone destruction in a model of myeloma bone disease. J Clin Invest. 2001;108:1833–1841.
43. Doran P, et al. Native osteoprotegerin gene transfer inhibits the development of murine osteolytic bone disease induced by tumor xenografts. Exp Hematol. 2004;32: 351–359.
44. Cruz JC, et al. Ibandronate decreases bone disease development and osteoclast stimulatory activity in an in vivo model of human myeloma. Exp Haematol. 2001;29:441–447.

45. Hjorth-Hansen H, et al. Marked osteoblastopenia and reduced bone formation in a model of multiple myeloma bone disease in severe combined immunodeficiency mice. J Bone Miner Res. 1999;14:256–263.
46. Rabin N, et al. A new xenograft model of myeloma bone disease demonstrating the efficacy of human mesenchymal stem cells expressing osteoprotegerin by lentiviral gene transfer. Leukemia. 2007;21:2181–2191.
47. Tsunenari T, et al. New xenograft model of multiple myeloma and efficacy of a humanized antibody against human interleukin-6 receptor. Blood. 1997;90:2437–2444.
48. Mitsiades CS, et al. Fluorescence imaging of multiple myeloma cells in a clinically relevant SCID/NOD in vivo model: biologic and clinical implications. Cancer Res. 2003;63: 6689–6696.
49. Tassone P, et al. A clinically relevant SCID-hu in vivo model of human multiple myeloma. Blood. 2005;106:713–716.
50. Feo-Zuppardi FJ, et al. Long-term engraftment of fresh human myeloma cells in SCID mice. Blood. 1992;80:2843–2850.
51. Ahsmann EJ, et al. The SCID mouse as a model for multiple myelom. Br J Haematol. 1995;89:319–327.
52. Pilarski L, Belch AR. Clonotypic myeloma cells able to xenograft myeloma to nonobese diabetic severe combined immunodeficient mice copurify with CD34 (+) hematopoietic progenitors. Clin Cancer Res. 2002;8:3198–3204.
53. McCune JM, et al. The SCID-hu mouse: murine model for the analysis of human hematolymphoid differentiation and function. Science. 1988;241:1632–1639.
54. Urashima M, et al. The development of a model for the homing of multiple myeloma cells to human bone marrow. Blood. 1997;90:754–765.
55. Yaccoby S, Barlogie B, Epstein J. Primary myeloma cells growing in SCID-hu mice: a model for studying the biology and treatment of myeloma and its manifestations. Blood. 1998;92:2908–2913.
56. Yaccoby S, Epstein J. The proliferative potential of myeloma plasma cells manifest in the SCID-hu host. Blood. 1999;94:3576–3582.
57. Yaccoby S, et al. Myeloma interacts with the bone marrow microenvironment to induce osteoclastogenesis and is dependent on osteoclast activity. Br J Haematol. 2002;116:278–290.
58. Yaccoby S, et al. Antimyeloma efficacy of thalidomide in the SCID-hu model. Blood. 2002;100:4162–4168.
59. Fujii R, Yaccoby S, Epstein J. Control of myeloma with the anti-angiogenic agent endostatin [abstract]. Blood. 2000;96:360A.
60. Tian E, et al. The role of the Wnt-signaling antagonist DKK1 in the development of osteolytic lesions in multiple myeloma. N Engl J Med. 2003;349:2483–2494.
61. Yaccoby S, et al. Inhibitory effects of osteoblasts and increased bone formation on myeloma in novel culture systems and a myelomatous mouse model. Haematologica. 2006;91: 192–199.
62. Yaccoby S, et al. Antibody-based inhibition of DKK1 suppresses tumor-induced bone resorption and multiple myeloma growth in vivo. Blood. 2007;109:2106–2111.
63. Qiang YW, Shaughnessy JDJ, Yaccoby S. Wnt3a signaling within bone inhibits multiple myeloma bone disease and tumor growth. Blood. 2008;112:374–382.
64. Yata K, Yaccoby S. The SCID-rab model: a novel in vivo system for primary human myeloma demonstrating growth of CD138-expressing malignant cells. Leukemia. 2004;18: 1891–1897.
65. Pennisi A, et al. The proteasome inhibitor, bortezomib suppresses primary myeloma and stimulates bone formation in myelomatous and nonmyelomatous bones in vivo. Am J Hematol. 2009;84:6–14.
66. Oyajobi BO, et al. A soluble murine receptor activator of NF-kB-human immunoglobulin fusion protein (RANK.Fc) inhibits bone resorption in a murine model of human multiple myeloma bone disease. J Bone Miner Res. 2000;15:S176 (Abstr).

67. Pearse RN, et al. Multiple myeloma disrupts the TRANCE/osteoprotegerin cytokine axis to trigger bone destruction and promote tumor progression. Proc Natl Acad Sci USA. 2001;98:11581–11586.
68. Oyajobi BO, Mundy GR. Receptor activator of NF-kappaB ligand, macrophage inflammatory protein-1alpha, and the proteosome: novel therapeutic targets in myeloma. Cancer. 2003;97 (3 Suppl):813–817.
69. Chesi M, et al. AID-dependent activation of a MYC transgene induces multiple myeloma in a conditional mouse model of post-germinal center malignancies. Cancer Cell. 2008;13: 167–180.

Chapter 9
RANK Ligand Is a Therapeutic Target
in Multiple Myeloma

William C. Dougall, Michelle Chaisson-Blake, Howard Yeh, and Susie Jun

Abstract Osteolytic bone disease is a frequent and severe complication of multiple myeloma (MM). MM cells interact with stromal cells in the bone marrow niche to create an environment that is favorable for tumor growth, in particular by inducing differentiation and activity of bone-resorbing osteoclasts, while concomitantly inhibiting differentiation and activity of bone-depositing osteoblasts. This results in a net loss of bone and subsequent skeletal morbidity including fracture, bone pain, and hypercalcemia. RANK ligand (RANKL), a member of the tumor necrosis factor (TNF) cytokine family, is required for differentiation, activation, and survival of osteoclasts and thus plays a critical role in cancer-induced bone disease. Under normal circumstances, RANKL activity is attenuated by its endogenous inhibitor, osteoprotegerin (OPG), a soluble TNF receptor family protein that prevents RANKL from binding to its receptor RANK, expressed on osteoclasts. However, in MM, both RANKL and OPG are dysregulated, resulting in excess RANKL available to stimulate osteoclastic bone resorption. An increased RANKL/OPG ratio is associated not only with the extent of bone disease in patients with MM but also with the prognosis for overall survival. In preclinical models of MM, pharmacologic inhibition of RANKL has been demonstrated to ablate osteoclasts and thus prevent MM-associated bone disease. In addition, RANKL inhibition led to decreased tumor burden in these models, demonstrating the dependence of MM on osteoclast activity. Clinical studies currently underway are evaluating the potential of denosumab, a fully human monoclonal antibody targeting RANKL, to prevent or treat cancer-induced bone disease in MM and other cancer types.

Keywords RANK · RANKL · Myeloma · Osteoclast · Denosumab

W.C. Dougall (✉)
Scientific Director, Amgen Inc., Seattle, WA, 98119-3105, USA
e-mail: dougallw@amgen.com

G.D. Roodman (ed.), *Myeloma Bone Disease*, Current Clinical Oncology,
DOI 10.1007/978-1-60761-554-5_9, © Springer Science+Business Media, LLC 2010

9.1 Introduction

Multiple myeloma (MM) is an incurable disseminated plasma cell malignancy that is characterized by the production of monoclonal immunoglobulin (M protein) detectable in serum and/or urine. In MM, the majority of tumor cells reside in the bone marrow [1]. One of the defining clinical characteristics of MM is diffuse and localized osteolytic bone disease. Typically, the severity of bone disease correlates with tumor burden and prognosis [2]. Up to 95% of patients exhibit skeletal complications including osteolytic lesions and subsequent skeletal fractures, osteopenia, hypercalcemia, and severe bone pain [3]. Thus, myeloma-induced bone disease results in significant morbidity and affects overall health-related quality of life [4]. Importantly, there is a reciprocal interaction of the bone and tumor, and as a result of interaction with the bone microenvironment components, myeloma cells may be protected from spontaneous and drug-induced apoptosis [1].

Current standard therapies have limitations based on toxicities. In most cases, myeloma patients will experience a relapse after initially responding to treatment. Despite newer therapies such as thalidomide, lenalidomide, and bortezomib, which have extended patient lives, myeloma remains an incurable disease. Intravenous (IV) bisphosphonates (BP) are used as supportive therapy to protect bone and delay skeletal-related events (SREs) such as fractures, spinal cord compression or surgery, or radiation to bone [5]. However, as patients are living longer with myeloma, more patients eventually experience some form of skeletal morbidity, and new bone-targeting treatments are needed to further delay or prevent SREs.

9.1.1 Myeloma-Associated Bone Disease

The development of MM is clearly influenced by the bone marrow microenvironment [6] such that the tumor-induced disruption of the bone matrix can support myeloma cell growth and protect cells from spontaneous or drug-induced apoptosis. The process of bone remodeling appears to become uncoupled in MM with suppression of bone formation and stimulation of bone destruction leading to a net effect of diffuse and localized bone loss [5]. The enhanced bone resorption and bone loss are apparently due to excessive osteoclast numbers and activity, but at the same time, osteoblast function is compromised. In addition to the effects on cells regulating bone mass, MM can induce angiogenesis and may suppress hematopoiesis and immune cell function, thereby leading to pancytopenia and increased risk for infections [7].

The ability of certain tumor types (i.e., prostate, breast, and MM) to grow avidly in bone suggests that bone may be a favorable milieu for tumor growth. The "vicious cycle" hypothesis proposes that tumor cells secrete factors to stimulate osteoclastogenesis and subsequent osteolysis, which then leads to the release of pro-tumor growth factors and cytokines from the bone microenvironment [8] (Fig. 9.1). These factors, in turn, may enhance tumor growth and survival, thereby resulting in a vicious cycle of bone breakdown and tumor proliferation. Based on this hypothesis, suppressing osteoclast formation and bone resorption may sufficiently alter the bone

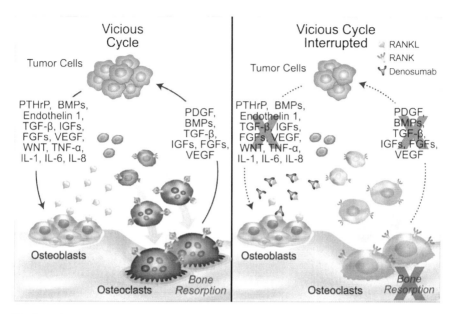

Fig. 9.1   Vicious cycle and mechanism of action for denosumab

marrow microenvironment by limiting the release of bone-derived factors available for tumor growth, resulting in an indirect anti-tumor or anti-myeloma effect.

In addition to indirectly supporting tumor growth via osteoclast-mediated bone resorption (i.e., the "vicious cycle"), recent observations suggest that direct interaction with osteoclasts may support myeloma cell growth independent of bone resorption [9, 10]. These studies have shown that osteoclasts in culture and in the absence of bone substrate will support long-term survival and proliferation of MM cells and confer resistance to dexamethasone-induced apoptosis [11]. The enhanced myeloma growth in co-cultures with osteoclasts may be due to paracrine factors, such as APRIL and BAFF, which are produced by osteoclasts [12].

Preclinical studies with pharmacologic inhibitors of osteoclast function have demonstrated that this reciprocal interaction between the bone and myeloma has consequences on myeloma pathophysiology. These experiments have demonstrated not only that myeloma bone disease depends upon osteoclast activity within the bone microenvironment but also that growth and survival of myeloma cells may depend upon osteoclast function.

9.2   Preclinical Aspects

9.2.1   Osteoclastogenesis Is Regulated by RANK/RANKL/OPG Proteins

Osteoclasts are cells of hematopoietic origin that are principally responsible for bone resorption. Relevant to MM-induced bone disease, the major driver

172   W.C. Dougall et al.

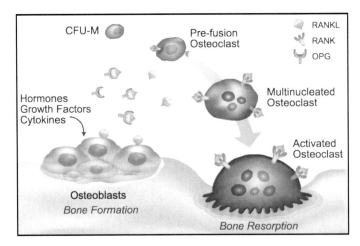

Fig. 9.2 RANK ligand is an essential mediator of osteoclast formation, function, and survival

contributing to these skeletal complications is increased osteoclast activity that leads to osteolysis. Osteoclast differentiation, activation, and survival are controlled through the trio of proteins consisting of RANK, its ligand RANKL, and osteoprotegerin (OPG) [13] (Fig. 9.2). RANK is a member of the tumor necrosis factor (TNF) receptor superfamily and is expressed on osteoclast precursors and mature osteoclasts. RANKL is a member of the TNF ligand family expressed on osteoblast-lineage cells and that binds to RANK, thereby activating downstream signaling pathways on RANK-expressing cells. Activation of these pathways leads to changes in expression of genes that control osteoclast precursor cell fusion and differentiation to form multinucleated osteoclasts. In addition, RANKL controls expression of genes related to osteoclast bone resorption, such as cathepsin K, MMP-9, and others. Another important element of RANKL/RANK signaling is to promote osteoclast survival. OPG, also a TNF receptor family member that can bind RANKL, does not function as a signaling receptor, but rather functions as a decoy receptor for RANKL and thereby limits osteoclastogenesis. Genetic studies in mice and rats have demonstrated that the ablation of the RANK or RANKL genes, or the overexpression of the OPG gene, results in a lack of osteoclasts in vivo [13]. Substantial evidence suggests that the pathologic bone resorption observed in myeloma-induced bone disease is ultimately governed by the ratio of RANKL to OPG proteins and the osteoclastic activity that results.

9.2.2 Expression of RANKL and OPG in Multiple Myeloma

RANKL and OPG are both produced by osteoblast-lineage cells derived from mesenchymal stem cells [14]. RANKL expression is higher in less-differentiated osteoblast precursor cells, which produce relatively little OPG. As differentiation of precursor cells into active osteoblasts proceeds, RANKL expression is suppressed while OPG expression is elevated. Both osteoblast differentiation and concomitant changes in RANKL and OPG expression have been shown to be regulated by the Wnt/β-catenin pathway [15]. In this pathway, binding of Wnt to co-receptors Frizzled and LRP5/6 leads to stabilization and nuclear accumulation of β-catenin, followed by activation of osteogenic transcription factors Runx2 and Osterix. This signaling pathway can be blocked by secreted factors, such as sFRPs and DKK-1, which prevent the binding of Wnt to either Frizzled or LRP5/6. These secreted factors, in particular DKK-1, have been associated with myeloma bone disease.

The association of DKK-1 and myeloma was first observed by Tian et al., who identified DKK1 in a microarray screen as a gene overexpressed in myeloma patients with bone lesions compared with those without bone lesions [16]. They further demonstrated a significant increase in bone marrow plasma levels of DKK-1 protein in myeloma patients with bone lesions. Subsequent studies confirmed the association between DKK-1 and myeloma patients with bone lesions. DKK-1 was shown to be elevated in MM relative to MGUS, and DKK-1 levels were correlated with the number of lytic lesions [17]. Another study by Terpos et al. found significant elevation of both DKK-1 and RANKL, along with serum markers of bone turnover (CTX and TRAP5b) in myeloma patients relative to controls [18]. In these patients, treatment with bortezomib resulted in significant decreases in both DKK-1 and RANKL along with normalization of bone turnover markers. In an in vitro model of osteoblast differentiation, addition of either recombinant DKK-1 protein or serum from myeloma patients was able to block the ability of Wnt-3a to upregulate OPG expression, while concomitantly relieving Wnt-mediated suppression of RANKL expression [19].

In addition to altering RANKL/OPG expression indirectly via suppressing osteoblast differentiation, MM cells may directly affect osteoclast activity by numerous other mechanisms. Immunohistochemical analysis has indicated increases in RANKL and decreases in OPG within the bone stroma of MM-involved bone [20, 21]. Conversely, flow cytometry analysis of MM patient samples has indicated that myeloma cells themselves can express low levels of RANKL [22–25], and RANKL expression has also been detected from T cells purified from MM patients with osteolytic bone disease [26]. MM cells also produce a number of cytokines, including TNF-α, IL-6, IL-8, and MIP1-α, which have been shown either to increase RANKL expression by bone marrow stromal cells or to augment the effects of RANKL to stimulate osteoclast activity. Adding to these observational data, a causal association between RANKL and the osteolytic lesions in MM has been defined using pharmacological inhibition of RANKL in rodent MM models.

9.2.3 Pharmacological Effect of RANKL Inhibition in Preclinical Models of Myeloma

The pathophysiological characteristics of human MM osteolytic bony lesions, including both excessive osteoclast activity and also reduced osteoblastic activity, can be recapitulated in mouse models using either syngeneic mouse MM cells or primary human patient MM cells in a SCID mouse containing a human bone explant. In either case, tumor cells lead to osteolytic lesions, loss of cancellous bone, and osteoblast suppression and have been used to demonstrate a role for RANKL in MM bone destruction.

The 5TMM murine MM models were derived from spontaneously developed myeloma in mice and from reintroducing 5T2 or 5T33 cells into C57BL/KalwRij animals, which caused changes in the bone marrow microenvironment, including osteolytic bone lesions [27]. In this model, treating mice that had established progressive MM disease (as measured by serum paraprotein) with the RANKL inhibitor Fc-OPG prevented MM-induced bone loss, lytic lesions, and tumor-induced osteoclast formation [28]. In support of the notion that RANKL inhibition has an indirect anti-myeloma effect, the significant suppression of tumor-induced osteoclasts by Fc-OPG was also associated with a 25% reduction in paraprotein (a surrogate for tumor progression). Additionally, Vanderkerken et al. demonstrated that administration of Fc-OPG at the time of 5T33MM inoculation resulted not only in reducing both serum paraprotein and MM cells in the bone marrow but also in significantly improving survival of MM-bearing animals [29]. Similar reductions in tumor-induced osteoclasts, osteolysis, and myeloma tumor burden were observed in the 5T2MM model after administering a different RANKL inhibitor, the OPG peptidomimetic (OP3-4) [30]. In the 5TGM1 model, another example of a syngeneic model of MM, RANKL inhibition both prevented myeloma bone disease and reduced tumor burden [31].

The Hu/SCID mouse is a unique model to study the interaction of MM and bone. In this model, human bone is explanted in the flanks of SCID animals and primary patient MM tumor cells are inoculated. In one such model, RANKL inhibition (using RANK-Fc) reduced both tumor-induced osteolysis and tumor burden, as measured by serum paraprotein levels and histology [21]. Similarly, reductions in osteolysis and tumor burden were observed after RANK-Fc treatment in a second Hu/SCID study [32]. Interestingly, Yaccoby also observed that osteoclast inhibition (using RANK-Fc or BPs) did not have a therapeutic benefit on plasma cell leukemias, which no longer require the bone microenvironment to grow.

These data suggest that inhibiting RANKL will prevent MM-induced bone lesions and can also result in an indirect anti-myeloma effect. Presumably, the tumor is supported by osteoclasts via the "vicious cycle" of bone destruction that promotes expansion or survival of myeloma restricted to the bone marrow. Additional mechanisms by which RANKL inhibition leads to reduced tumor burden are also possible via inhibiting factors produced by osteoclasts directly and not as a result of bone resorption [10].

9.3 Clinical Correlations of RANKL, OPG, and Myeloma Disease

Alterations in RANKL and OPG have been demonstrated in several independent studies of MM patients, at both the local level in bone marrow and systemically [25, 33, 34]. In all of these studies, the overall combined effect of either increased

RANKL or decreased OPG expression is consistent with a net increase in the amount of RANKL available to stimulate osteoclastic bone resorption [35]. In the first study, the OPG serum levels of 225 patients with myeloma were compared with 40 healthy age- and sex-matched controls [36]. Patients with MM were found to have OPG serum levels that were 18% lower than controls. Among myeloma patients, OPG serum levels were inversely correlated with the number of radiographically confirmed osteolytic lesions and World Health Organization (WHO) performance status. A positive correlation with the bone turnover marker cTX was also noted. Similar findings were confirmed by Lipton et al. who assessed OPG serum levels in 112 healthy controls and 111 patients with various hematologic malignancies [37]. OPG serum levels were 29% lower in patients with MM ($n = 34$) than in healthy controls.

A study by Standal et al. analyzed local OPG concentrations in plasma samples obtained from bone marrow aspirates of 33 patients with MM and 27 healthy controls [38]. OPG protein concentrations within the bone marrow microenvironment in this study were 27% lower in patients with MM than in healthy controls. Notably, OPG concentrations were twofold higher in the bone marrow plasma compared with serum and were found to be positively correlated with each other.

Lastly, Terpos et al. measured soluble RANKL (sRANKL)/OPG ratios and bone remodeling markers in 121 patients with newly diagnosed MM to evaluate their role in bone disease and survival [2]. The study reported that serum levels of sRANKL were elevated in patients with MM and were correlated with bone disease. The sRANKL/OPG ratio was increased and correlated with markers of bone resorption, osteolytic lesions, and markers of disease activity. While the changes in sRANKL were consistent with the extent of bone disease, a recent paper has highlighted the analytical challenges of immunodetection of RANKL in human serum [39].

Collectively, these expression analysis studies indicate that several mechanisms may alter the ratio of RANKL/OPG in MM, and they highlight that the RANKL/OPG ratio has a role in the biology of plasma cell growth and influences survival in myeloma patients.

9.3.1 RANKL Inhibition as Treatment of Myeloma Bone Disease

Denosumab is a fully human monoclonal antibody that specifically targets RANKL (Fig. 9.1). Denosumab is currently being tested in the clinical setting, following preclinical studies that suggested that RANKL inhibition can reduce bone resorption and may have therapeutic potential to decrease tumor burden in patients with MM.

9.3.2 Phase 1 Study on Pharmacodynamics of Denosumab in Multiple Myeloma Subjects

A randomized, double-blind, active-controlled, dose-escalation study was conducted in 54 patients with MM- or breast cancer-related bone metastases [40]. The subjects were stratified based on tumor type. The objectives of this study were to

evaluate the safety and pharmacodynamic and pharmacokinetic profiles of denosumab when administered subcutaneously (SC) and to determine the dosing regimen
for future studies. Twenty MM patients received denosumab and five received
pamidronate, the active control. Twenty-four breast cancer patients received denosumab and five received pamidronate. Dose levels of 0.1, 0.3, 1.0, and 3.0 mg/kg
denosumab were evaluated.

In this study, the pattern of adverse events with single SC doses of denosumab
was consistent with that observed for advanced cancer patients receiving systemic
therapy in all dose levels. Decreases in urinary N-telopeptide of type I colla-
gen/creatinine (uNTx/Cr) levels were rapid, sustained, and dose-dependent in both
disease strata. Administration of 1 and 3 mg/kg doses suppressed uNTx/Cr by 70%
for each of the doses 28 days after denosumab was administered and by 70 and
73%, respectively, 84 days after denosumab was administered in patients with MM.
Similar results were seen in the breast cancer stratum.

The ≥1.0 mg/kg dose maintained denosumab serum concentrations at >1,000
ng/ml in most patients who had MM or breast cancer at 3 months after dosing and
was associated with marked suppression of bone resorption (uNTx/Cr, >50% suppression). All patients who received a dose of 0.3 mg/kg or less had serum levels
of denosumab that were <6 ng/ml at week 12 and had escape from bone turnover
suppression by week 12, with uNTx/Cr levels returning toward baseline values.

9.3.3 Phase 2 Studies in Multiple Myeloma Subjects

Data are available from a completed phase 2 study in patients with MM or advanced
cancer with bone metastasis previously treated with intravenous bisphosphonates
[41] and from an ongoing proof-of-concept study evaluating the effect of denosumab
on MM [42].

9.3.4 Denosumab in Multiple Myeloma and Other Advanced Cancer Patients Previously Receiving IV BPs

This study was restricted to advanced cancer and myeloma patients who were
receiving IV BPs for treatment of bone metastases and lytic bone disease and had
moderate or high levels of bone resorption as determined by bone marker assessments of uNTX >50 uNTx/Cr within 4 weeks before study entry [41]. Elevated
levels of bone turnover markers, such as uNTx, represent excessive bone resorption
and are predictive of SREs, cancer progression, and death [43–47]. The primary
objective of this study was to determine whether denosumab would further increase
the proportion of patients with uNTx <50 uNTx/Cr in myeloma bone disease and
advanced cancer patients with bone metastases at week 13.

Results indicated that a significantly higher proportion of patients treated with
denosumab achieved uNTx/Cr <50 uNTx/Cr at week 13 than those treated with
IV BP. The pattern remained similar when patients were stratified by cancer
type (breast, prostate or myeloma and other solid tumors) and level of uNTx/Cr,

with a greater proportion of the combined denosumab groups demonstrating uNTx/Cr <50 nM BCE/mM cr. Furthermore, suppression of uNTx/Cr levels was more rapid and sustained longer for each denosumab treatment group compared with the IV BP treatment group. These results demonstrate the biologic activity of denosumab and suggest that denosumab can further suppress markers of bone turnover despite previous use of IV BPs in patients with cancer-related bone disease, irrespective of tumor type and baseline levels of uNTx. The Kaplan–Meier curves of time to first on-study SRE were also similar for denosumab- and IV BP-treated cohorts during the 6 month treatment period.

Safety results showed that there were no unexpected laboratory parameter changes for calcium, serum creatinine, liver enzymes, or electrolytes in denosumab cohorts. Also, the incidence of serious adverse events appeared to be similar for all denosumab and IV BP cohorts, with no serious adverse events attributed to denosumab or IV BPs.

9.3.5 Denosumab as Anti-myeloma Therapy in Treating Patients with Advanced Multiple Myeloma

Based on the preclinical hypothesis described earlier [21, 28], a proof-of-concept, single-arm study investigated whether RANKL inhibition with denosumab could reduce serum M-protein levels in relapsed or plateau-phase myeloma patients [42]. The primary objective was to estimate the objective response rate (complete response or partial response) in each myeloma cohort. All patients received denosumab monthly, with loading doses on days 8 and 15 of month one until disease progression or patient discontinuation.

Results of this study demonstrated that no patients in either cohort met the protocol-defined objective response criteria of complete or partial response, but that denosumab effectively inhibited the RANKL pathway regardless of previous exposure to bisphosphonates, as evidenced by suppressed levels of the bone turnover marker serum C-telopeptide (sCTx). Bone turnover marker suppression suggests that RANKL inhibition can represent an alternative bone-targeting agent to bisphosphonates for treating skeletal morbidities. In addition, 11 patients (21%) who relapsed within 3 months of study entry maintained stable disease for up to 16.5 months (median duration: 2.6 months). Nineteen patients (46%) with plateau-phase myeloma maintained stable disease for up to 18.3 months (median duration: 10.2 months). The safety profile of denosumab therapy in this heavily pretreated population was consistent with that observed in advanced cancer patients receiving systemic therapy, and no neutralizing anti-denosumab antibody was observed in either cohort.

9.3.6 Phase 3 Studies on Bone Metastasis-Related Complications

Three large, head-to-head, active-controlled phase 3 pivotal studies are ongoing to evaluate the use of denosumab compared with zoledronic acid to reduce the risk of SREs in patients with bone metastases. Among them, a multiple myeloma subset is being evaluated in one study, which combined subjects with multiple myeloma, non-small cell lung cancer, and other solid tumors with bone metastases (not including breast and prostate cancer).

The osteoclastic component of all bone metastases, irrespective of radiographic appearance or tumor origin, is critical to the development of clinical consequences (e.g., SREs and pain). This is seen across a broad range of cancers through elevated bone resorption with bone metastases, by histomorphometric evidence of increased osteoclast activity, and through the already demonstrated clinical effect of anti-resorptive therapy. Because RANKL is the central mediator in osteoclast activation and differentiation, inhibition of the RANKL pathway is hypothesized to have efficacy at preventing the occurrence of adverse SREs in multiple myeloma and other bone metastases. The ongoing trials into the ability of denosumab to reduce SREs in patients with bone disease should provide insight into this hypothesis.

9.4 Conclusion

Patient expression analysis has suggested that MM causes an imbalance in RANKL and OPG and that this can influence MM-induced bone disease. Phase 1 and 2 clinical studies of denosumab have demonstrated that RANKL inhibition will reduce MM-induced bone resorption. In preclinical studies of MM, RANKL inhibition not only prevented tumor-induced osteolysis but also reduced MM tumor burden. Since osteoclast-mediated bone resorption releases growth factors from the bone matrix, the host bone microenvironment induces a vicious cycle of bone destruction and tumor proliferation and survival, and one prediction of this vicious cycle hypothesis is that targeting the host bone microenvironment by osteoclast inhibition would reduce tumor growth and survival. Preclinical studies with RANKL inhibition have provided experimental support for this hypothesis and suggest that targeting the bone microenvironment and reducing tumor-induced bone resorption with a RANKL inhibitor may sensitize tumor cells to the effects of chemotherapy or other novel anti-myeloma agents (e.g., IMiDs and bortezomib).

Acknowledgment The authors would like to acknowledge Vidya Setty, MPH, MBA for expert editorial assistance.

References

1. Dalton WS. The tumor microenvironment: focus on myeloma. Cancer Treat Rev. May 2003;29(Suppl 1):11–19.
2. Terpos E, Szydlo R, Apperley J F, et al. Soluble receptor activator of nuclear factor kappaB ligand-osteoprotegerin ratio predicts survival in multiple myeloma: proposal for a novel prognostic index. Blood. August 1, 2003;102(3):1064–1069.
3. Kyle RA, Gertz MA, Witzig TE, et al. Review of 1027 patients with newly diagnosed multiple myeloma. Mayo Clin Proc. January 2003;78(1):21–33.
4. Cook R. Economic and clinical impact of multiple myeloma to managed care. J Manag Care Pharm. September 2008;14(7 Suppl):19–25.

5. Roodman GD. Novel targets for myeloma bone disease. Expert Opin Ther Targets. November 2008;12(11):1377–1387.
6. Mitsiades CS, Mitsiades N, Munshi NC, Anderson KC. Focus on multiple myeloma. Cancer Cell. Nov 2004;6(5):439–444.
7. Podar K, Chauhan D, Anderson KC. Bone marrow microenvironment and the identification of new targets for myeloma therapy. Leukemia. Jan 2009;23(1):10–24.
8. Mundy GR. Metastasis to bone: causes, consequences and therapeutic opportunities. Nat Rev Cancer. Aug 2002;2(8):584–593.
9. Abe M, Hiura K, Wilde J, et al. Osteoclasts enhance myeloma cell growth and survival via cell-cell contact: a vicious cycle between bone destruction and myeloma expansion. Blood. Oct 15 2004;104(8):2484–2491.
10. Yaccoby S, Wezeman MJ, Henderson A, et al. Cancer and the microenvironment: myeloma-osteoclast interactions as a model. Cancer Res. March 15, 2004;64(6):2016–2023.
11. Yaccoby S. The phenotypic plasticity of myeloma plasma cells as expressed by dedifferentiation into an immature, resilient, and apoptosis-resistant phenotype. Clin Cancer Res. Nov 1 2005;11(21):7599–7606.
12. Yaccoby S, Pennisi A, Li X, et al. Atacicept (TACI-Ig) inhibits growth of TACI(high) primary myeloma cells in SCID-hu mice and in coculture with osteoclasts. Leukemia. February 2008;22(2):406–413.
13. Boyle WJ, Simonet WS, Lacey DL. Osteoclast differentiation and activation. Nature. May 15, 2003;423(6937):337–342.
14. Gori F, Hofbauer LC, Dunstan CR, Spelsberg TC, Khosla S, Riggs BL. The expression of osteoprotegerin and RANK ligand and the support of osteoclast formation by stromal-osteoblast lineage cells is developmentally regulated. Endocrinology. December 2000;141(12):4768–4776.
15. Pinzone JJ, Hall BM, Thudi NK, et al. The role of Dickkopf-1 in bone development, homeostasis, and disease. Blood. January 15, 2009;113(3):517–525.
16. Tian E, Zhan F, Walker R, et al. The role of the Wnt-signaling antagonist DKK1 in the development of osteolytic lesions in multiple myeloma. N Engl J Med. December 25, 2003;349(26):2483–2494.
17. Kaiser M, Mieth M, Liebisch P, et al. Serum concentrations of DKK-1 correlate with the extent of bone disease in patients with multiple myeloma. Eur J Haematol. June 2008;80(6):490–494.
18. Terpos E, Heath DJ, Rahemtulla A, et al. Bortezomib reduces serum dickkopf-1 and receptor activator of nuclear factor-kappaB ligand concentrations and normalises indices of bone remodelling in patients with relapsed multiple myeloma. Br J Haematol. December 2006;135(5):688–692.
19. Qiang YW, Chen Y, Stephens O, et al. Myeloma-derived Dickkopf-1 disrupts Wnt-regulated osteoprotegerin and RANKL production by osteoblasts: a potential mechanism underlying osteolytic bone lesions in multiple myeloma. Blood. July 1, 2008;112(1):196–207.
20. Giuliani N, Bataille R, Mancini C, Lazzaretti M, Barille S. Myeloma cells induce imbalance in the osteoprotegerin/osteoprotegerin ligand system in the human bone marrow environment. Blood. December 15, 2001;98(13):3527–3533.
21. Pearse RN, Sordillo EM, Yaccoby S, et al. Multiple myeloma disrupts the TRANCE/osteoprotegerin cytokine axis to trigger bone destruction and promote tumor progression. Proc Natl Acad Sci USA. September 25, 2001;98(20):11581–11586.
22. Farrugia AN, Atkins GJ, To LB, et al. Receptor activator of nuclear factor-kappaB ligand expression by human myeloma cells mediates osteoclast formation in vitro and correlates with bone destruction in vivo. Cancer Res. September 1, 2003;63(17):5438–5445.
23. Heider U, Langelotz C, Jakob C, et al. Expression of receptor activator of nuclear factor kappaB ligand on bone marrow plasma cells correlates with osteolytic bone disease in patients with multiple myeloma. Clin Cancer Res. April 2003;9(4):1436–1440.
24. Lai FP, Cole-Sinclair M, Cheng WJ, et al. Myeloma cells can directly contribute to the pool of RANKL in bone bypassing the classic stromal and osteoblast pathway of osteoclast stimulation. Br J Haematol. July 2004;126(2):192–201.

25. Sezer O, Heider U, Zavrski I, Kuhne CA, Hofbauer LC. RANK ligand and osteoprotegerin in myeloma bone disease. Blood. March 15, 2003;101(6):2094–2098.

26. Giuliani N, Colla S, Sala R, et al. Human myeloma cells stimulate the receptor activator of nuclear factor-kappa B ligand (RANKL) in T lymphocytes: a potential role in multiple myeloma bone disease. Blood. December 15, 2002;100(13):4615–4621.

27. Vanderkerken K, Asosingh K, Croucher P, Van Camp B. Multiple myeloma biology: lessons from the 5TMM models. Immunol Rev. August 2003;194:196–206.

28. Croucher PI, Shipman CM, Lippitt J, et al. Osteoprotegerin inhibits the development of osteolytic bone disease in multiple myeloma. Blood. December 15, 2001;98(13): 3534–3540.

29. Vanderkerken K, De Leenheer E, Shipman C, et al. Recombinant osteoprotegerin decreases tumor burden and increases survival in a murine model of multiple myeloma. Cancer Res. January 15, 2003;63(2):287–289.

30. Heath DJ, Vanderkerken K, Cheng X, et al. An osteoprotegerin-like peptidomimetic inhibits osteoclastic bone resorption and osteolytic bone disease in myeloma. Cancer Res. January 1, 2007;67(1):202–208.

31. Oyajobi BO, Mundy GR. Receptor activator of NF-kappaB ligand, macrophage inflammatory protein-1alpha, and the proteasome: novel therapeutic targets in myeloma. Cancer. February 1, 2003;97(3 Suppl):813–817.

32. Yaccoby S, Pearse RN, Johnson CL, Barlogie B, Choi Y, Epstein J. Myeloma interacts with the bone marrow microenvironment to induce osteoclastogenesis and is dependent on osteoclast activity. Br J Haematol. February 2002;116(2):278–290.

33. Hofbauer LC, Schoppet M. Serum measurement of osteoprotegerin–clinical relevance and potential applications. Eur J Endocrinol. December 2001;145(6):681–683.

34. Dougall WC, Chaisson M. The RANK/RANKL/OPG triad in cancer-induced bone diseases. Cancer Metast Rev. December 2006;25(4):541–549.

35. Roodman GD, Dougall WC. RANK ligand as a therapeutic target for bone metastases and multiple myeloma. Cancer Treat Rev. February 2008;34(1):92–101.

36. Seidel C, Hjertner O, Abildgaard N, et al. Serum osteoprotegerin levels are reduced in patients with multiple myeloma with lytic bone disease. Blood. October 1, 2001;98(7):2269–2271.

37. Lipton A, Ali SM, Leitzel K, et al. Serum osteoprotegerin levels in healthy controls and cancer patients. Clin Cancer Res. July 2002;8(7):2306–2310.

38. Standal T, Seidel C, Hjertner O, et al. Osteoprotegerin is bound, internalized, and degraded by multiple myeloma cells. Blood. October 15, 2002;100(8):3002–3007.

39. Bowsher RR, Sailstad JM. Insights in the application of research-grade diagnostic kits for biomarker assessments in support of clinical drug development: bioanalysis of circulating concentrations of soluble receptor activator of nuclear factor kappaB ligand. J Pharm Biomed Anal. December 15, 2008;48(5):1282–1289.

40. Body JJ, Facon T, Coleman RE, et al. A study of the biological receptor activator of nuclear factor-kappaB ligand inhibitor, denosumab, in patients with multiple myeloma or bone metastases from breast cancer. Clin Cancer Res. February 15, 2006;12(4):1221–1228.

41. Fizazi K, Lipton A, Mariette X, et al. Randomized phase II trial of denosumab in patients with bone metastases from prostate cancer, breast cancer, or other neoplasms after intravenous bisphosphonates. J Clin Oncol April 1, 2009;27(10):1564–1571.

42. Vij R, Horvath N, Spencer A, et al. An open-label, phase 2 trial of denosumab in the treatment of relapsed (R) or plateau-phase (PP) multiple myeloma (MM). Blood. 2007;110:1054A ASH 2007. Abstract 3604.

43. Brown JE, Cook RJ, Major P et al. Bone turnover markers as predictors of skeletal complications in prostate cancer, lung cancer, and other solid tumors. J Natl Cancer Inst. January 5, 2005;97(1):59–69.

44. Brown JE, Thomson CS, Ellis SP, Gutcher SA, Purohit OP, Coleman RE. Bone resorption predicts for skeletal complications in metastatic bone disease. Br J Cancer. December 1, 2003;89(11):2031–2037.

45. Coleman RE, Major P, Lipton A, et al. Predictive value of bone resorption and formation markers in cancer patients with bone metastases receiving the bisphosphonate zoledronic acid. J Clin Oncol. August 1, 2005;23(22):4925–4935.
46. Costa L, Demers LM, Gouveia-Oliveira A, et al. Prospective evaluation of the peptide-bound collagen type I cross-links N-telopeptide and C-telopeptide in predicting bone metastases status. J Clin Oncol. February 1, 2002;20(3):850–856.
47. Rajpar S, Laplanche A, Tournay E, Massard C, Gross-Goupil M, Fizazi K. Urinary N-telopeptide (uNTX) is a strong independent prognostic factor in patients (pts) with castration-resistant prostate cancer (CRPC) and bone metastases. Proc Am Soc Clin Oncol. 2008;26.

Chapter 10
Osteoclast Activation in Multiple Myeloma

Sonia Vallet and Noopur Raje

Abstract Osteolytic bone disease affects more than 80% of multiple myeloma (MM) patients with a negative impact on both quality of life and overall survival. The pathogenesis of osteolytic disease resides in increased osteoclast (OC) activation along with osteoblast (OB) inhibition resulting in altered bone remodeling. OC number and activity in MM are enhanced mainly via cytokine deregulation within the bone marrow (BM) milieu and an imbalance of the OC/OB axis. Several novel agents are currently under investigation for their positive effect on bone remodeling via OC inhibition or OB activation. In addition to restoring bone remodeling, these drugs may inhibit tumor growth in vivo. Therefore, targeting bone disease is a promising therapeutic strategy not only with the goal of alleviating morbidity from bone disease but also resultant anti-tumor activity.

Keywords Osteolysis · MM niche · Osteoclast activation · Osteoblasts

10.1 Introduction

Osteolytic lesions are a pathognomonic feature of multiple myeloma (MM). More than 80% of MM patients develop osteolytic bone disease (OBD), frequently complicated by skeletal-related events (SRE) such as severe bone pain, vertebral compression fractures, and pathologic fractures resulting in a need for radiation or surgical fixation. Importantly, pathologic fractures affect 40–50% of MM patients increasing the risk of death by more than 20% compared to the patients without fractures [1, 2]. Therefore, OBD reduces not only patients' quality of life but also survival.

N. Raje (✉)
Harvard Medical School, Massachusetts General Hospital Cancer Center, Boston,
MA 02114, USA
e-mail: nraje@partners.org

G.D. Roodman (ed.), *Myeloma Bone Disease*, Current Clinical Oncology,
DOI 10.1007/978-1-60761-554-5_10, © Springer Science+Business Media, LLC 2010

The pathogenesis of OBD in MM is primarily associated with generalized osteoclast (OC) activation. Bone marrow (BM) biopsies from MM patients show a correlation between tumor burden, OC number, and resorption surface [3, 4]. Although enhanced OC function is a key player in the development of OBD, a decrease in trabecular thickness and low calcification rate in BM biopsy specimens of MM patients with osteolysis suggest that osteoblast (OB) activity is also impaired [5]. Therefore, the bone remodeling balance in MM is disrupted by a deregulation of the OC/OB axis.

Several novel agents are aimed at restoring bone homeostasis targeting either OC or OB activity. Interestingly, inhibition of osteolysis leads to reduced tumor growth in vivo [6, 7]. Therefore, novel agents targeting bone disease are promising therapeutic strategies for the treatment of MM. Optimal drug development requires further clarification of the pathogenesis of osteolysis as well as understanding the role of the microenvironment in the progression of myeloma.

10.2 Bone Marrow Niche in Multiple Myeloma

The cross talk between MM cells and their local bone marrow microenvironment is tightly regulated. Neighborhood cells termed the cancer niche provide the microenvironment for the propagation of tumor cells [8–13]. Malignant cells in turn shape their local microenvironment to create a permissive niche for their survival [14–16]. MM is an exquisitely niche-dependent cancer and can serve as a model to identify niche-directed therapeutic strategies. Stromal, endothelial, immune, and bone cells as well as extracellular matrix components, like osteopontin and fibronectin constitute the MM niche that supports tumor growth and survival (Fig. 10.1). Under normal physiologic states, OC and OB result in balanced bone resorption and formation maintaining normal homeostasis. In MM the OC/OB axis is disrupted favoring bone resorption with the development of pathognomonic osteolytic lesions [17]. OCs, bone marrow stromal cells (BMSC), and endothelial cells promote cell growth, survival, homing, and drug resistance via chemokine secretion and cell-to-cell contact. The main cytokines involved in OC and BMSC interactions with MM cells are interleukin-6 (IL-6), receptor activator of NF-kB ligand (RANKL)/osteoprotegerin (OPG), B-cell-activating factor (BAFF), chemokine (C-C motif) ligand 3 (CCL3)/macrophage inflammatory protein (MIP)-1α, and vascular endothelial growth factor (VEGF). Cell adhesion is mediated by integrin signaling, mainly very late antigen (VLA)-4/vascular cell adhesion molecule (VCAM)-1 and lymphocyte function-associated antigen (LFA)-1/intercellular adhesion molecule (ICAM)-1 that activates drug resistance mechanisms (CAM-DR) [12, 18–22]. Another recently described MM-derived factor is dickkopf (DKK)-1, a WNT/β-catenin signaling antagonist [23]. Highly expressed in BM plasma of MM patients with osteolytic lesions, DKK1 is apparently involved in early stages of bone disease. DKK1 and other cytokines have inhibitory effects on OB and thus promote MM bone disease. Indeed, OBs as well as immune system cells have opposing

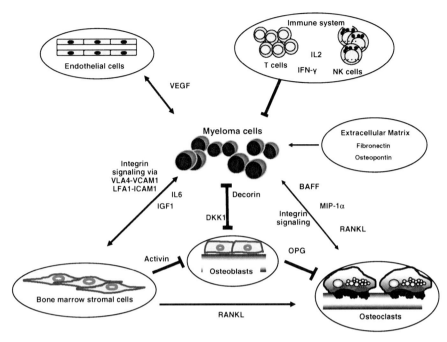

Fig. 10.1 Multiple myeloma (MM) niche. Malignant plasma cells depend on their microenvironment for growth and survival. Both cellular and extracellular components constitute the MM niche. Endothelial cells, bone marrow stromal cells (BMSC), and osteoclasts (OC) support MM cells via cytokine secretion and adhesive interactions. The cytokines promoting MM cell survival and proliferation are interleukin-6 (IL-6), B-cell-activating factor (BAFF), chemokine (C-C motif) ligand 3 (CCL3)/macrophage inflammatory protein (MIP)-1α, and vascular endothelial growth factor (VEGF). Moreover, cell adhesion mediated by very late antigen (VLA)-4/vascular cell adhesion molecule (VCAM)-1 and lymphocyte function-associated antigen (LFA)-1/intercellular adhesion molecule (ICAM)-1 activates drug resistance mechanisms (CAM-DR). In turn MM promote osteoclast development and angiogenesis, respectively, via deregulation of the receptor activator of NF-kB ligand (RANKL)/osteoprotegerin (OPG) ratio and release of VEGF. OBs and immune system cells on the other hand inhibit MM cells growth. A possible mediator of this inhibition is an OB-derived extracellular matrix component, decorin that induces MM cell apoptosis. MM cell indeed inhibit OB differentiation via direct secretion of DKK1 and indirectly stimulating BMSC production of activin A. Finally, several extracellular matrix components, like osteopontin and fibronectin, participate also in the MM niche and enhance tumor cell survival

effects on MM cells compared to OCs and BMSCs. Although OBs secrete MM growth factors such as IL-6, they have an overall inhibitory effect on MM cell proliferation [24]. In vivo up-regulation of OBs stimulating the β-catenin signaling pathway results in significant tumor growth inhibition [7]. Although the mechanism is still to be clarified, small leucine-rich proteoglycans are probably involved. Decorin, in particular, is an OB-derived extracellular matrix component regulating bone formation and mineralization. Decorin induces MM cell apoptosis via p21 activation and inhibits angiogenesis and osteoclastogenesis [25].

These data suggest that the OC, OB, and BMSC interactions in the MM niche regulate tumor growth. Importantly, tumor cells shape their local microenvironment by recruiting OCs, promoting angiogenesis, and inhibiting OBs differentiation to create a permissive niche for their survival. Ultimately, the interactions in the MM niche deregulate bone homeostasis leading to development of osteolysis and tumor development. These interactions are a relevant but underexploited therapeutic target in MM. Here we will focus mainly on osteoclast activation in the context of MM bone disease.

10.3 Mechanisms of Osteoclast Activation

Bone is a dynamic organ that undergoes extensive remodeling throughout life. Regulation of bone homeostasis relies mainly on the OC/OB balance that is notably disrupted in MM. Indeed, MM cells directly promote OC differentiation and function and indirectly affect OC activity by inhibition of OB differentiation and stimulation of BMSC synthesis of OC-activating factors (OAF) (Fig. 10.2).

10.3.1 Osteoclastogenesis

OCs are terminally-differentiated cells of the monocytic–macrophagic lineage. OC differentiation is a complex multistep process regulated by cytokines and direct interactions with OBs. Three major stages have been identified in osteoclastogenesis: progenitor cell proliferation, cell-to-cell fusion into multinucleated precursors, and OC activation.

Monocyte colony-stimulating factor (M-CSF) and RANKL are important growth factors in OC differentiation, both produced by BMSC, OBs, and T lymphocytes. M-CSF activates the mitogen-activated protein kinase (MAPK) pathway and regulates mainly OC precursor proliferation and survival. RANKL promotes OC differentiation, survival, and activity via TNF receptor-associated factor (TRAF)-6 activation and induction of nuclear factor of activated T cells, cytoplasmic, calcineurin-dependent (NFATc)-1. Other important transcription factors activated during OC differentiation are PU.1 and c-fos. RANKL activity is normally balanced by its soluble decoy receptor, OPG secreted by OBs. The balance between the OPG and RANKL is an important regulator of bone resorption.

The generation of multinucleated cells require chemotaxis and cell fusion signals. Specifically, mononuclear OC precursor cells secrete CCL3, CCL5, monocyte-chemotactic protein (MCP)-1, and other chemotactic factors that stimulate cell-to-cell migration via chemokine (CC motif) receptor (CCR)1, CCR2, and CCR5 signaling expressed on pre-OC cell surface. Disruption of these signaling sequences leads to generation of tartrate-resistant acidic phosphatase (TRAP)-positive mononuclear cells with limited bone resorption ability.

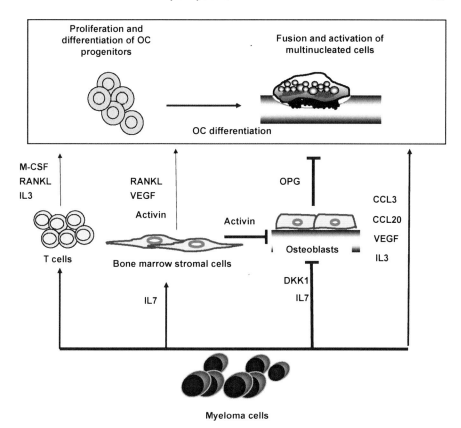

Fig. 10.2 Osteoclast activation in multiple myeloma (MM). Osteoclast (OC) differentiation consists of several stages: progenitor cell proliferation, cell-to-cell fusion into multinucleated precursors, and OC activation. (MM) cells enhance OC development by direct secretion of OC-activating factors, such as IL-3, CCL20, CCL3, and VEGF and, indirectly, by affecting bone marrow stromal cells (BMSC) and T lymphocyte production of catabolic cytokines. Malignant plasma cells deregulate the RANKL/OPG balance by up-regulating RANKL expression in BMSC and T lymphocytes. The concomitant inhibition of OPG production is related to osteoblast (OB) impairment mediated by MM-derived DKK1 and IL7 as well as BMSC-derived activin. Other OC-activating factors are T lymphocyte-derived IL-3 and BMSC-derived VEGF and activin, induced by interactions with MM cells

OC activation and bone resorption depend on adhesion to the bone surface mediated by alphaVbeta3 integrin, acidification of the resorption site, and release of cathepsins and extracellular matrix degradation enzymes.

In the bone remodeling process OCs and OBs activities are coupled. OC formation and activation require the presence of RANKL-secreting OBs. OCs also regulate the OB maturation via bidirectional Ephrin/Eph signaling. OCs express ephrinB2 that acts on the receptor EphB4 on OBs to promote their differentiation, while reverse signaling via ephrinB2 in OC precursor cells inhibits OC differentiation [26].

Besides OBs, T lymphocytes also modulate osteoclastogenesis via release of osteoclast-activating factors like IL-6, IL-1, and IL-7 and OC inhibitory cytokines, IL-4, IL-13, IL-10; underscoring the important link between immune system and bone.

10.3.2 RANKL/OPG Ratio in MM

Deregulation of the RANKL/OPG ratio results in bone loss in cancer and inflammatory disease [27, 28]. In MM patients BM levels of RANKL are increased while OPG expression is reduced compared to normal control and MGUS [29]. Importantly, low serum levels of OPG correlated with advanced osteolytic bone disease in MM [30]. Discordant data on direct RANKL secretion by MM cells have been reported, however, in coculture systems malignant plasma cells up-regulated RANKL expression and strongly down-regulated OPG production in OB, BMSCs, and T lymphocytes [29, 31–33]. Further decrease in OPG levels is related to OB loss and direct OPG degradation by MM cells via CD138 [34]. The relevance of the RANKL/OPG pathway in mediating OC activation in MM has been further confirmed in several murine models of MM-OBD. Treatment with OPG and OPG-like molecules prevented both bone destruction and MM growth in vivo [35, 36]. Interestingly, specific anti-MM strategies like thalidomide and autologous bone marrow transplantation inhibited bone resorption by normalizing the RANKL/OPG ratio [37, 38]. Therefore, the RANKL/OPG axis is an important target in the development of novel therapeutic strategies for MM bone disease.

10.3.3 CCL3/CCR1 Pathway in MM

CCL3 is a chemokine binding to G-protein coupled receptors, CCR1 and CCR5, to activate AKT and MAPK signaling pathways. High BM serum levels of CCL3 correlate with osteolytic lesions and survival in MM patients [39]. CCL3 is secreted by OCs and MM cells. Interestingly, fibroblast growth factor receptor 3 (FGFR3) overexpression in MM with t(4,14) results in up-regulation of CCL3 expression [40]. The CCL3/CCR1 pathway has multiple roles in MM, like growth and survival stimulation, and chemotaxis induction on malignant plasma cells [19]. It also induces osteoclastogenesis by promoting OC precursor cell migration and fusion into multinucleated TRAP positive cells [41]. The dual activity of CCL3 has been targeted in vivo with different strategies, both antisense sequence and neutralizing antibody against CCL3 effectively inhibited tumor growth and restored bone remodeling in mouse model of MM bone disease [6, 42]. Importantly, CCR1 inhibition was also associated with impairment of osteoclastogenesis and OC-induced tumor cell proliferation in vitro, suggesting that the CCL3/CCR1 pathway is a relevant target in MM bone disease [43].

10.3.4 Other OC-Activating Factors in MM

Other than RANKL and CCL3, several OC-activating factors (OAF) such as IL-1, IL-6, IL-3, IL-7, CCL20, and activin are highly expressed in BM serum of MM patients [44].

IL-3 is secreted by both malignant plasma cells and T lymphocytes in MM and stimulates OC differentiation in combination with RANKL [45, 46]. Interestingly, IL-3 is also a growth factor for MM cells and indirectly inhibits OBs differentiation via stimulation of CD45+ monocytic–macrophagic cell population [47].

IL-7 is secreted by MM cells and stimulates RANKL production by T lymphocytes, therefore promoting OC differentiation [31]. Moreover, IL-7 mediates MM-induced OB inhibition via down-regulation of runt-related transcription factor (RUNX)2 activity [48].

Activin, a transforming growth factor (TGF)β family member, has been recently identified as a key player in the pathogenesis of osteolytic bone disease in MM. Activin modulates bone remodeling by a dual activity as OCs promoter and inhibitor of OB differentiation. In MM, high activin A levels are associated with advanced bone disease. BMSC and OCs are the main sources of activin and MM cells further up-regulate BMSC expression of activin.

10.3.5 MM-Induced OC Differentiation via BMSC and OB

MM cells stimulate OC differentiation by secreting OAF and, indirectly, by stimulating BMSC secretion of RANKL and activin and by inhibiting OBs differentiation.

MM to BMSC adhesion leads to RANKL and VEGF secretion via p38 MAPK activation [49, 50]. The sequestrosome p62 is a recently discovered upstream regulator of p38 MAPK and NF-kB signaling pathway activated in BMSC by MM cell adhesion. Inhibition of p62 in BMSC represses OC differentiation and MM cell proliferation, therefore p62 is a novel promising target in MM-OBD [51].

MM-derived DKK1 inhibits wingless (Wnt)3a-induced OPG expression in OBs and stimulates RANKL secretion [52]. Moreover, OB inhibition by MM cells may result in reduced OPG production producing an unbalanced OC differentiation.

10.4 Targeting Osteoclasts in Multiple Myeloma Bone Disease

Current treatment strategies in MM have resulted in improved patients' overall survival but patients continue to relapse and no definitive cure is achieved. Given improved survival of MM patients, treatment of OBD has taken on a new relevance as the focus is now largely on quality of life. The therapeutic options for MM-OBD are mainly based on bisphosphonates (BPs), radiotherapy, and surgery, which are discussed in detail in other chapters. These therapies aim at preventing SRE and reducing the development of new osteolytic lesions. Interestingly, several studies

Table 10.1 Novel agents in MM-OBD

Agent	Mechanism of action	Manufacturer	Notes
Denosumab	RANKL neutralizing antibody	Amgen	• Subcutaneous administration • Phase III randomized clinical trials compared to bisphosphonates
MLN3897	CCR1 inhibition	Millennium Pharmaceuticals	• Oral administration
BAFF-antibody	BAFF neutralizing antibody	Ely Lilly	• Intravenous administration • Phase II study in multiple myeloma patients in combination with Velcade
RAP011/ACE011	Decoy receptor neutralizing activin A	Acceleron Pharma	• Subcutaneous administration
BHQ880	DKK1 neutralizing antibody	Novartis	• Intravenous administration • Phase I/II clinical trial in relapsed/refractory multiple myeloma patients in combination with zoledronic acid

using novel bone-targeting agents suggest that restoring bone homeostasis may lead to tumor growth inhibition. Therefore, these promising results set the stage for clinical evaluation of novel strategies targeting MM via improvement of bone disease. A list of novel anti-catabolic and anabolic agents is provided in Table 10.1.

10.4.1 Bisphosphonates

Bisphosphonates represent the standard of care in cancer-related bone disease and osteoporosis. The anti-catabolic effects of BPs result from enhanced OC apoptosis partly due to inhibition of the mevalonate pathway [53]. In the clinical setting, treatment with either pamidronate or zoledronic acid significantly reduces pain related to bone metastasis and prevent SRE, but they do not cure existing osteolytic lesions [54]. In vitro data also suggest that high concentration of BPs may have a direct cytotoxic effect on tumor cells as well as inhibit tumor–stromal cells interactions [55]. Recently, it has been shown that zoledronic acid may improve disease-free survival in breast cancer patients when combined with adjuvant endocrine therapies [56]. These data suggest that tumor growth may be negatively affected by normalization of the bone structure. The most serious adverse events associated with BPs are renal impairment and osteonecrosis of the jaw (ONJ) [57]. ONJ is characterized by exposed bone, severe localized pain, and increased risk of secondary infections.

A possible explanation suggest that OB inhibition by high long-lasting concentrations of BPs bound to the bone matrix impairs bone remodeling [58, 59]. Therefore, novel treatment approaches alternative to BPs are needed.

10.4.2 Denosumab

The RANKL/OPG pathway is critical to the pathogenesis of OBD in MM and both OPG-like molecules and neutralizing antibody against RANKL effectively inhibit osteolysis in murine models of MM-OBD [60]. Denosumab, a RANKL neutralizing antibody *(AMG162,* Amgen Pharmaceutical), has been successfully used in MM and breast cancer patients to inhibit bone resorption markers. Compared to BPs, subcutaneous administrations of denosumab induce a sustained inhibition of bone resorption markers lasting about 80 days vs. 30 days of BPs. Denosumab displayed a limited toxicity, consisting mainly of asthenia and peripheral edema [61]. Interestingly, a recent randomized clinical trial showed that denosumab inhibited bone resorption and prevented SREs also in patients refractory to BPs therapy [62]. An ongoing phase III trial is comparing the effectiveness of zoledronic acid with denosumab. These data suggest that RANKL inhibition may be a valid treatment alternative to BPs.

10.4.3 MLN3897

The CCL3/CCR1 pathway mediates OC differentiation and is involved in MM cell survival and migration, making it an appealing therapeutic target. In vitro and in vivo data showed that inhibition of CCL3 by antisense strategies prevents the development of osteolytic lesions and inhibits tumor growth [6]. Similar results have been shown with MLN3897 (Millennium Pharmaceuticals), a specific orally available CCR1 inhibitor. MLN3897 inhibits osteoclastogenesis and overcomes the proliferative advantage conferred by OC to MM cells [43]. Future clinical trials using CCR1 inhibition strategies in patients with MM-OBD will confirm these promising preliminary results.

10.4.4 BAFF Neutralizing Antibody

OC and MM cells interact by stimulating each others' growth and survival and a critical mediator in this interplay is the TNF family member, B-cell-activating factor (BAFF). BAFF is a MM growth factor derived from OC and BMSC and mediates both MM cell survival and MM-BMSC adhesion [22, 63]. In vivo neutralizing antibodies against BAFF (Ely Lilly) significantly inhibits tumor burden and, importantly, reduces the number of lytic lesions and OC differentiation [64]. Based on these results, a clinical trial combining BAFF neutralizing antibody with bortezomib is currently ongoing.

10.4.5 RAP-011

Activin is a novel cytokine up-regulated in MM patients with advanced bone disease. It has a dual activity on bone remodeling, both stimulating OC differentiation and inhibiting OB formation. Activin can be targeted by a chimeric antibody RAP-011 (Acceleron Pharma, Cambridge, MA), derived from the fusion of the extracellular domain of activin receptor IIA and the constant domain of the murine IgG2a [65]. Inhibition of activin A via both RAP-011 and neutralizing antibody against activin leads to increased OB differentiation and inhibits OC development in vitro. In murine models of osteoporosis and MM-OBD, RAP-011 treatment improved bone density and prevented osteolytic lesions. Moreover, RAP-011 effectively reduced tumor growth [66]. The humanized counterpart of RAP-011, ACE-011 effectively inhibited bone resorption markers and stimulated bone formation parameters in postmenopausal women. Ongoing clinical trials are evaluating its role in the MM setting.

10.4.6 DKK1 Antagonists

As recently shown, DKK1 plays a key role in mediating OB inhibition in MM [23], therefore treatment strategies to block DKK1 activity have been developed. In vitro assays demonstrate that DKK1 inhibition via specific neutralizing antibody promote OBs differentiation and function and reverse the negative effect of MM cells on OBs formation [67, 68]. Moreover, in vivo studies using both murine and humanized models of MM-induced bone disease showed increased bone formation, OBs number, and improvement of osteolytic lesions by DKK1 inhibition [67, 69, 70]. Importantly, blocking DKK1 resulted also in reduction of tumor growth, mainly as indirect effect via modification of the tumor microenvironment [67]. Therefore, DKK1 inhibition via neutralizing antibody restores bone homeostasis and may have an inhibitory effect on tumor growth. Currently ongoing clinical trials combining DKK1 neutralizing antibody and BPs will confirm these promising preclinical results.

10.4.7 Thalidomide Analogues

Thalidomide derivatives with immunomodulatory functions like Revlimid or lenalidomide and Actimid or pomalidomide display a direct inhibitory effect on MM growth [71], moreover they affect the microenvironment by regulating the immune response and inhibiting angiogenesis [72, 73]. Recent studies also suggest a role for these agents as inhibitors of OC development. Both Revlimid and Actimid down-regulate PU.1 expression in OC precursor cells. PU.1 is an early transcription factor involved in monocytic cell commitment to OC differentiation [74, 75]. Lenalidomide also inhibits RANKL secretion by BMSCs and the RANKL/OPG balance is restored in patients treated with lenalidomide. Immunomodulatory derivatives of thalidomide (IMiDs) therefore have a broad range of effects affecting tumor growth directly and indirectly by alteration of the tumor microenvironment.

10.4.8 Bortezomib

Bortezomib is a proteasome and NF-kB signaling pathway inhibitor with potent anti-MM activity. Bortezomib also inhibits MM–BMSC interactions, impairs osteo-clastogenesis, and stimulates mesenchymal stem cell differentiation to OB, and therefore actively modulates bone remodeling in MM [76–78]. The anabolic effects of bortezomib are associated with RUNX2 up-regulation via inhibition of proteasomal degradation. RUNX2 is a critical transcription factor in early OB differentiation and modulates the expression of the OB-specific transcription factor, osterix [78, 79]. The anti-OC effects of bortezomib are mediated by p38 MAPK inhibition at early timepoints and, at later timepoints, by impairment of NF-kB signaling and AP1 inhibition [77]. These effects have been confirmed in the clinical setting by up-regulation of OB activation markers and down-regulation of bone-resorption markers in patients treated with bortezomib [80].

10.4.9 Signaling Pathways Inhibitors

Several signaling pathways are involved in MM cell growth and survival, but they also modulate MM-BMSC interactions and OC differentiation. Therefore, specific inhibition of these pathways leads to both anti-tumor effects and alterations in the MM niche.

MAPK inhibitors, like extracellular signal-regulated kinases (ERK) and p38 MAPK inhibitors, block early OC differentiation and in "in vivo" models of MM, they control tumor growth and reduce OCs number [49, 81].

Heat shock protein (HSP)90 inhibitors, in particular SNX-2112, showed a broad range of effects on the MM microenvironment [82]. Importantly, the anti-OC effects of SNX-2112 were mediated by down-regulation of ERK signaling and the transcription factors c-fos and PU.1.

10.5 Future Perspectives

Although OCs are a critical player in the pathogenesis of bone disease, other cell types such as OBs and BMSCs are affected in MM and contribute to the development of osteolysis. Therefore, effective therapeutic strategies to overcome MM-induced bone disease should target the OB/OC axis, combining bone-anabolic with anti-catabolic effects. Current clinical trials are studying the benefits of combination strategies such as BAFF inhibitors and bortezomib, or DKK1 neutralizing antibodies and bisphosphonates. Novel agents with dual activity on bone remodeling such as ACE-011 may also result in improvement of bone disease besides prevention of osteolytic lesions.

Importantly, OC, OBs, and BMSCs along with immune cells and endothelial cells constitute the bone marrow niche that regulates tumor cell growth, survival, and chemoresistance. Recent in vitro and in vivo data suggest that manipulating the niche by increasing OBs and decreasing OCs may inhibit tumor growth [7, 24]. Therefore, agents restoring bone balance in MM represents a novel strategy to overcome osteolytic disease and, more provocatively, to create a hostile niche for MM tumor growth.

References

1. Saad F, Lipton A, Cook R, Chen YM, Smith M, Coleman R. Pathologic fractures correlate with reduced survival in patients with malignant bone disease. Cancer. 2007;110:1860–1867.
2. Sonmez M, Akagun T, Topbas M, et al. Effect of pathologic fractures on survival in multiple myeloma patients: a case control study. J Exp Clin Cancer Res. 2008;27:11.
3. Valentin-Opran A, Charhon SA, Meunier PJ, Edouard CM, Arlot ME. Quantitative histology of myeloma-induced bone changes. Br J Haematol. 1982;52:601–610.
4. Taube T, Beneton MN, McCloskey EV, Rogers S, Greaves M, Kanis JA. Abnormal bone remodelling in patients with myelomatosis and normal biochemical indices of bone resorption. Eur J Haematol. 1992;49:192–198.
5. Bataille R, Chappard D, Marcelli C, et al. Mechanisms of bone destruction in multiple myeloma: the importance of an unbalanced process in determining the severity of lytic bone disease. J Clin Oncol. 1989;7:1909–1914.
6. Choi SJ, Oba Y, Gazitt Y, et al. Antisense inhibition of macrophage inflammatory protein 1-alpha blocks bone destruction in a model of myeloma bone disease. J Clin Invest. 2001;108:1833–1841.
7. Edwards CM, Edwards JR, Lwin ST, et al. Increasing Wnt signaling in the bone marrow microenvironment inhibits the development of myeloma bone disease and reduces tumor burden in bone in vivo. Blood. 2008;111:2833–2842.
8. Gupta GP, Massague J. Cancer metastasis: building a framework. Cell. 2006;127:679–695.
9. Kalluri R, Zeisberg M. Fibroblasts in cancer. Nat Rev Cancer. 2006;6:392–401.
10. Calabrese C, Poppleton H, Kocak M, et al. A perivascular niche for brain tumor stem cells. Cancer Cell. 2007;11:69–82.
11. Ame-Thomas P, Maby-El Hajjami H, Monvoisin C, et al. Human mesenchymal stem cells isolated from bone marrow and lymphoid organs support tumor B-cell growth: role of stromal cells in follicular lymphoma pathogenesis. Blood. 2007;109:693–702.
12. Hideshima T, Mitsiades C, Tonon G, Richardson PG, Anderson KC. Understanding multiple myeloma pathogenesis in the bone marrow to identify new therapeutic targets. Nat Rev Cancer. 2007;7:585–598.
13. Dierks C, Grbic J, Zirlik K, et al. Essential role of stromally induced hedgehog signaling in B-cell malignancies. Nat Med. 2007;13:944–951.
14. Chauhan D, Uchiyama H, Akbarali Y, et al. Multiple myeloma cell adhesion-induced interleukin-6 expression in bone marrow stromal cells involves activation of NF-kappa B. Blood. 1996;87:1104–1112.
15. Roodman GD. Mechanisms of bone metastasis. N Engl J Med. 2004;350:1655–1664.
16. Giuliani N, Rizzoli V, Roodman GD. Multiple myeloma bone disease: Pathophysiology of osteoblast inhibition. Blood. 2006;108:3992–3996.
17. Roodman GD. New potential targets for treating myeloma bone disease. Clin Cancer Res. 2006;12:6270s–6273s.

18. Damiano JS, Cress AE, Hazlehurst LA, Shtil AA, Dalton WS. Cell adhesion mediated drug resistance (CAM-DR): role of integrins and resistance to apoptosis in human myeloma cell lines. Blood. 1999;93:1658–1667.
19. Lentzsch S, Gries M, Janz M, Bargou R, Dorken B, Mapara MY. Macrophage inflammatory protein 1-alpha (MIP-1 alpha) triggers migration and signaling cascades mediating survival and proliferation in multiple myeloma (MM) cells. Blood. 2003;101:3568–3573.
20. Abe M, Hiura K, Wilde J, et al. Osteoclasts enhance myeloma cell growth and survival via cell-cell contact: a vicious cycle between bone destruction and myeloma expansion. Blood. 2004;104:2484–2491.
21. Podar K, Anderson KC. The pathophysiologic role of VEGF in hematologic malignancies: therapeutic implications. Blood. 2005;105:1383–1395.
22. Tai YT, Li XF, Breitkreutz I, et al. Role of B-cell-activating factor in adhesion and growth of human multiple myeloma cells in the bone marrow microenvironment. Cancer Res. 2006;66:6675–6682.
23. Tian E, Zhan F, Walker R, et al. The role of the Wnt-signaling antagonist DKK1 in the development of osteolytic lesions in multiple myeloma. N Engl J Med. 2003;349: 2483–2494.
24. Yaccoby S, Wezeman MJ, Zangari M, et al. Inhibitory effects of osteoblasts and increased bone formation on myeloma in novel culture systems and a myelomatous mouse model. Haematologica. 2006;91:192–199.
25. Li X, Pennisi A, Yaccoby S. Role of decorin in the antimyeloma effects of osteoblasts. Blood. 2008;112:159–168.
26. Zhao C, Irie N, Takada Y, et al. Bidirectional ephrinB2-EphB4 signaling controls bone homeostasis. Cell Metab. 2006;4:111–121.
27. Mancino AT, Klimberg VS, Yamamoto M, Manolagas SC, Abe E. Breast cancer increases osteoclastogenesis by secreting M-CSF and upregulating RANKL in stromal cells. J Surg Res. 2001;100:18–24.
28. Moschen AR, Kaser A, Enrich B, et al. The RANKL/OPG system is activated in inflammatory bowel disease and relates to the state of bone loss. Gut. 2005;54:479–487.
29. Giuliani N, Bataille R, Mancini C, Lazzaretti M, Barille S. Myeloma cells induce imbalance in the osteoprotegerin/osteoprotegerin ligand system in the human bone marrow environment. Blood. 2001;98:3527–3533.
30. Seidel C, Hjertner O, Abildgaard N, et al. Serum osteoprotegerin levels are reduced in patients with multiple myeloma with lytic bone disease. Blood. 2001;98:2269–2271.
31. Giuliani N, Colla S, Sala R, et al. Human myeloma cells stimulate the receptor activator of nuclear factor-kappa B ligand (RANKL) in T lymphocytes: a potential role in multiple myeloma bone disease. Blood. 2002;100:4615–4621.
32. Lai FP, Cole-Sinclair M, Cheng WJ, et al. Myeloma cells can directly contribute to the pool of RANKL in bone bypassing the classic stromal and osteoblast pathway of osteoclast stimulation. Br J Haematol. 2004;126:192–201.
33. Giuliani N, Colla S, Morandi F, Barille-Nion S, Rizzoli V. Lack of receptor activator of nuclear factor-kB ligand (RANKL) expression and functional production by human multiple myeloma cells. Haematologica. 2005;90:275–278.
34. Standal T, Seidel C, Hjertner O, et al. Osteoprotegerin is bound, internalized, and degraded by multiple myeloma cells. Blood. 2002;100:3002–3007.
35. Pearse RN, Sordillo EM, Yaccoby S, et al. Multiple myeloma disrupts the TRANCE/ osteoprotegerin cytokine axis to trigger bone destruction and promote tumor progression. Proc Natl Acad Sci USA. 2001;98:11581–11586.
36. Croucher PI, Shipman CM, Lippitt J, et al. Osteoprotegerin inhibits the development of osteolytic bone disease in multiple myeloma. Blood. 2001;98:3534–3540.
37. Terpos E, Politou M, Szydlo R, et al. Autologous stem cell transplantation normalizes abnormal bone remodeling and sRANKL/osteoprotegerin ratio in patients with multiple myeloma. Leukemia. 2004;18:1420–1426.

38. Terpos E, Mihou D, Szydlo R, et al. The combination of intermediate doses of thalidomide with dexamethasone is an effective treatment for patients with refractory/relapsed multiple myeloma and normalizes abnormal bone remodeling, through the reduction of sRANKL/osteoprotegerin ratio. Leukemia. 2005;19:1969–1976.
39. Terpos E, Politou M, Szydlo R, Goldman JM, Apperley JF, Rahemtulla A. Serum levels of macrophage inflammatory protein-1 alpha (MIP-1alpha) correlate with the extent of bone disease and survival in patients with multiple myeloma. Br J Haematol. 2003;123:106–109.
40. Masih-Khan E, Trudel S, Heise C, et al. MIP-1alpha (CCL3) is a downstream target of FGFR3 and RAS-MAPK signaling in multiple myeloma. Blood. 2006;108:3465–3471.
41. Han JH, Choi SJ, Kurihara N, Koide M, Oba Y, Roodman GD. Macrophage inflammatory protein-1alpha is an osteoclastogenic factor in myeloma that is independent of receptor activator of nuclear factor kappaB ligand. Blood. 2001;97:3349–3353.
42. Oyajobi BO, Franchin G, Williams PJ, et al. Dual effects of macrophage inflammatory protein-1alpha on osteolysis and tumor burden in the murine 5TGM1 model of myeloma bone disease. Blood. 2003;102:311–319.
43. Vallet S, Raje N, Ishitsuka K, et al. MLN3897, a novel CCR1 inhibitor, impairs osteoclastogenesis and inhibits the interaction of multiple myeloma cells and osteoclasts. Blood. 2007;110:3744–3752.
44. Giuliani N, Lisignoli G, Colla S, et al. CC-Chemokine ligand 20/macrophage inflammatory protein-3alpha and CC-chemokine receptor 6 are overexpressed in myeloma microenvironment related to osteolytic bone lesions. Cancer Res. 2008;68:6840–6850.
45. Lee JW, Chung HY, Ehrlich LA, et al. IL-3 expression by myeloma cells increases both osteoclast formation and growth of myeloma cells. Blood. 2004;103:2308–2315.
46. Giuliani N, Morandi F, Tagliaferri S, et al. Interleukin-3 (IL-3) is overexpressed by T lymphocytes in multiple myeloma patients. Blood. 2006;107:841–842.
47. Ehrlich LA, Chung HY, Ghobrial I, et al. . IL-3 is a potential inhibitor of osteoblast differentiation in multiple myeloma. Blood. 2005;106:1407–1414.
48. Giuliani N, Colla S, Morandi F, et al. Myeloma cells block RUNX2/CBFA1 activity in human bone marrow osteoblast progenitors and inhibit osteoblast formation and differentiation. Blood. 2005;106:2472–2483.
49. Ishitsuka K, Hideshima T, Neri P, et al. p38 mitogen-activated protein kinase inhibitor LY2228820 enhances bortezomib-induced cytotoxicity and inhibits osteoclastogenesis in multiple myeloma; therapeutic implications. Br J Haematol. 2008;141:598–606.
50. Nguyen AN, Stebbins EG, Henson M, et al. Normalizing the bone marrow microenvironment with p38 inhibitor reduces multiple myeloma cell proliferation and adhesion and suppresses osteoclast formation. Exp Cell Res. 2006;312:1909–1923.
51. Hiruma Y, Kurihara N, Jelinek DF, Roodman D. Increased signaling through p62 in the marrow microenvironment increases myeloma cell growth and osteoclast formation. Blood. 2008;112:239.
52. Qiang YW, Chen Y, Stephens O, et al. Myeloma-derived Dickkopf-1 disrupts Wnt-regulated osteoprotegerin and RANKL production by osteoblasts: a potential mechanism underlying osteolytic bone lesions in multiple myeloma. Blood. 2008;112:196–207.
53. Weinstein RS, Roberson PK, Manolagas SC. Giant osteoclast formation and long-term oral bisphosphonate therapy. N Engl J Med. 2009;360:53–62.
54. Berenson JR, Lichtenstein A, Porter L, et al. Efficacy of pamidronate in reducing skeletal events in patients with advanced multiple myeloma. Myeloma Aredia Study Group. N Engl J Med. 1996;334:488–493.
55. Aparicio A, Gardner A, Tu Y, Savage A, Berenson J, Lichtenstein A. In vitro cytoreductive effects on multiple myeloma cells induced by bisphosphonates. Leukemia. 1998;12:220–229.
56. Gnant M, Mlineritsch B, Schippinger W, et al. Endocrine therapy plus zoledronic acid in premenopausal breast cancer. N Engl J Med. 2009;360:679–691.
57. Kyle RA, Yee GC, Somerfield MR, et al. American Society of Clinical Oncology 2007 clinical practice guideline update on the role of bisphosphonates in multiple myeloma. J Clin Oncol. 2007;25:2464–2472.

58. Raje N, Woo SB, Hande K, et al. Clinical, radiographic, and biochemical characterization of multiple myeloma patients with osteonecrosis of the jaw. Clin Cancer Res. 2008;14:2387–2395.
59. Orriss IR, Key ML, Colston KW, Arnett TR. Inhibition of osteoblast function in vitro by aminobisphosphonates. J Cell Biochem. 2009;106:109–118.
60. Vanderkerken K, De Leenheer E, Shipman C, et al. Recombinant osteoprotegerin decreases tumor burden and increases survival in a murine model of multiple myeloma. Cancer Res. 2003;63:287–289.
61. Body JJ, Greipp P, Coleman RE, et al. A phase I study of AMGN-0007, a recombinant osteoprotegerin construct, in patients with multiple myeloma or breast carcinoma related bone metastases. Cancer. 2003;97:887–892.
62. Fizazi K, Lipton A, Mariette X, et al. Randomized phase II trial of denosumab in patients with bone metastases from prostate cancer, breast cancer, or other neoplasms after intravenous bisphosphonates. J Clin Oncol. 2009;27:1564–1571.
63. Abe M, Kido S, Hiasa M, et al. BAFF and APRIL as osteoclast-derived survival factors for myeloma cells: a rationale for TACI-Fc treatment in patients with multiple myeloma. Leukemia. 2006;20:1313–1315.
64. Neri P, Kumar S, Fulciniti MT, et al. Neutralizing B-cell activating factor antibody improves survival and inhibits osteoclastogenesis in a severe combined immunodeficient human multiple myeloma model. Clin Cancer Res. 2007;13:5903–5909.
65. Pearsall RS, Canalis E, Cornwall-Brady M, et al. A soluble activin type IIA receptor induces bone formation and improves skeletal integrity. Proc Natl Acad Sci USA. 2008;105:7082–7087.
66. Vallet S, Mukherjee S, Vaghela N, et al. Restoration of bone balance via activin a inhibition results in anti-myeloma activity. Blood. 2008;112:240.
67. Fulciniti M, Tassone P, Hideshima T, et al. . Anti-DKK1 mAb (BHQ880) as a potential therapeutic for multiple myeloma. Blood. 2007;110:551.
68. Pozzi S, Yan H, Vallet S, et al. Preclinical validation of a novel Dkk-1 neutralizing antibody for the treatment of multiple myeloma related bone disease. ASBMR 30th annual meeting. 2008:Su239.
69. Yaccoby S, Ling W, Zhan F, Walker R, Barlogie B, Shaughnessy JD Jr. Antibody-based inhibition of DKK1 suppresses tumor-induced bone resorption and multiple myeloma growth in vivo. Blood. 2007;109:2106–2111.
70. Heath DJ, Chantry AD, Buckle CH, et al. Inhibiting Dickkopf-1 (Dkk1) removes suppression of bone formation and prevents the development of osteolytic bone disease in multiple myeloma. J Bone Miner Res, 2009;24:425–436.
71. Mitsiades N, Mitsiades CS, Poulaki V, et al. Apoptotic signaling induced by immunomodulatory thalidomide analogs in human multiple myeloma cells: therapeutic implications. Blood. 2002;99:4525–4530.
72. Davies FE, Raje N, Hideshima T, et al. Thalidomide and immunomodulatory derivatives augment natural killer cell cytotoxicity in multiple myeloma. Blood. 2001;98:210–216.
73. Lentzsch S, LeBlanc R, Podar K, et al. Immunomodulatory analogs of thalidomide inhibit growth of Hs Sultan cells and angiogenesis in vivo. Leukemia. 2003;17:41–44.
74. Anderson G, Gries M, Kurihara N, et al. Thalidomide derivative CC-4047 inhibits osteoclast formation by down-regulation of PU.1. Blood. 2006;107:3098–3105.
75. Breitkreutz I, Raab MS, Vallet S, et al. Lenalidomide inhibits osteoclastogenesis, survival factors and bone-remodeling markers in multiple myeloma. Leukemia. 2008;22:1925–1932.
76. Zangari M, Esseltine D, Lee CK, et al. Response to bortezomib is associated to osteoblastic activation in patients with multiple myeloma. Br J Haematol. 2005;131:71–73.
77. von Metzler I, Krebbel H, Hecht M, et al. Bortezomib inhibits human osteoclastogenesis. Leukemia. 2007;21:2025–2034.
78. Mukherjee S, Raje N, Schoonmaker JA, et al. Pharmacologic targeting of a stem/progenitor population in vivo is associated with enhanced bone regeneration in mice. J Clin Invest. 2008;118:491–504.

79. Giuliani N, Morandi F, Tagliaferri S, et al. The proteasome inhibitor bortezomib affects osteoblast differentiation in vitro and in vivo in multiple myeloma patients. Blood. 2007;110:334–338.

80. Terpos E, Heath DJ, Rahemtulla A, et al. Bortezomib reduces serum dickkopf-1 and receptor activator of nuclear factor-kappaB ligand concentrations and normalises indices of bone remodelling in patients with relapsed multiple myeloma. Br J Haematol. 2006;135:688–692.

81. Breitkreutz I, Raab MS, Vallet S, et al. Targeting MEK1/2 blocks osteoclast differentiation, function and cytokine secretion in multiple myeloma. Br J Haematol. 2007;139:55–63.

82. Okawa Y, Hideshima T, Steed P, et al. SNX-2112, a selective Hsp90 inhibitor, potently inhibits tumor cell growth, angiogenesis, and osteoclastogenesis in multiple myeloma and other hematologic tumors by abrogating signaling via Akt and ERK. Blood. 2009;113:846–855.

Chapter 11
Potential Role of IMiDs and Other Agents as Therapy for Myeloma Bone Disease

Suzanne Lentzsch

Abstract Multiple myeloma (MM) is a plasma cell malignancy characterized by the frequent development of bone lesions (Lentzsch et al. Hematol Oncol Clin North Am 21:1035–1049, 2007). The development of osteolytic lesions is attributable to increased bone resorption caused by stimulation of osteoclast formation and activity (Barille-Nion and Bataille Leuk Lymphoma 44:1463–1467, 2003), (Giuliani et al. Exp Hematol 32:685–691, 2004), and (Roodman Blood Cells Mol Dis 32:290–292, 2004). The increased osteoclast activity is accompanied by decreased osteoblast function resulting in imbalanced bone remodeling, which increases bone resorption and decreases bone formation (Bataille et al. J Clin Oncol 7:1909–1914, 1989) and (Bataille et al. Br J Haematol 76:484–487, 1990). Bisphosphonate therapy targets the inhibition of osteoclast activity. But unfortunately bisphosphonates are associated with side effects such as renal toxicity and osteonecrosis of the jaw. Therefore new drugs capable of targeting activated osteoclasts without completely arresting bone resorption and remodeling are needed. In this chapter, the author discusses potential new drugs which target osteoclast formation and activity and which also lack severe side effects and provide a potential effective treatment for bone disease in MM.

Keywords IMiDs · PU.1 · NF-κB · RANKL · MIP-1α · Signaling pathways

11.1 Introduction

Multiple myeloma (MM) is an incurable plasma cell malignancy characterized by the development of osteolytic lesions. More than 80% of MM patients develop osteopenia or osteolytic lesions which result in >50% of all patients suffering

S. Lentzsch (✉)
Assistant Professor of Medicine, Division of Hematology/Oncology, University of Pittsburgh, Pittsburgh, PA, USA
e-mail: lentzschs@upmc.edu

G.D. Roodman (ed.), *Myeloma Bone Disease*, Current Clinical Oncology, DOI 10.1007/978-1-60761-554-5_11, © Springer Science+Business Media, LLC 2010 pathologic fractures during the course of their disease [1]. The development of osteolytic lesions is due to increased bone resorption that is caused by the stimulation of osteoclast (OCL) formation and activity [2–4]. The increased OCL activity is accompanied by decreased or absent osteoblast function resulting in uncoupling of normal bone remodeling in which increased bone resorption is no longer linked to new bone formation [5, 6]. Bisphosphonate therapy targets the inhibition of OCL activity resulting in diminished bone resorption. Unfortunately, bisphosphonate therapy can be associated with severe side effects such as renal toxicity and osteonecrosis of the jaw which is believed to be linked with drug-induced irreversible cessation of bone remodeling. Additionally, the use of bisphosphonates in the face of significant impairment of renal function is difficult and may be contraindicated. New drugs capable of targeting activated OCLs or inhibiting OCL formation without completely arresting bone resorption and remodeling are needed. Over the last year, several drugs have been shown to be potent OCL inhibitors, such as the immunomodulatory drugs (IMiDs), e.g., thalidomide, or non-steroidal anti-inflammatory drugs (NSAIDs) such as etodolac derivatives SDX-308 and SDX-101. In addition, the broader knowledge and deeper insight into the pathophysiology of increased OCL activity in MM provide more targets for the inhibition of OCL formation/activity.

11.2 Effects of IMiDs on OCLs

IMiDs such as lenalidomide and pomalidomide are immunomodulatory drugs which are derivatives of thalidomide. Both drugs have been shown to be highly effective in the treatment of MM [7, 8]. Anderson et al. were the first to report that pomalidomide, which is a derivative of thalidomide and has similar actions to lenalidomide, inhibited OCL development by affecting the lineage commitment of OCL precursors [9]. Pomalidomide downregulated the expression of PU.1, a transcription factor critical for the development of OCLs. The downregulation of PU.1 in CD34$^+$ cells resulted in a complete shift of lineage differentiation toward myeloid progenitors and away from OCLs. The group later showed that neutrophil maturation was also inhibited due to downregulation of PU.1 [10]. The results of Anderson et al. are in accordance with previous results reporting the function of PU.1. It is known that PU.1 knock-out mice develop osteopetrosis due to a complete shutdown of OCL activity [11]. Anderson et al. showed that the downregulation of PU.1 inhibited OCL maturation and also completely inhibited bone resorption activity. The group did not observe any toxic effects on hematopoietic progenitors as determined by colony formation assays. The inhibition of formation of mature multinucleated OCLs in marrow cultures was accompanied by the production of a population of small cells that overgrew the cultures and lacked the features of OCLs. The group showed that pomalidomide acted especially at the early stage of OCL differentiation, and significant inhibition of OCL formation was observed at concentrations of 1 μM, which is similar or even lower than that achieved in vivo after therapeutic administration of this agent. In this study, the authors reported that thalidomide exhibited similar but less potent effects than pomalidomide, suggesting that thalidomide is less potent than pomalidomide in the inhibition of OCL formation [9].

Breitkreutz et al. showed that lenalidomide also inhibited OCL formation through similar mechanisms, such as downregulation of PU.1 expression. In this study lenalidomide inhibited OCL differentiation in a dose-dependent manner. The median percentage of OCLs identified by flow cytometry analysis using anti-αVβ3-integrin antibodies decreased from 69% without lenalidomide to 50% when lenalidomide was added at 2 μM to the culture system and to 39% when lenalidomide was added at 10 μM. Lenalidomide also reduced tartrate-resistant acid phosphatase positive (TRAP$^+$) OCLs and bone resorption. In accordance with the reports from Anderson et al., lenalidomide did not alter the numbers of mature OCLs. This group also found that lenalidomide strongly inhibited the B cell activation factor (BAFF) and a proliferation producing ligand (APRIL) that are also major MM growth and survival factors and may be produced by OCLs [12]. They concluded that the reduction of OCL formation seems to break a vicious cycle between MM cells and OCLs, leading to further reduction of tumor burden and bone resorption. Unfortunately, the inhibitory effect on OCLs induced by IMiDs was not associated with the stimulating effect on osteoblast activity or bone formation in the preclinical setting. In addition, there are no data available from clinical trials supporting the role of IMiDs on osteoblast activity in the clinical setting.

Two clinical phase II trials have studied the effects of thalidomide on bone disease in patients with MM. Terpos et al. showed that thalidomide in combination with dexamethasone reduced bone resorption in 35 patients with relapsed and refractory MM [13]. Patients received thalidomide at a dose of 200 mg/day and dexamethasone 40 mg/day for 4 days every 15 days until maximum response was achieved. Patients had the option to continue on treatment until disease progression if they showed response or stable disease. All patients received zoledronic acid at the time of diagnosis and continued to receive zoledronic acid at a dose of 4 mg every 28 days while on study. In this study, the treatment produced a significant reduction of the bone resorption markers CTX and TRACP-5b in the third month of treatment. This continued until the sixth month of treatment. The treatment also reduced soluble receptor activator of nuclear factor-κB ligand (sRANKL) levels and sRANKL/OPG ratio at 6 months after treatment initiation. Furthermore, there was strong correlation between the changes of sRANKL/OPG ratio and changes of TRACP-5b and CTX, suggesting that the reduction of bone resorption by thalidomide is most likely due to reduction of RANKL levels. Terpos et al. showed further that despite the reduction of bone resorption and response of MM to treatment, there was no effect on bone formation as assessed by serum levels of bone alkaline phosphatase (bALP) and osteocalcin (OC) [13]. Another study by Tosi et al. showed that thalidomide reduced bone resorption in newly diagnosed MM patients [14]. In this study the patients received a combination of thalidomide 100 mg/day for 14 days which was subsequently increased to 200 mg/day and dexamethasone 40 mg/day 4 days on and 4 days off during odd cycles and only day 1–4 on even cycles. Again, zoledronic acid was given 4 mg every 28 days for 4 months. Tosi et al. observed a significant reduction in the urinary NTX and serum CTX bone resorption markers. The reduction of bone resorption markers was only associated with a detection of a MM response. The reduction of bone resorption markers was also associated with a reduction of bone pain in 60% of the patients. However, in accordance with the studies from Terpos et al., markers of bone formation such as bALP and OC were not increased and showed a slight reduction, suggesting that the combined regimen might also have negative effects on osteoblasts possibily due to dexamethasone.

There is only limited information on the effect of IMiDs on bone metabolism. Breitkreutz et al. published data on 20 MM patients showing that lenalidomide significantly decreased RANKL and RANKL/OPG ratio and significantly increased OPG [12].

11.3 Inhibition of OCL Activity by Targeting Nuclear Factor-κB (NF-κB) Signaling

SDX-308 is a NSAID lacking COX inhibitory effects [15]. Due to the lack of the COX inhibitory activity, SDX-308 has a more favorable safety profile than its parent substance S-etodolac. It was shown by Yasui et al. that SDX-308 has potent anti-myeloma activity [16]. They showed that SDX-308 induced cytotoxicity in dexamethasone–doxorubicin–melphalan-resistant MM cell lines as well as in bortezomib-resistant lymphoma/leukemia cell lines and in primary patient MM cells. Further, the presence of IL-6, IGF-1, and bone marrow stromal cells could not overcome the growth inhibitory effects of SDX-308 on MM cells. The anti-myeloma effect was associated with a lack of cytotoxicity at high concentrations of SDX-308 on normal peripheral blood mononuclear cells or bone marrow mononuclear cells, suggesting selective cytotoxicity against tumor cells.

Feng et al. investigated SDX-101 and SDX-308 for their capacity to inhibit OCL formation. The investigators used a human bone marrow culture system to assess OCL formation and showed that the development of OCLs derived from healthy bone marrow and MM bone marrow was completely inhibited by SDX-308 at concentrations as low as 3 µM. The inhibition of OCL formation was accompanied by complete suppression of bone resorption [17]. Time course experiments showed that SDX-308 did not preferentially affect a particular stage of OCL development in human bone marrow cultures from healthy donors and MM patients. They found that SDX-308 had no toxic effects on hematopoietic progenitors as determined in colony formation assays using purified CD34$^+$ cells. Since RANKL-induced NF-κB activation and plays a central role in OCL formation [18], Feng et al. examined the effects of SDX-308 on NF-κB activity in OCLs. They showed that SDX-308 inhibited constitutive and RANKL-induced NF-κB activation in the murine OCL RAW 264.7 cells by blocking phosphorylation and nuclear translocation of p65 as well as by blocking phosphorylation of IκB-α. They used RAW 264.7 cells transiently transfected with NF-κB luciferase reporter gene and measured the RANKL-stimulated luciferase activity. SDX-308 significantly suppressed

RANKL-induced NF-κB activation, suggesting that SDX-308 not only inhibits OCL formation but also inhibits activity of mature OCLs (Fig. 11.1). This result suggests that SDX-308 may be a promising candidate for the treatment of MM since it is both directly cytotoxic to MM and suppresses OCL formation and function, and might thereby restore osteoblast function (Fig. 11.2). Despite the fact that SDX-308 has fewer unwanted side effects due to significant COX-1 and COX-2 inhibitions, it still might exert some adverse side effects associated with NSAIDs. These side effects include gastrointestinal side effects such as nausea, vomiting, dyspepsia, gastric ulceration, bleeding, or diarrhea, as well as renal side effects such as fluid retention and hypertension. Therefore, SDX-308 should be carefully tested in future phase I trials.

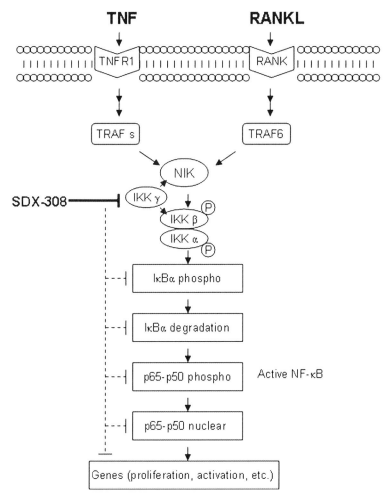

Fig. 11.1 Effects of SDX-308 on TNF-α and RANKL-activated NF-κB pathways. (Figure provided by Feng and Lentzsch [40])

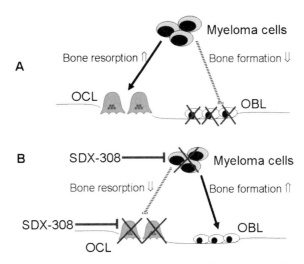

Fig. 11.2 (**a**) Imbalance between bone resorption and bone formation in MM. MM cells induce the activation of OCLs resulting in increased bone resorption. At the same time, osteoblast activity is inhibited, resulting in decreased bone formation. (**b**) SDX-308 inhibits the proliferation and survival of MM cells and OCLs, and therefore disturbs the signal between the myeloma cells and the OCLs. This results in decreased bone resorption. Since fewer MM cells secrete inhibitory cytokines to osteoblasts, the osteoblast activity could be restored resulting in increased bone formation

A similar mechanism of OCL inhibition by decreasing NF-κB activation was reported by Sung et al. They showed that zerumbone abolishes RANKL-induced NF-κB activation in mouse monocytes, an OCL precursor cell. Zerumbone also suppressed RANKL-induced differentiation of these cells to OCLs and also decreased osteoblasts in tumor-bearing athymic nude mice [19].

11.4 Targeting RANKL for Inhibition of OCL Activity

RANKL is responsible for OCL-mediated bone resorption in a broad range of hematological conditions and plays a key role in MM bone disease. Denosumab (AMG 162) is a fully human monoclonal antibody that binds RANKL with high affinity and specificity and inhibits RANKL–RANK interaction. This interaction mimics the endogenous effects of OPG that is a sRANKL decoy receptor. A phase I clinical trial in healthy postmenopausal women and patients with MM or breast cancer showed that single and multiple subcutaneous injections of denosumab caused rapid and sustained suppression of bone resorption markers with a favorable safety profile [20]. A phase II trial of denosumab as a single agent in patients with plateau phase or progressive MM showed that denosumab significantly inhibited skeletal-related events but did not significantly decrease the tumor burden [21]. A phase III trial of denosumab in patients with bone metastases and osteoporosis is ongoing, but preliminary results showed that denosumab had little or no toxicity.

11.5 Targeting MIP-1α for Inhibition of OCL Activity

Macrophage inflammatory protein (MIP-1α) belongs to the RANTES (Regulated upon Activation, Normal T cell Expressed, and Secreted) family of chemokines and is a chemoattractant and activator of phagocytes [22]. MIP-1α is also a chemotactic factor for OCL precursors and can induce differentiation of OCL progenitors and contributes to OCL formation [23–26]. MIP-1α is produced and secreted by MM cells, and the levels correlate with the severity of MM bone disease [23, 27–29]. MIP-1α antibodies or blocking antibodies against the receptor CCR5, and transfection of MM cells with antisense constructs to MIP-1α, blocked enhanced bone resorption in murine models of MM bone disease [23, 30]. Furthermore, MIP-1α can enhance RANKL expression in stromal cells and thereby indirectly increase osteoclastogenesis [23].

Vallet et al. investigated a novel MIP-1α receptor inhibitor (MLN3897). MLN3897 is a specific antagonist of the chemokine receptor CCR1. MLN3897 demonstrated a significant impairment of OCL formation (by 40%) and function (by 70%) associated with decreased precursor cell multinucleation and downregulation of c-fos signaling. OCLs secrete high levels of MIP-1α which triggers MM cell migration, and conversely, MLN3897 abrogated its effects by inhibiting Akt signaling. MLN3897 inhibited MM cell-to-OCL adhesion and thereby inhibited MM cell survival and proliferation. The authors concluded that this drug shows novel biologic potency for inhibition of MIP-1α in both osteoclastogenesis and MM cell growth, providing the preclinical rationale for clinical trials of MLN3897 to treat bone disease in MM [31].

11.6 Targeting Signaling Pathways Relevant for OCL Activity and OCL Formation

11.6.1 Targeting ERK Signaling

The extracellular signal-regulated protein kinase (ERK1/2) pathway mediates OCL differentiation and maturation. Breitkreutz et al. investigated whether the inhibition of ERK1/2 prevents OCL differentiation and downregulation of OCL function. For this purpose they used AZD6244, a mitogen-activated or extracellular signal-regulated protein kinase (MEK) inhibitor. AZD6244 blocked OCL differentiation and formation in a dose-dependent manner, as evidenced by decreased αVβ3-integrin expression and the number of TRAP⁺ cells. Functional activity of OCLs on dentine disc cultures showed inhibition of OCL-induced bone resorption. Critical MM growth and survival factors produced by OCLs including BAFF and APRIL, as well as MIP-1α, were significantly inhibited. In addition to ERK1/2 inhibition, nuclear factor of activated T cells, cytoplasmic 1 (NFATc1) and c-fos were both downregulated, suggesting that AZD6244 targets a later stage of OCL differentiation. The authors concluded that AZD6244

inhibits OCL differentiation and bone resorption, providing the preclinical rationale for the evaluation of AZD6244 as a potential new therapy for patients
with MM.

Vanderkerken et al. investigated the inhibition of p38α mitogen-activated protein
kinase (MAPK) and observed the inhibition of the development of osteolytic bone
disease, reduced tumor burden, and increased survival in a murine model of MM
as determined by SCIO-469, a selective p38α MAPK. They found that SCIO-469
decreased constitutive p38α MAPK phosphorylation of both 5T2MM and 5T33MM
cells in vitro. Treatment of 5T2MM-injected mice with SCIO-469 reduced development of bone disease and decreased MM tumor burden. They postulate that targeting
p38α MAPK with SCIO-469 might decrease myeloma burden and help prevent
development of MM bone disease [32].

The same group also investigated geranylgeranyl transferase II (GGTase II) for
its ability to prevent MM bone disease. GGTase II is an enzyme that plays a key
role in the isoprenylation of proteins. They found that the GGTase II inhibitor
blocks bone resorption by significantly inhibiting OCL number and OCL surface area in their 5T2MM model of MM. They further showed that 3-PEHPC, a
novel GGTase II inhibitor, prevented bone loss and development of osteolytic bone
lesions [33].

KD5170 is a histone deacetylase (HDAC) inhibitor which has been shown in
vitro to inhibit not only OCL formation but also proliferation of MM cells by
interfering with the vicious cycle between MM cells and OCLs [34]. In addition,
recently another HDAC inhibitor, PXD101 was also shown to inhibit OCL formation synergistically with bortezomib [35]. Okawa et al. showed that SNX-2112, a
selective heat shock protein 90 (HSP90), markedly inhibited OCL formation via the
downregulation of ERK/c-fos and PU.1 [36].

Bortezomib has been shown to inhibit maturation and function of OCLs at
concentrations of 2.5 and 5 nM, and that bortezomib acted on osteoclastogenesis
at low concentrations by interfering with TRAF6 production [37]. Other proteasome inhibitors such as MG-132 and MG-262 reduce both OCL differentiation and
activity of mature OCLs in vitro [38, 39].

11.7 Conclusions

Novel anti-myeloma agents such as IMiDs, bortezomib, and more recent MEK1/2
and HDAC inhibitors decrease bone resorption either directly through the inhibition
of OCL formation or indirectly through the modification of interactions between
malignant plasma cells and OCLs. Thus, agents which directly target tumor-derived
factors or tumor-induced factors that increase bone destruction in MM patients
should be in clinical trials within the next few years. These agents in combination with agents that effect tumor growth will have a major effect on MM bone
disease.

References

1. Melton LJ 3rd, Chrischilles EA, Cooper C, Lane AW, Riggs BL. How many women have osteoporosis? JBMR Anniversary Classic. JBMR. 1992;7(9). J Bone Miner Res. 2005;20:886–892.
2. Barille-Nion S, Bataille R. New insights in myeloma-induced osteolysis. Leuk Lymphoma. 2003;44:1463–1467.
3. Giuliani N, Colla S, Rizzoli V. New insight in the mechanism of osteoclast activation and formation in multiple myeloma: focus on the receptor activator of NF-kappaB ligand (RANKL). Exp Hematol. 2004;32:685–691.
4. Roodman GD. Pathogenesis of myeloma bone disease. Blood Cells Mol Dis. 2004;32: 290–292.
5. Bataille R, Chappard D, Marcelli C, et al. Mechanisms of bone destruction in multiple myeloma: the importance of an unbalanced process in determining the severity of lytic bone disease. J Clin Oncol. 1989;7:1909–1914.
6. Bataille R, Chappard D, Marcelli C, et al. Osteoblast stimulation in multiple myeloma lacking lytic bone lesions. Br J Haematol. 1990;76:484–487.
7. Dimopoulos M, Spencer A, Attal M, et al. Lenalidomide plus dexamethasone for relapsed or refractory multiple myeloma. N Engl J Med. 2007;357:2123–2132.
8. Weber DM, Chen C, Niesvizky R, et al. Lenalidomide plus dexamethasone for relapsed multiple myeloma in North America. N Engl J Med. 2007;357:2133–2142.
9. Anderson G, Gries M, Kurihara N, et al. Thalidomide derivative CC-4047 inhibits osteoclast formation by down-regulation of PU.1. Blood. 2006;107:3098–3105.
10. Pal R, Monaghan SA, Mapara MY, et al. Immunomodulatory Derivatives (IMiDs) Induce PU.1 Downregulation, Myeloid Maturation Arrest and Neutropenia. Blood. 2010;115:605–614.
11. Tondravi MM, McKercher SR, Anderson K, et al. Osteopetrosis in mice lacking haematopoietic transcription factor PU.1. Nature. 1997;386:81–84.
12. Breitkreutz I, Raab MS, Vallet S, et al. Lenalidomide inhibits osteoclastogenesis, survival factors and bone-remodeling markers in multiple myeloma. Leukemia. 2008;22:1925–1932.
13. Terpos E, Mihou D, Szydlo R, et al. The combination of intermediate doses of thalidomide with dexamethasone is an effective treatment for patients with refractory/relapsed multiple myeloma and normalizes abnormal bone remodeling, through the reduction of sRANKL/osteoprotegerin ratio. Leukemia. 2005;19:1969–1976.
14. Tosi P, Zamagni E, Cellini C, et al. First-line therapy with thalidomide, dexamethasone and zoledronic acid decreases bone resorption markers in patients with multiple myeloma. Eur J Haematol. 2006;76:399–404.
15. Demerson CA, Humber LG, Abraham NA, Schilling G, Martel RR, Pace-Asciak C. Resolution of etodolac and antiinflammatory and prostaglandin synthetase inhibiting properties of the enantiomers. J Med Chem. 1983;26:1778–1780.
16. Yasui H, Hideshima T, Ikeda H, et al. Novel etodolac analog SDX-308 (CEP-18082) induces cytotoxicity in multiple myeloma cells associated with inhibition of beta-catenin/TCF pathway. Leukemia. 2007;21:535–540.
17. Feng R, Anderson G, Xiao G, et al. SDX-308, a nonsteroidal anti-inflammatory agent, inhibits NF-{kappa}B activity, resulting in strong inhibition of osteoclast formation/activity and multiple myeloma cell growth. Blood. 2007;109:2130–2138.
18. Yasuda H, Shima N, Nakagawa N, et al. Osteoclast differentiation factor is a ligand for osteoprotegerin/osteoclastogenesis-inhibitory factor and is identical to TRANCE/RANKL. Proc Natl Acad Sci USA. 1998;95:3597–3602.
19. Sung B, Murakami A, Oyajobi BO, Aggarwal BB. Zerumbone abolishes RANKL-induced NF-kappaB activation, inhibits osteoclastogenesis, and suppresses human breast cancer-induced bone loss in athymic nude mice. Cancer Res. 2009;69:1477–1484.

20. Body JJ, Facon T, Coleman RE, et al. A study of the biological receptor activator of nuclear factor-kappaB ligand inhibitor, denosumab, in patients with multiple myeloma or bone metastases from breast cancer. Clin Cancer Res. 2006;12:1221–1228.
21. Vij R, Horvath N, Spencer A, et al. An open-label, phase 2 trial of denosumab in the treatment of Relapsed (R) or Plateau-Phase (PP) Multiple Myeloma (MM). Blood. 2007;110:3604.
22. Cook DN. The role of MIP-1 alpha in inflammation and hematopoiesis. J Leukoc Biol. 1996;59:61–66.
23. Abe M, Hiura K, Wilde J, et al. Role for macrophage inflammatory protein (MIP)-1alpha and MIP-1beta in the development of osteolytic lesions in multiple myeloma. Blood. 2002;100:2195–2202.
24. Fuller K, Owens JM, Chambers TJ. Macrophage inflammatory protein-1 alpha and IL-8 stimulate the motility but suppress the resorption of isolated rat osteoclasts. J Immunol. 1995;154:6065–6072.
25. Kukita T, Nomiyama H, Ohmoto Y, et al. Macrophage inflammatory protein-1 alpha (LD78) expressed in human bone marrow: its role in regulation of hematopoiesis and osteoclast recruitment. Lab Invest. 1997;76:399–406.
26. Lentzsch S, Gries M, Janz M, Bargou R, Dorken B, Mapara MY. Macrophage inflammatory protein 1-alpha (MIP-1 alpha) triggers migration and signaling cascades mediating survival and proliferation in multiple myeloma (MM) cells. Blood. 2003;101:3568–3573.
27. Choi SJ, Cruz JC, Craig F, et al. Macrophage inflammatory protein 1-alpha is a potential osteoclast stimulatory factor in multiple myeloma. Blood. 2000;96:671–675.
28. Hashimoto T, Abe M, Oshima T, et al. Ability of myeloma cells to secrete macrophage inflammatory protein (MIP)-1alpha and MIP-1beta correlates with lytic bone lesions in patients with multiple myeloma. Br J Haematol. 2004;125:38–41.
29. Uneda S, Hata H, Matsuno F, et al. Macrophage inflammatory protein-1 alpha is produced by human multiple myeloma (MM) cells and its expression correlates with bone lesions in patients with MM. Br J Haematol. 2003;120:53–55.
30. Choi SJ, Oba Y, Gazitt Y, et al. Antisense inhibition of macrophage inflammatory protein 1-alpha blocks bone destruction in a model of myeloma bone disease. J Clin Invest. 2001;108:1833–1841.
31. Vallet S, Raje N, Ishitsuka K, et al. MLN3897, a novel CCR1 inhibitor, impairs osteoclastogenesis and inhibits the interaction of multiple myeloma cells and osteoclasts. Blood. 2007;110:3744–3752.
32. Vanderkerken K, Medicherla S, Coulton L, et al. Inhibition of p38alpha mitogen-activated protein kinase prevents the development of osteolytic bone disease, reduces tumor burden, and increases survival in murine models of multiple myeloma. Cancer Res. 2007;67:4572–4577.
33. Lawson MA, Coulton L, Ebetino FH, Vanderkerken K, Croucher PI. Geranylgeranyl transferase type II inhibition prevents myeloma bone disease. Biochem Biophys Res Commun. 2008;377:453–457.
34. Feng R, Ma H, Hassig CA, et al. KD5170, a novel mercaptoketone-based histone deacetylase inhibitor, exerts antimyeloma effects by DNA damage and mitochondrial signaling. Mol Cancer Ther. 2008;7:1494–1505.
35. Feng R, Oton A, Mapara MY, Anderson G, Belani C, Lentzsch S. The histone deacetylase inhibitor, PXD101, potentiates bortezomib-induced anti-multiple myeloma effect by induction of oxidative stress and DNA damage. Br J Haematol. 2007;139:385–397.
36. Okawa Y, Hideshima T, Steed P, et al. SNX-2112, a selective Hsp90 inhibitor, potently inhibits tumor cell growth, angiogenesis, and osteoclastogenesis in multiple myeloma and other hematologic tumors by abrogating signaling via Akt and ERK. Blood. 2009;113:846–855.
37. Hongming H, Jian H. Bortezomib inhibits maturation and function of osteoclasts from PBMCs of patients with multiple myeloma by downregulating TRAF6. Leuk Res. 2009;33:115–122.
38. von Metzler I, Krebbel H, Hecht M, et al. Bortezomib inhibits human osteoclastogenesis. Leukemia. 2007;21:2025–2034.

39. Zavrski I, Krebbel H, Wildemann B, et al. Proteasome inhibitors abrogate osteoclast differentiation and osteoclast function. Biochem Biophys Res Commun. 2005;333:200–205.
40. Feng R, Lentzsch S. Treatment of multiple myeloma with SDX-308. Drug News Perspect. 2007 Sep;20(7):431–435.

Chapter 12
Proteasome Inhibitors and the Wnt Signaling Pathway in Myeloma Bone Disease

Claire M. Edwards and Gregory R. Mundy

Abstract One of the major clinical features of multiple myeloma is the development of a unique osteolytic bone disease, characterized by progressive and devastating bone destruction, bone pain, pathological fractures and hypercalcemia. As our understanding of the molecular mechanisms involved in the development of myeloma bone disease increases, new approaches have been identified for the treatment of this devastating bone disease. These include the ubiquitin–proteasome system and the Wnt signaling pathway, both of which represent novel therapeutic targets for the treatment of myeloma bone disease.

Keywords Multiple myeloma · Bone disease · Proteasome inhibition · Wnt signaling · Dkk1

12.1 Introduction

One of the most common features of multiple myeloma is the development of a progressive and destructive osteolytic bone disease, which is a major cause of morbidity for patients with multiple myeloma. This osteolytic bone disease is characterized by severe bone pain, pathological fractures, hypercalcemia and spinal cord compression. Myeloma sometimes presents with a generalized osteoporosis, which substantially increases the risk of developing a pathological fracture. Myeloma bone disease is a significant clinical problem, for which there is, as yet, no effective cure. Bisphosphonates are potent inhibitors of osteoclastic bone resorption, and are the standard therapy for myeloma-induced bone disease, however, they are limited by their inability to repair existing bone lesions. Novel therapeutic targets for the treatment of myeloma bone disease have been identified, which include the

C.M. Edwards (✉)
Departments of Cancer Biology and Clinical Pharmacology/Medicine,
Vanderbilt Center for Bone Biology, Vanderbilt University Medical Center, Nashville, TN, USA
e-mail: claire.edwards@vanderbilt.edu

G.D. Roodman (ed.), *Myeloma Bone Disease*, Current Clinical Oncology,
DOI 10.1007/978-1-60761-554-5_12, © Springer Science+Business Media, LLC 2010

RANK/RANKL/OPG system, proteasome inhibitors, and Wnt signaling, and their efficacy in myeloma bone disease is currently under investigation in preclinical models of myeloma.

In order to develop novel therapeutic strategies, it is important to identify the cellular and molecular processes involved in the development of myeloma bone disease. In normal bone remodeling, bone resorption and bone formation are tightly coupled, with bone formation occurring at sites of prior bone resorption. Patients with multiple myeloma have abnormal bone remodeling, where resorption and formation become uncoupled, with the end result being an increase in bone resorption and a decrease in bone formation. Histomorphometric studies have demonstrated that bone resorption is increased in patients with multiple myeloma, with an increase in both the number and activity of osteoclasts [1–3]. The increase in resorption is thought to be an early event in the development of myeloma bone disease [3]. Although early stages of multiple myeloma have been associated with an increase in osteoblast recruitment, a very marked impairment of bone formation due to reduced osteoblast number and activity is a common feature in the later stages of the osteolytic bone disease [3–5]. This has been confirmed in recent studies which demonstrate that markers of bone formation are decreased in patients with multiple myeloma [6, 7].

The majority of patients with multiple myeloma have discrete osteolytic lesions occurring in areas of myeloma cell infiltration. Myeloma cells are found in close association with sites of active bone resorption, and the interactions between myeloma cells, osteoclasts, and osteoblasts are crucial both for the development of the osteolytic bone disease and for myeloma cell growth and survival in the bone marrow [8, 9]. Myeloma cells secrete a number of osteoclast-activating factors which can promote osteoclast formation and activation, including lymphotoxin, TNF-α, IL-1, IL-3, and IL-6 [10–13]. While in vitro studies have demonstrated a role for these factors in the development of myeloma bone disease, their role in vivo remains unclear. Cell–cell contact between myeloma cells and bone marrow stromal cells is critically important in the development of myeloma bone disease and plays a key role in the abnormal regulation of factors implicated in myeloma bone disease, including RANKL, OPG, and Dkk1. Over recent years, our understanding of the osteoclastogenic and osteoblastic factors involved in the development of myeloma bone disease has dramatically increased. Factors which have been implicated include RANKL, OPG, MIP-1α, Dkk1, and sFRP-2. Many of these factors have been demonstrated to be dysregulated in patients with multiple myeloma, and all play a role in either bone resorption or bone formation. Thus, these factors represent potential therapeutic targets for the treatment of myeloma bone disease.

12.2 Targeting the Ubiquitin Proteasome System in Multiple Myeloma

The proteasome is the main nonlysosomal intracellular machinery in eukaryotic cells for proteolytic degradation of cytoplasmic and nuclear proteins involved in a number of key biological processes, including cell cycle progression, transcriptional activation, signal transduction, and apoptosis. Proteins that are targeted for degradation are covalently attached to multiple molecules of ubiquitin by the sequential actions of specific ubiquitin ligases. The ubiquitinated protein is then escorted to the proteasome, where it undergoes degradation, and the ubiquitin is released and recycled. Proteasomes are large multisubunit protease complexes that are located in the nucleus and the cytosol. The 26S proteasome complex contains a 20S proteasome core, which contains multiple peptidase activities, including chymotrypsin-like, trypsin-like, and caspase-like activities. The regulatory unit of the 26S proteasome is the 19S unit, which consists of polypeptide subunits including ATPases, a de-ubiquitinating enzyme and polyubiquitin-binding subunits. Once a protein has been ubiquitinated, it is recognized by the 19S subunit in an ATP-dependent-binding step and the 19S subunit regulates entry of ubiquitinated proteins into the 20S core. The overall process of ubiquitination and proteasomal degradation is known as the ubiquitin–proteasome system.

The ubiquitin–proteasome pathway is essential for normal cellular function, and is important for the breakdown of misfolded proteins in response to cellular stress. The ubiquitin–proteasome pathway has been implicated in several forms of malignancy, in the pathogenesis of several genetic diseases, and in diseases associated with muscle wasting. Inhibition of proteasome function prevents the normal elimination of misfolded proteins, leading to an accumulation of these proteins resulting in cell death. Thus, proteasome inhibitors have emerged as novel anticancer agents, limited primarily by their inherent mechanism of action and the ubiquitous nature of the proteasome resulting in toxicity from proteasome inhibition in normal nonmalignant cells. In multiple myeloma, the malignant plasma cells are highly sensitive to proteasome inhibitors when compared with normal lymphocytes, and the use of proteasome inhibitors has emerged as a highly effective therapeutic approach for the treatment of patients with myeloma. Of particular interest is the discovery that additional cell types within the bone marrow are also sensitive to proteasome inhibition, including osteoblasts. Therefore, proteasome inhibitors have the potential to directly target both the tumor and bone disease directly in multiple myeloma.

Initial in vitro studies identified myeloma cells as highly sensitive to proteasome inhibitors, undergoing apoptosis in response to these agents. Subsequent preclinical studies confirmed the powerful antimyeloma effect of proteasome inhibitors, in particular, the dipeptide boronic acid bortezomib. Bortezomib was initially found to reduce myeloma tumor burden in a human plasmacytoma xenograft model, with an effect on both tumor growth and angiogenesis. Data accrued from phase I and phase II clinical trials demonstrated the remarkable therapeutic efficacy and acceptable toxicity profiles of bortezomib in patients with advanced or refractory myeloma. This led to its fast-tracked approval by the FDA for use in relapsed refractory myeloma, which was subsequently extended to include patients with progressive myeloma after previous treatment. More recently, bortezomib has been approved for treatment of newly diagnosed myeloma when used in combination with melphalan and prednisolone. Despite the success of bortezomib, it is associated with off-target toxicities and drug resistance, and therefore there are extensive attempts to delineate the precise molecular mechanism of action and validate novel proteasome inhibitors for their use in multiple myeloma.

12.3 Proteasome Inhibition in Myeloma Bone Disease

The tremendous impact that proteasome inhibition as a therapeutic strategy is having in the clinical management of myeloma is all the more relevant because of the accumulating evidence for a direct effect of proteasome inhibition to prevent myeloma bone disease. The initial evidence for this came from Garrett et al., who demonstrated that proteasome inhibitors could act directly on osteoblasts to stimulate osteoblast differentiation and bone formation in vitro and in vivo [14]. Other studies have also suggested that proteasome inhibitors may have direct effects to inhibit osteoclastic bone resorption. These preclinical studies are supported by clinical studies to suggest that bortezomib treatment is associated with increases in markers of bone formation. Although, to date, there are no studies which directly investigate the effect of bortezomib on myeloma bone disease by studying skeletal-related events, all evidence points toward a direct effect of bortezomib to prevent myeloma bone disease. Since tumor burden and bone disease are inextricably linked in multiple myeloma, the ideal therapeutic agents are those which target both aspects of the vicious cycle, such as proteasome inhibitors.

12.3.1 Preclinical Studies

Garret and colleagues provided the first evidence that proteasome inhibitors may have direct effects to promote osteoblast differentiation and bone formation [14]. They demonstrated that a series of structurally distinct proteasome inhibitors could stimulate bone formation in cultures of neonatal murine calvarial bones. The proteasome inhibitors PS1 and epoxomicin were demonstrated to increase trabecular bone volume and bone formation rates in vivo, with similar effects to well-characterized bone anabolic agents. The bone anabolic effects were observed at concentrations as low as 10 nM, which is similar to the concentrations used to induce myeloma cell apoptosis in vitro, suggesting that osteoblasts may also be highly sensitive to proteasome inhibition in vivo. In support of this, Garret et al. also demonstrated a positive correlation between inhibition of proteasome activity and stimulation of bone formation. Further mechanistic studies demonstrated that the effect of proteasome inhibitors to stimulate bone formation was mediated via BMP-2, and that this was dependent upon inhibition of the proteolytic processing of Gli-3. More recently, the bone anabolic effect of the proteasome inhibitor bortezomib has been directly linked to the Wnt signaling antagonist Dkk1. Oyajobi and colleagues demonstrate that bortezomib can directly stimulate new bone formation in mouse calvarial cultures, and that this anabolic effect can be inhibited by Dkk1 [15]. In vitro studies suggest that proteasome inhibitors can decrease the expression of Dkk1 in osteoblasts and bone marrow stromal cells. Taken together, these studies clearly demonstrate that proteasome inhibitors, including bortezomib, have direct effects on osteoblasts, both in vitro and in vivo, to stimulate new bone formation.

In addition to direct effects on osteoblasts, a recent study has suggested that bortezomib targets mesenchymal stem cells in vivo, and stimulates these multipotent

cells to undergo osteoblastic differentiation resulting in an increase in bone formation [16]. In vitro studies confirmed the effect of bortezomib to increase osteoblast
differentiation and concomitantly decrease adipocyte differentiation. This effect of
bortezomib is mediated by stabilization of activity of Runx-2, a critical transcription
factor required for osteoblastic differentiation. Mukherjee et al. also demonstrated
that bortezomib increased trabecular bone volume and bone formation in ovariec-
tomized mice, providing the first evidence that bortezomib could increase bone
volume in a disease state in vivo [16]. In support of an effect of bortezomib on
osteoblast progenitor cells, as opposed to mature osteoblasts, Giuliani and coworkers demonstrated that bortezomib could induce osteoblast differentiation in human
mesenchymal stem cells, and that this was associated with an increase in Runx2
expression [17]. Bortezomib was not found to have any effect on the proliferation or apoptosis of more mature osteoblast-like cells. Qiang and colleagues have
recently demonstrated that the effect of bortezomib to induce osteoblast differentiation from osteoprogenitor cells and mesenchymal stem cells is dependent upon the
stabilization of β-catenin and subsequent increase in β-catenin/TCF signaling [18].

Although their focus was primarily on the effect of proteasome inhibitors on
osteoblasts or mesenchymal stem cells, both Garret et al. and Mukherjee et al.
found no effect of proteasome inhibition on osteoclast formation in vitro. This
is in contrast to studies by Zavrski et al., who demonstrated that the proteasome
inhibitors MG-132 and MG-262 both inhibited RANKL-mediated osteoclast formation and bone resorption at nanomolar concentrations [19]. These effects on
osteoclasts correlated with inhibition of NFkB activity, which is known to be critical for osteoclast formation and activity. Furthermore, Von Metzler and colleagues
have also observed that bortezomib prevented osteoclast differentiation and subsequent bone resorption in a dose- and time-dependent manner [20]. Hongming and
Jian have recently demonstrated that bortezomib inhibits osteoclast differentiation
from peripheral blood mononuclear cells from patients with multiple myeloma, by
reducing TRAF6 expression [21]. It is unclear why such different effects of proteasome inhibition on osteoclast activity would be observed, however, these may reflect
differences in the compounds and/or concentrations used. Of note, Garret et al.
observed a slight reduction in osteoclast number in vivo following treatment with
proteasome inhibitors; however, this did not reach statistical significance. Given the
magnitude of new bone formed in response to treatment with proteasome inhibitors,
it is unlikely that this is due solely to an inhibition of osteoclastic bone resorption.
However, it is of interest that proteasome inhibition may not only directly promote
osteoblast differentiation and bone formation, but may also inhibit osteoclastic bone
resorption.

The potential for proteasome inhibitors to target both tumor burden and
osteoblastic bone formation has tremendous therapeutic implications for the treatment of myeloma bone disease. The effect of bortezomib on myeloma bone disease
in vivo was examined in a preclinical murine model of myeloma, the SCID-rab
model [22]. In this model, human myeloma cells are engrafted into fetal rabbit
bones implanted into immune-compromised mice. Bortezomib treatment was associated with a reduction in tumor burden and an increase in bone mineral density. Of

interest, when the results were subdivided into responders and nonresponders with respect to the effect of bortezomib to reduce tumor burden, bortezomib treatment was found to have a greater effect to increase bone mineral density in responders. The effect of bortezomib treatment was compared with that of melphalan, which has direct antimyeloma effects but no direct effect on bone. Only bortezomib prevented myeloma bone disease suggesting that these effects of bortezomib were not a consequence of reduced tumor burden but a direct effect on bone cells. The increase in bone mineral density was associated with an increase in osteoblast number and bone formation rates, and a significant reduction in TRAP-positive osteoclasts. Bortezomib was found to have a similar effect, to promote osteoblastogenesis and inhibit osteoclastogenesis in normal nonmyeloma-bearing mice. Since myeloma growth and survival is dependent upon critical factors within the bone marrow microenvironment, modulation of this environment by bortezomib has the potential to indirectly reduce tumor burden by rendering this environment inhospitable for myeloma growth. Using the well-characterized 5TGM1 murine model of myeloma, Edwards et al. have recently demonstrated that myeloma cells exhibit a greater response to proteasome inhibition when located within the bone microenvironment, as compared with extraosseous sites [23]. Their results also suggest that myeloma cells may be more sensitive to proteasome inhibitors when located within the bone marrow. Taken together, these studies demonstrate the effect of bortezomib to prevent myeloma bone disease and the critical role for the bone marrow microenvironment in the dramatic response to bortezomib in multiple myeloma.

12.3.2 Clinical Studies

The use of bortezomib in the treatment of multiple myeloma was initially a direct result of the powerful antimyeloma effect of these compounds. The emergence of preclinical evidence to suggest that bortezomib may also have direct effects to prevent myeloma bone disease has led to a number of clinical studies, which have reported effects of bortezomib on markers of both bone formation and bone resorption. To date, there are no clinical studies which have directly investigated the effect of bortezomib on myeloma bone disease by measuring skeletal-related events, such as bone volume or fracture.

Shimazaki et al. observed that treatment of a patient with refractory myeloma with bortezomib-combined therapy (bortezomib plus incadronate and dexamethasone) resulted in an increase in serum bone-specific alkaline phosphatase (BAP) and total alkaline phosphatase (ALP), indicating an effect of this combined treatment on osteoblast differentiation [24]. Zangari et al. also observed significant increases in ALP in patients responding to bortezomib treatment [25]. Subsequent analysis of two large bortezomib trials (Study of Uncontrolled Multiple Myeloma managed with Proteasome Inhibition Therapy (SUMMIT) and Assessment of Proteasome Inhibition for Extending Remission (APEX)) demonstrated that response to bortezomib was associated with a significant increase in ALP, which occurred within the first three cycles of therapy and correlated with a reduction in tumor burden. In three patients treated with single-agent bortezomib following relapse after transplantation, response to bortezomib was associated with an increase in ALP, BAP, and parathyroid hormone (PTH), suggesting that the response to bortezomib may be due to osteoblast activation. The marker of osteoblast differentiation, alkaline phosphatase, was also found to predict the quality and duration of response to bortezomib treatment in multiple myeloma. Analysis of the APEX study determined that at least a 25% increase in ALP from baseline at week 6 was the strongest predictor of response to bortezomib and time to disease progression [26].

Heider and colleagues analyzed serum markers of osteoblast activity in patients receiving either bortezomib alone, bortezomib in combination with dexamethasone or patients receiving a different non-bortezomib therapy [27]. A significant increase in BAP and osteocalcin was observed in patients treated with bortezomib. In contrast to previous studies, the increase in BAP was observed in both those patients who did respond to bortezomib and in those patients who did not have a significant reduction in tumor burden. Those patients receiving a non-bortezomib therapy had no increase in either BAP or osteocalcin. Taken together, these data suggest that the effects of bortezomib to increase markers of bone formation are specific to proteasome inhibition and are not merely due to a reduction in tumor burden, indicating a direct effect of bortezomib to increase bone formation in patients with multiple myeloma. Ozaki and colleagues also observed an increase in ALP, BAP, and osteocalcin in patients with relapsed or refractory myeloma receiving bortezomib and dexamethasone [28]. Furthermore, radiographic examination demonstrated an improvement in bone lesions, providing evidence that bortezomib may be able to repair existing lesions.

In contrast to those studies investigating only serum markers of bone formation, Giuliani and colleagues investigated the effect of single-agent bortezomib treatment of patients with relapsed or refractory myeloma by analysis of bone marrow biopsies [17]. They observed an increase in the number of osteoblasts lining the bone surface in those patients who responded to bortezomib treatment, although bortezomib treatment was not able to restore osteoblast number to that of healthy nonmyeloma controls. An increase in osteoid surface was also observed, and an increase in Runx2-positive osteoblasts, supporting preclinical evidence for a role for Runx2 in the osteoblastic response to bortezomib.

In addition to the measurement of serum markers of bone formation, Terpos and colleagues investigated the effect of bortezomib treatment on additional markers of bone remodeling, including factors associated with myeloma bone disease, sRANKL and Dkk1, and markers of osteoclastic bone remodeling C-terminal cross-linking telopeptide of collagen type-I (CTX) and TRACP-5b. Bortezomib treatment was found to increase BAP and osteocalcin, and to decrease serum Dkk1, sRANKL, CTX, and TRACP-5b, and these changes were observed irrespective of response to therapy. This study suggests that bortezomib can normalize bone remodeling, and that bortezomib may target both osteoblasts and osteoclasts [29]. Further evidence of an effect of bortezomib on osteoclastic bone resorption in vivo is provided by Uy and colleagues, who investigated the effects of bortezomib in patients with myeloma who received bortezomib before and after autologous stem cell transplantation

[30]. Bortezomib treatment was found to decrease urinary N-terminal cross-linking telopeptide of collagen type-1 (NTX), and these effects were in the absence of bisphosphonate treatment and not associated with changes in tumor burden. Boissy et al. demonstrate that bortezomib treatment causes an immediate decrease in CTX and NTX in patients with multiple myeloma, but that these concentrations begin to increase after 3 days, suggesting that osteoclast activity is recovering [31].

Proteasome inhibitors represent an important therapeutic advance in the treatment of myeloma (Fig. 12.1), made all the more exciting by their potential to have direct effects to target both the tumor and the bone disease. Preclinical studies provide compelling evidence to suggest that bortezomib can regulate remodeling, with both direct effects to promote bone formation and inhibit osteoclastic bone resorption. These are strongly supported by clinical data linking bortezomib to markers of both bone formation and bone resorption. Interpretation of the clinical data is complicated by the multiple drug regimens. Furthermore, it is difficult to delineate direct effects on myeloma bone disease from indirect effects as a result of reduction in tumor burden, as have been previously demonstrated with bisphosphonates. Future studies investigating bortezomib as a single agent, and designed to specifically evaluate the effect of bortezomib on bone mineral density and skeletal-related

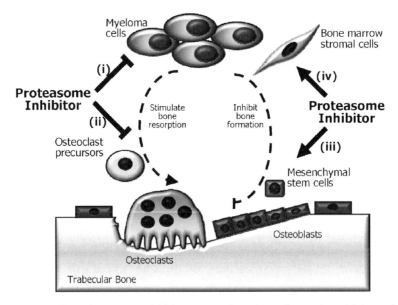

Fig. 12.1 The effect of proteasome inhibitors on myeloma bone disease. In multiple myeloma, osteoclastic bone resorption is increased, whereas osteoblastic bone formation is suppressed, resulting in the development of an osteolytic bone disease. Proteasome inhibitors have several proposed mechanisms of action to prevent myeloma bone disease. (i) Directly inducing myeloma cell apoptosis. (ii) Inhibition of osteoclastic bone resorption. (iii) Acting on osteoblasts and mesenchymal stem cells to promote osteoblastic differentiation and bone formation. (iv) Acting on bone marrow stromal cells to regulate RANKL and Dkk1 expression

events will provide critical information as to the potential for bortezomib to directly treat myeloma bone disease.

12.4 Wnt Signaling Pathway in Bone Biology

Wnts are secreted glycoproteins that activate receptor-mediated signaling pathways, which play critical roles in cell development and differentiation both in embryogenesis and in adults [32]. Canonical Wnt signaling is transduced by two transmembrane protein receptor families; frizzled proteins and lipoprotein receptor-related proteins 5 and 6 (LRP5/6). In the absence of Wnts, glycogen synthase kinase-3β, axin, adenomatous polyposis coli (APC), and casein kinase Iα (CKIα) form a complex which phosphorylates β-catenin and targets it for degradation by the proteasome. Activation of the canonical Wnt signaling pathway occurs when Wnt binds to one of the frizzled protein receptors. This ligand–receptor complex then binds to LRP5/6 which results in the removal of axin from its complex, so preventing β-catenin phosphorylation. This results in the translocation of β-catenin to the nucleus and activation of downstream target genes.

There are two classes of extracellular antagonists of the Wnt signaling pathway, with distinct inhibitory mechanisms, acting either by binding directly to Wnt (secreted FRPs, WIF-1) or by binding to part of the Wnt receptor complex (Dickkopf (Dkk) family). Dkk1 binds to LRP5/6 and so prevents LRP5/6 from interacting with the Wnt-frizzled complex. The Wnt signaling pathway plays a key role in many cellular processes, and the activity of the pathway is the result of a fine balance between extracellular ligands and antagonists coupled with the complex regulation of the intracellular components of the pathway. Dysregulation of the Wnt signaling pathway is a feature of many degenerative disorders and malignancies.

The Wnt signaling pathway plays a key role in the regulation of bone mass [33]. Inactivating mutations in the gene for LRP5 result in osteoporosis-pseudoglioma syndrome in humans, whereas "gain of function" mutations in LRP5 are associated with a syndrome of hereditary high bone density [34, 35]. In vivo genetic mouse models provide evidence for the function of the Wnt signaling pathway and its soluble antagonists in bone biology. Overexpression of β-catenin in osteoblasts has been demonstrated to induce osteoblast proliferation and a high bone mass phenotype [36]. Transgenic mice overexpressing the soluble antagonist of Wnt, Dkk1 in osteoblasts develop severe osteopenia, whereas deletion of a single allele of Dkk1 caused an increase in bone mass [37, 38]. LRP5-deficient mice have a low bone mass, whereas mice which express a mutant form of LRP5 which is unable to bind to Dkk1 exhibit a high bone mass phenotype [36, 39]. Several Wnt ligands have been associated with the differentiation of mesenchymal stem cells down the osteoblast lineage, and an increase in β-catenin is associated with osteoblast formation. Dkk1 is expressed by osteoblasts and bone marrow stromal cells, and has been demonstrated to inhibit bone formation in osteoblasts in vitro [40]. Dkk1 is thought to counteract the effects of Wnt on osteoblast formation by switching mesenchymal stem cell differentiation from osteoblastic differentiation in favor of adipogenesis [41, 42]. The importance of Wnt signaling in the regulation of bone mass has raised the possibility that this signaling pathway may be important in diseases associated with abnormal bone formation, including multiple myeloma.

12.5 Wnt Signaling in Myeloma Bone Disease

The first evidence for a role for the Wnt signaling pathway, and specifically Dkk1, in myeloma bone disease came from a study by Tian and colleagues, which demonstrated that patients with multiple myeloma had increased expression of Dkk1 that correlated with the extent of the osteolytic bone disease [43]. This work has paved the way for extensive studies into the role of Dkk1 and Wnt signaling in myeloma bone disease, addressing the regulation of Wnt signaling in myeloma, the therapeutic potential of manipulating this pathway for the treatment of myeloma bone disease, and the complex balance of Wnt signaling in myeloma cells versus the tumor microenvironment.

12.5.1 Dkk1 Expression

Tian et al. initially identified Dkk1 as overexpressed in patients with multiple myeloma by cDNA microarray [43]. Further analysis revealed an increase in both serum and bone marrow plasma Dkk1 concentrations which correlated with osteolytic bone lesions. Low expression of Dkk1 was observed in patients with monoclonal gammopathy of undetermined significance (MGUS) and in myeloma patients with no focal lesions by MRI, whereas high levels of Dkk1 expression were detected in myeloma patients with one or more osteolytic lesions by MRI. Despite the correlation with myeloma bone disease, an increase in Dkk1 expression was not detected in patients with advanced disease, which was attributed to a dependence upon microenvironmental interactions which are most prominent during early stages of disease development.

Since the initial observation by Tian et al. there have been several studies which have investigated Dkk1 expression in patients with multiple myeloma. Politou et al. found a significant increase in serum Dkk1 in newly diagnosed patients with myeloma, as compared with MGUS or healthy controls, whereas no difference was detected between MGUS and controls [44]. Further analysis of Dkk1 concentrations following autologous stem cell transplantation demonstrated that Dkk1 concentrations were decreased, whereas markers of bone formation were elevated. Gene expression analysis from patients with newly diagnosed multiple myeloma, MGUS, or controls demonstrated a strong correlation between overexpression of Dkk1 and osteolytic bone disease, as assessed by radiography [45]. In support of the initial study by Tian and colleagues, a larger study has demonstrated a significant correlation between serum Dkk1 concentration and the number of osteolytic bone lesions [46].

In addition to a clear association with osteolytic bone disease, several studies have also examined serum Dkk1 concentrations in response to antimyeloma treatment. Terpos et al. demonstrated a significant reduction in Dkk1 concentrations in patients with relapsed myeloma, following treatment with bortezomib [29]. Heider and colleagues demonstrated a significant decrease in serum Dkk1 following treatment with bortezomib, lenalidomide, or adriamycin and dexamethasone plus high-dose chemotherapy followed by autologous stem cell transplantation. In addition, treatment with thalidomide also decreased serum Dkk1, however, this did not reach significance. In all cases, a significant decrease in Dkk1 was only observed in those patients who responded to the antimyeloma treatment [47].

The initial study by Tian and colleagues, combined with the critical role of Wnt signaling in the regulation of bone mass, suggested a major role for Dkk1 in the pathogenesis of myeloma bone disease. Tian et al. demonstrated that osteoblast differentiation was blocked by bone marrow serum from patients with myeloma, and the inhibitory effect was found to be due to Dkk1 [43].

In most normal human tissues, Dkk1 is expressed at low levels, however it is expressed by bone marrow stromal cells and osteoblasts. Dkk1 is expressed by human myeloma cells, and it is this expression that is thought to result in the high serum concentrations of Dkk1 detected in patients with multiple myeloma. Dkk1 is also expressed at both the mRNA and protein level in the majority of myeloma cell lines and in primary myeloma cells isolated from patients with multiple myeloma [48]. The regulation of Dkk1 expression in myeloma cells is poorly understood. Dkk1 is known to be a direct transcriptional target of β-catenin, and thought to mediate a negative feedback loop in the Wnt signaling pathway [49]. Colla and colleagues demonstrated that osteoclasts both support myeloma cell survival and decrease Dkk1 expression by modulation of the JNK pathway [50]. In contrast to the observations from clinical trials, they demonstrated that treatment with thalidomide and lenalidomide increased expression of Dkk1 by myeloma cells. Furthermore, they observed that oxidative stress could stimulate Dkk1 expression, and that this was the mechanism for the effect of lenalidomide. Taken together these results suggest that modulation of the JNK pathway be a novel approach for regulation of Dkk1 in multiple myeloma.

In addition to Dkk1, Oshima and colleagues have identified a role for another antagonist of the Wnt signaling pathway, sFRP-2, in myeloma bone disease [51]. Initial studies demonstrated that conditioned media from human myeloma cell lines and primary myeloma cells could inhibit osteoblastic differentiation in vitro. The cells were found to constitutively produce sFRP-2, and when sFRP-2 was depleted from the conditioned media, the effect on osteoblast differentiation was blocked, demonstrating a role for myeloma cell-derived sFRP-2 in the suppression of bone formation.

12.5.2 Mechanism of Action of Dkk1 in Multiple Myeloma

Dkk1 is now thought to play a critical role in the suppression of osteoblasts that is a major part of myeloma bone disease. Tian and coworkers found that osteoblast differentiation was blocked by bone marrow serum from patients with myeloma, and the inhibitory effect was found to be the result of Dkk1 in the serum [43]. Subsequent studies demonstrated that plasma from patients with myeloma could inhibit canonical Wnt signaling in osteoblasts, and that this plasma contained high concentrations of Dkk1. Furthermore, recombinant Dkk1 could inhibit Wnt-3A-induced β-catenin accumulation and BMP-2-mediated osteoblast differentiation [52]. Qiang and colleagues also demonstrated that myeloma-derived Dkk1 disrupted Wnt3A-mediated OPG and RANKL expression in osteoblasts [53] (Fig. 12.2). Primary myeloma cells were found to decrease Wnt-3A-induced OPG expression by osteoblasts. Serum from patients with myeloma was found to suppress Wnt-3A-mediated OPG expression, and this effect was prevented by pretreatment with a neutralizing antibody to Dkk1. Serum from myeloma patients containing high

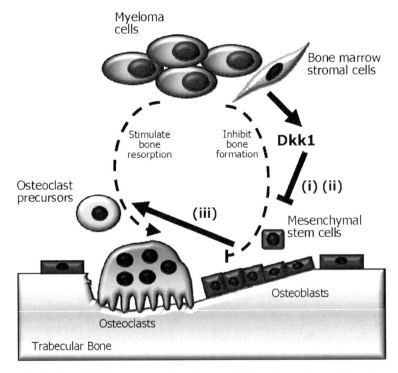

Fig. 12.2 The role of Dkk1 in myeloma bone disease. Myeloma is associated with an increase in Dkk1, both from myeloma cells and bone marrow stromal cells. (i) Dkk1 acts to suppress osteoblas-togenesis by inhibiting osteoblast differentiation from mesenchymal stem cells. (ii) Dkk1 regulates RANKL and OPG expression by osteoblasts. (iii) The upregulation of RANKL and downregulation of OPG result in an increase in osteoclast formation and bone resorption

Dkk1 concentrations was found to block Wnt3a-mediated inhibition of RANKL in osteoblasts, whereas serum containing low Dkk1 concentrations had no effect, suggesting a role for Dkk1 in regulating both RANKL and OPG expressions in osteoblasts. In contrast to these studies, Giuliani and colleagues found that although myeloma cells or bone marrow plasma from myeloma patients could inhibit canonical Wnt signaling in murine osteoprogenitor cells, and express high concentrations of soluble Wnt antagonists Dkk1 and sFRP3, it did not block canonical Wnt signaling in human mesenchymal stem cells or osteoprogenitor cells [54].

Gunn et al. have reported that conditioned media from mesenchymal stem cells can promote myeloma cell proliferation and increase expression of Dkk1 by myeloma cells. Dkk1 then acts back on the mesenchymal stem cells to prevent their osteoblastic differentiation and maintain them in an immature state, where they express higher levels of IL-6 and therefore have greater potential to stimulate myeloma cell proliferation, thus creating a relationship between mesenchymal stem cells and myeloma cells resulting in an increase in myeloma proliferation and a decrease in osteoblastogenesis [55]. In addition to the expression of factors permissive for myeloma growth, it has recently been demonstrated that expression of Dkk1 is increased within the bone marrow microenvironment in myeloma. Garderet and colleagues identified an increase in Dkk1 expression in mesenchymal stem cells from patients with myeloma as compared with normal controls [56]. In addition, Corre et al. also identified an increase in Dkk1 expression in mesenchymal stem cells from patients with multiple myeloma. Furthermore, these mesenchymal stem cells could both promote myeloma growth and had impaired osteoblastic differentiation capacity [57]. Taken together, these studies suggest that the increase in Dkk1 in myeloma directly prevents osteoblastic differentiation and indirectly promotes myeloma growth by maintaining mesenchymal stem cells in an immature state which are more supportive of myeloma survival. Furthermore, these studies suggest that myeloma cells may not be the sole source for Dkk1 within the myeloma bone marrow microenvironment.

12.5.3 Wnt Signaling in Myeloma Cells

Activation of the Wnt signaling pathway through β-catenin plays a critical oncogenic role in many human malignancies and expression of β-catenin has been demonstrated in myeloma cell lines and in malignant plasma cells from patients with multiple myeloma [54, 58]. However, published data are conflicting as to the function of the Wnt signaling pathway in myeloma cells. Derksen et al. demonstrated that stimulation of the canonical Wnt signaling pathway increases proliferation of human myeloma cell lines [58]. More recently, a small molecule inhibitor of the β-catenin/TCF interaction was found to inhibit myeloma cell proliferation, both in vitro and in a xenograft model of myeloma [59]. In contrast, Qiang et al. have demonstrated that although activation of Wnt signaling results in an increase in β-catenin activity in myeloma cells, this is not associated with a proliferative effect [60]. In addition, they showed that activation of Wnt signaling with Wnt-3A results in morphological changes and an increase in invasion and migration of myeloma cells. Importantly, they also demonstrated that these effects were mediated through the Wnt/RhoA pathway and were independent of signaling through β-catenin [60, 61]. Edwards et al. have demonstrated that increasing Wnt signaling by treatment with lithium chloride increased the growth of myeloma cells when the cells were inoculated at an extraosseous subcutaneous site [62]. This effect was associated with an increase in β-catenin expression, and expression of the β-catenin target gene axin2, and was abrogated by overexpression of a dominant-negative TCF4, confirming that lithium chloride was increasing myeloma growth in vivo. Interestingly, in vitro studies confirmed that LiCl significantly increased β-catenin activity of myeloma cells, but had no effect on proliferation. While these differences may reflect the well-known limitations of using myeloma cell lines in vitro, they may also suggest a dependence of the Wnt signaling pathway upon environmental factors that are not present in in vitro systems. In contrast, Qiang et al. demonstrate that overexpression of Wnt3A in myeloma cells has no effect on proliferation, either in vitro, or at the subcutaneous site [63]. This may suggest that there are subtle, yet important differences in the cellular response, dependent upon the precise molecular mechanism by which the Wnt signaling pathway is activated. Importantly, in both these studies, when the tumor cells were present within the bone marrow microenvironment, activation of Wnt signaling resulted in a reduction in tumor burden and prevention of myeloma bone disease. Edwards et al. demonstrated that despite the effect of lithium chloride to increase extraosseous myeloma growth, increasing Wnt signaling within the bone marrow microenvironment prevented the development of myeloma bone disease and inhibited myeloma growth within bone [62]. This was associated with an increase in osteoblastic bone formation, and increased expression of β-catenin in osteoblasts. Qiang et al. observed that either overexpression of Wnt3A by myeloma cells or treatment of myeloma-bearing mice with Wnt3A resulted in a reduction in tumor burden and prevented myeloma bone disease [63].

12.5.4 Targeting the Wnt Signaling Pathway in Myeloma Bone Disease

It is clear that Dkk1 plays a critical role in the pathogenesis of myeloma bone disease, and therefore Dkk1 and the Wnt signaling pathway represent therapeutic targets for the treatment of myeloma bone disease. Yaccoby and colleagues tested the effect of antibody-based inhibition of Dkk1 in the SCID-rab model of myeloma [64]. Mice were engrafted with primary myeloma cells which were known to express differing levels of Dkk1 and were treated with an anti-Dkk1 neutralizing antibody. Treatment with anti-Dkk1 was found to increase bone mineral density in myeloma-bearing mice, and this was associated with an increase in osteoblasts and a reduction in osteoclasts, and a reduction in tumor burden. Bone mineral density was also increased in nonmyeloma-bearing mice. In a similar study, the effect of anti-Dkk1 was investigated in the 5T2MM murine model of myeloma [65]. 5T2 myeloma cells were found to express Dkk1, and treatment of 5T2MM myeloma-bearing mice was associated with an increase in osteoblast number, bone formation rate, and trabecular bone volume. Surprisingly, anti-Dkk1 treatment had no significant effect on tumor burden. In addition to directly targeting Dkk1, several studies have investigated other components of the Wnt signaling pathway in the treatment of myeloma bone disease. Sukhedo et al. used a novel small molecule compound which acts to disrupt the interaction between β-catenin and TCF and so inhibit Wnt signaling [59]. Inhibition of Wnt signaling was found to inhibit tumor growth and prolong survival in a xenograft model of myeloma, however, the effects of this small molecule have not been evaluated in an in vivo model of myeloma bone disease. Edwards et al. used a systemic pharmacological approach, by treatment with lithium chloride, which acts to inhibit glycogen synthase kinase 3beta and so activate β-catenin [62]. Lithium chloride was found to significantly prevent myeloma bone disease and reduce tumor burden within bone in the 5TGM1 murine model of myeloma. Qiang et al. demonstrated that systemic Wnt3A treatment could prevent the development of myeloma bone disease and reduce tumor burden in a SCID mouse model of myeloma [63]. These data highlight the importance of the local microenvironment in the effect of Wnt signaling on the development of myeloma bone disease, and demonstrate that, despite potential direct effects to increase tumor growth at extraosseous sites, increasing Wnt signaling in the bone marrow microenvironment can prevent the development of myeloma bone disease. Overall, targeting the Wnt signaling pathway is an attractive therapeutic approach for the treatment of multiple myeloma. However, concerns are raised due to the inconclusive role of Wnt signaling in myeloma growth and survival, and the potential for increasing extramedullary tumor growth.

12.6 Conclusions

Multiple myeloma is a fatal hematological malignancy and so it is essential to develop new therapeutic approaches for the treatment of both the tumor and the associated osteolytic bone disease. For many years now, our efforts have been focused on inhibitors of osteoclastic bone resorption, and this has proven to be effective, with the development of potent bisphosphonates and the discovery and subsequent targeting of the RANK/RANKL system. However, more recently, our understanding of the biology of myeloma bone disease has increased and it has become clear that while the osteoclast is the major destructive cell in myeloma bone disease, a major component of this bone disease is a lack of new bone formation, which is not restored by inhibitors of osteoclastic bone resorption. Proteasome inhibitors represent an important therapeutic advance for the treatment of multiple myeloma, due not only to their potent antimyeloma effects but also to their direct effects on osteoblasts to promote bone formation, and thus their potential to repair existing bone lesions. In a similar manner, targeting the Wnt signaling pathway in myeloma has the potential to increase bone formation and therefore prevent myeloma bone disease. The future direction for the treatment of myeloma bone disease may lie in a combination of inhibition of bone resorption and stimulation of bone formation to restore the balance of bone remodeling in patients with myeloma, and so protect against this destructive bone disease.

Acknowledgments This work was supported by NCI through P01 CA-40035 (GRM), the International Myeloma Foundation (CME) and by the Elsa U. Pardee Foundation (CME).

References

1. Valentin OA, Charhon SA, Meunier PJ, Edouard CM, Arlot ME. Quantitative histology of myeloma-induced bone changes. Br J Haematol. 1982;52:601–610.
2. Taube T, Beneton MNC, McCloskey EV, Rogers S, Greaves M, Kanis JA. Abnormal bone remodelling in patients with myelomatosis and normal biochemical indices of bone resorption. Eur J Haematol. 1992;49:192–198.
3. Bataille R, Chappard D, Marcelli C, et al. Recruitment of new osteoblasts and osteoclasts is the earliest critical event in the pathogenesis of human multiple myeloma. J Clin Invest. 1991;88:62–66.
4. Evans CE, Galasko CS, Ward C. Does myeloma secrete an osteoblast inhibiting factor? J Bone Joint Surg Br. 1989;71(2):288–290.
5. Bataille R, Delmas PD, Chappard D, Sany J. Abnormal serum bone Gla protein levels in multiple myeloma. Crucial role of bone formation and prognostic implications. Cancer. 1990;66(1):167–172.
6. Abildgaard N, Rungby J, Glerup H, et al. Long-term oral pamidronate treatment inhibits osteoclastic bone resorption and bone turnover without affecting osteoblastic function in multiple myeloma. Eur J Haematol. 1998;61(2):128–134.
7. Woitge HW, Horn E, Keck AV, Auler B, Seibel MJ, Pecherstorfer M. Biochemical markers of bone formation in patients with plasma cell dyscrasias and benign osteoporosis. Clin Chem. 2001;47(4):686–693.
8. Mundy GR. Myeloma bone disease. Eur J Cancer. 1998;34:246–251.
9. Mundy GR, Raisz LG, Cooper RA, Schechter GP, Salmon S. Evidence for the secretion of an osteoclast stimulating factor in myeloma. N Engl J Med. 1974;291:1041–1046.
10. Garrett IR, Durie BG, Nedwin GE, et al. Production of lymphotoxin, a bone-resorbing cytokine, by cultured human myeloma cells. N Engl J Med. 1987;317(9):526–532.
11. Kawano M, Hirano T, Matsuda T, et al. Autocrine generation and requirement of BSF-2/IL-6 for human multiple myelomas. Nature. 1988;332:83–85.
12. Lee JW, Chung HY, Ehrlich LA, et al. IL-3 expression by myeloma cells increases both osteoclast formation and growth of myeloma cells. Blood. 2004;103(6):2308–2315.
13. Lichtenstein A, Berenson J, Norman D, Chang MP, Carlile A. Production of cytokines by bone marrow cells obtained from patients with multiple myeloma. Blood. 1989;74(4):1266–1273.
14. Garrett IR, Chen D, Gutierrez G, et al. Selective inhibitors of the osteoblast proteasome stimulate bone formation in vivo and in vitro. J Clin Invest. 2003;111(11):1771–1782.
15. Oyajobi BO, Garrett IR, Gupta A, et al. Stimulation of new bone formation by the proteasome inhibitor, bortezomib: implications for myeloma bone disease. Br J Haematol. 2007;139(3):434–438.
16. Mukherjee S, Raje N, Schoonmaker JA, et al. Pharmacologic targeting of a stem/progenitor population in vivo is associated with enhanced bone regeneration in mice. J Clin Invest. 2008;118(2):491–504.
17. Giuliani N, Morandi F, Tagliaferri S, et al. The proteasome inhibitor bortezomib affects osteoblast differentiation in vitro and in vivo in multiple myeloma patients. Blood. 2007;110(1):334–338.

18. Qiang YW, Hu B, Chen Y, et al. Bortezomib induces osteoblast differentiation via Wnt-independent activation of {beta}-catenin/TCF signaling. Blood. 2009;113(18):4319–4330.
19. Zavrski I, Krebbel H, Wildemann B, et al. Proteasome inhibitors abrogate osteoclast differentiation and osteoclast function. Biochem Biophys Res Commun. 2005;333(1):200–205.
20. von Metzler I, Krebbel H, Hecht M, et al. Bortezomib inhibits human osteoclastogenesis. Leukemia. 2007;21(9):2025–2034.
21. Hongming H, Jian H. Bortezomib inhibits maturation and function of osteoclasts from PBMCs of patients with multiple myeloma by downregulating TRAF6. Leuk Res. 2009;33(1):115–122.
22. Pennisi A, Li X, Ling W, Khan S, Zangari M, Yaccoby S. The proteasome inhibitor, bortezomib suppresses primary myeloma and stimulates bone formation in myelomatous and nonmyelomatous bones in vivo. Am J Hematol. 2008;84(1):6–14.
23. Edwards CM, Lwin ST, Fowler JA, et al. Myeloma cells exhibit an increase in proteasome activity and an enhanced response to proteasome inhibition in the bone marrow microenvironment in vivo. Am J Hematol. 2009;84(5):268–272.
24. Shimazaki C, Uchida R, Nakano S, et al. High serum bone-specific alkaline phosphatase level after bortezomib-combined therapy in refractory multiple myeloma: possible role of bortezomib on osteoblast differentiation. Leukemia. 2005;19(6):1102–1103.
25. Zangari M, Esseltine D, Lee CK, et al. Response to bortezomib is associated to osteoblastic activation in patients with multiple myeloma. Br J Haematol. 2005;131(1):71–73.
26. Zangari M, Esseltine D, Cavallo F, et al. Predictive value of alkaline phosphatase for response and time to progression in bortezomib-treated multiple myeloma patients. Am J Hematol. 2007;82(9):831–833.
27. Heider U, Kaiser M, Muller C, et al. Bortezomib increases osteoblast activity in myeloma patients irrespective of response to treatment. Eur J Haematol. 2006;77(3):233–238.
28. Ozaki S, Tanaka O, Fujii S, et al. Therapy with bortezomib plus dexamethasone induces osteoblast activation in responsive patients with multiple myeloma. Int J Hematol. 2007;86(2):180–185.
29. Terpos E, Heath DJ, Rahemtulla A, et al. Bortezomib reduces serum dickkopf-1 and receptor activator of nuclear factor-kappaB ligand concentrations and normalises indices of bone remodelling in patients with relapsed multiple myeloma. Br J Haematol. 2006;135(5): 688–692.
30. Uy GL, Trivedi R, Peles S, et al. Bortezomib inhibits osteoclast activity in patients with multiple myeloma. Clin Lymphoma Myeloma. 2007;7(9):587–589.
31. Boissy P, Andersen TL, Lund T, Kupisiewicz K, Plesner T, Delaisse JM. Pulse treatment with the proteasome inhibitor bortezomib inhibits osteoclast resorptive activity in clinically relevant conditions. Leuk Res. 2008;32(11):1661–1668.
32. Moon RT, Kohn AD, DeFerrari GV, Kaykas A. Wnt and b-catenin signalling: disease and therapies. Nat Rev Genet. 2004;5(9):691–701.
33. Westendorf JJ, Kahler RA, Schroeder TM. Wnt signaling in osteoblasts and bone diseases. Gene. 2004;341:19–39.
34. Gong Y, Slee RB, Fukai N, et al. LDL receptor-related protein 5 (LRP5) affects bone accrual and eye development. Cell. 2001;107(4):513–523.
35. Boyden LM, Mao J, Belsky J, et al. High bone density due to a mutation in LDL-receptor-related protein 5. N Engl J Med. 2002;346(20):1513–1521.
36. Kato M, Patel M, Levasseur R, et al. Cbfa1-independent decrease in osteoblast proliferation, osteopenia, and persistant embryonic eye vascularization in mice deficient in LRP5, a Wnt coreceptor. J Cell Biol. 2002;157(2):303–314.
37. Li J, Sarosi I, Cattley RC, et al. Dkk1-mediated inhibition of Wnt signaling in bone results in osteopenia. Bone. 2006;39(4):754–766.
38. Morvan F, Boulukos K, Clement-Lacroix P, et al. Deletion of a single allele of the Dkk1 gene leads to an increase in bone formation and bone mass. J Bone Miner Res. 2006;21(6): 934–945.

39. Babij P, Zhao W, Small C, et al. High bone mass in mice expressing a mutant LRP5 gene. J Bone Miner Res. 2003;18(6):960–974.
40. Rawadi G, Vayssiere B, Dunn F, Baron R, Roman-Roman S. BMP-2 controls alkaline phosphatase expression and osteoblast mineralization by a Wnt autocrine loop. J Bone Miner Res. 2003;18(10):1842–1853.
41. Christodoulides C, Laudes M, Cawthorn WP, et al. The Wnt antagonist Dickkopf-1 and its receptors are coordinately regulated during early human adipogenesis. J Cell Sci. 2006;119 (Pt 12):2613–2620.
42. Cheng SL, Shao JS, Cai J, Sierra OL, Towler DA. Msx2 exerts bone anabolism via canonical Wnt signaling. J Biol Chem. 2008;283(29):20505–20522.
43. Tian E, Zhan F, Walker R, et al. The role of the Wnt-signaling antagonist in the development of osteolytic lesions in multiple myeloma. N Engl J Med. 2003;349(26):2483–2494.
44. Politou MC, Heath DJ, Rahemtulla A, et al. Serum concentrations of Dickkopf-1 protein are increased in patients with multiple myeloma and reduced after autologous stem cell transplantation. Int J Cancer. 2006;119(7):1728–1731.
45. Haaber J, Abildgaard N, Knudsen LM, et al. Myeloma cell expression of 10 candidate genes for osteolytic bone disease. Only overexpression of DKK1 correlates with clinical bone involvement at diagnosis. Br J Haematol. 2008;140(1):25–35.
46. Kaiser M, Mieth M, Liebisch P, et al. Serum concentrations of DKK-1 correlate with the extent of bone disease in patients with multiple myeloma. Eur J Haematol. 2008;80(6):490–494.
47. Heider U, Kaiser M, Mieth M, et al. Serum concentrations of DKK-1 decrease in patients with multiple myeloma responding to anti-myeloma treatment. Eur J Haematol. 2009;82(1):31–38.
48. Qian J, Xie J, Hong S, et al. Dickkopf-1 (DKK1) is a widely expressed and potent tumor-associated antigen in multiple myeloma. Blood. 2007;110(5):1587–1594.
49. Chamorro MN, Schwartz DR, Vonica A, Brivanlou AH, Cho KR, Varmus HE. FGF-20 and DKK1 are transcriptional targets of beta-catenin and FGF-20 is implicated in cancer and development. EMBO J. 2005;24(1):73–84.
50. Colla S, Zhan F, Xiong W, et al. The oxidative stress response regulates DKK1 expression through the JNK signaling cascade in multiple myeloma plasma cells. Blood. 2007;109(10):4470–4477.
51. Oshima T, Abe M, Asano J, et al. Myeloma cells suppress bone formation by secreting a soluble Wnt inhibitor, sFRP-2. Blood. 2005;106(9):3160–3165.
52. Qiang YW, Barlogie B, Rudikoff S, Shaughnessy JD Jr. Dkk1-induced inhibition of Wnt signaling in osteoblast differentiation is an underlying mechanism of bone loss in multiple myeloma. Bone. 2008;42(4):669–680.
53. Qiang YW, Chen Y, Stephens O, et al. Myeloma-derived Dickkopf-1 disrupts Wnt-regulated osteoprotegerin and RANKL production by osteoblasts: a potential mechanism underlying osteolytic bone lesions in multiple myeloma. Blood. 2008;112(1):196–207.
54. Giuliani N, Morandi F, Tagliaferri S, et al. Production of Wnt inhibitors by myeloma cells: potential effects on canonical Wnt pathway in the bone microenvironment. Cancer Res. 2007;67(16):7665–7674.
55. Gunn WG, Conley A, Deininger L, Olson SD, Prockop DJ, Gregory CA. A crosstalk between myeloma cells and marrow stromal cells stimulates production of DKK1 and interleukin-6: a potential role in the development of lytic bone disease and tumor progression in multiple myeloma. Stem Cells. 2006;24(4):986–991.
56. Garderet L, Mazurier C, Chapel A, et al. Mesenchymal stem cell abnormalities in patients with multiple myeloma. Leuk Lymphoma. 2007;48(10):2032–2041.
57. Corre J, Mahtouk K, Attal M, et al. Bone marrow mesenchymal stem cells are abnormal in multiple myeloma. Leukemia. 2007;21(5):1079–1088.
58. Derksen PW, Tjin E, Meijer HP, et al. Illegitimate WNT signaling promotes proliferation of multiple myeloma cells. Proc Natl Acad Sci USA. 2004;101(16):6122–6127.
59. Sukhdeo K, Mani M, Zhang Y, et al. Targeting the beta-catenin/TCF transcriptional complex in the treatment of multiple myeloma. Proc Natl Acad Sci USA. 2007;104(18):7516–7521.

60. Qiang YW,, Endo Y,, Rubin JS,, Rudikoff S. Wnt signaling in B-cell neoplasia. Oncogene. 2003;22(10):1536–1545.
61. Qiang YW,, Walsh K,, Yao L,et al. Wnts induce migration and invasion of myeloma plasma cells. Blood. 2005;106(5):1786–1793.
62. Edwards CM,, Edwards JR,, Lwin ST,et al. Increasing Wnt signaling in the bone marrow microenvironment inhibits the development of myeloma bone disease and reduces tumor burden in bone in vivo. Blood. 2008;111(5):2833–2842.
63. Qiang YW, Shaughnessy JD Jr, Yaccoby S. Wnt3a signaling within bone inhibits multiple myeloma bone disease and tumor growth. Blood. 2008;112(2):374–382.
64. Yaccoby S, Ling W, Zhan F, Walker R, Barlogie B, Shaughnessy JD Jr. Antibody-based inhibition of DKK1 suppresses tumor-induced bone resorption and multiple myeloma growth in vivo. Blood. 2007;109(5):2106–2111.
65. Heath DJ, Chantry AD, Buckle CHet al. Inhibiting Dickkopf-1 (Dkk1) removes suppression of bone formation and prevents the development of osteolytic bone disease in multiple myeloma. J Bone Miner Res. 2009;24(3):425–436.

Chapter 13
Mechanisms Involved in Osteoblast Suppression in Multiple Myeloma

Nicola Giuliani

Abstract Multiple myeloma (MM) is a plasma cell malignancy characterized by a high capacity to induce osteolytic bone lesions and bone destruction. Histomorphometric studies have demonstrated that MM patients with high plasma cell infiltrates are characterized by a lower number of osteoblasts and a decreased bone formation that contributes together with osteoclast activation, to the development of bone lesions.

Osteoblastic cells differentiate from mesenchymal stem cells through a tightly regulated mechanism involving several growth and transcription factors. Runx2 is critically involved in this process along with a large number of nuclear co-regulators. Wnt signaling has been recently identified as a critical pathway involved in the regulation of osteoblast formation. The impairment of osteogenic differentiation in mesenchymal cells occurs in multiple myeloma due to the capacity of malignant plasma cells to suppress the osteogenic differentiation of mesenchymal cells either through cell contact or the release of soluble factors such as interleukin (IL-7), hepatocyte growth factor (HGF), IL-3, and Wnt inhibitors. Runx2 and the Wnt pathway could be therapeutic targets in the treatment of MM bone disease to counterbalance the block of osteogenic differentiation induced by MM cells.

Keywords Multiple myeloma · Osteoblast · Pathophysiology · Bone disease

13.1 Introduction

Multiple myeloma (MM) is a plasma cell malignancy characterized by its high capacity to induce osteolytic bone lesions and bone destruction [1]. Histomorphometric studies have demonstrated that MM patients with bone lesions

N. Giuliani (✉)
Department of Internal Medicine and Biomedical Science,
Hematology and BMT Center, University of Parma, Parma, 43100, Italy
e-mail: nicola.giuliani@unipr.it; n_giuliani@yahoo.com

G.D. Roodman (ed.), *Myeloma Bone Disease*, Current Clinical Oncology,
DOI 10.1007/978-1-60761-554-5_13, © Springer Science+Business Media, LLC 2010

have uncoupled or severely imbalanced bone remodeling in which bone resorption and formation are no longer balanced but instead bone resorption is markedly increased and bone formation is either decreased or absent. In contrast, MM patients without bone lesions display balanced bone remodeling with increased osteoclastogenesis and normal or increased bone formation rates [2]. Clinical studies have shown that MM patients with advanced bone lesions may have a reduction of bone formation markers, such as alkaline phosphatase and osteocalcin, together with increased bone resorption markers [3]. Similarly, marked osteoblastopenia and reduced bone formation have been also reported in murine models of MM [4]. These data suggest that MM cells suppress osteoblast formation and differentiation and thereby inhibit bone formation. Increased knowledge of the signaling pathways involved in the regulation of osteoblast formation and differentiation have provided a better understanding of the pathophysiological mechanisms involved in MM-induced osteoblast inhibition and permitted identification of several potential therapeutics targets for the treatment of MM bone disease.

13.2 Osteoblast Formation: Role of Runx2 and Wnt Pathways

Under physiological conditions osteoblast formation from mesenchymal cells is tightly regulated either by systemic hormones such as PTH, estrogens, and glucocorticoids or by local growth factors, including the bone morphogenetic protein (BMP) family, transforming growth factor-β (TGF-β), and fibroblast growth factor 2 (FGF-2) [5]. Moreover, these factors activate specific intracellular signal pathways that modify the expression and activity of several transcription factors in mesenchymal and osteoprogenitor cells, which result in osteoblastic differentiation [5, 6]. In the last several years most of these transcription factors have been identified. Runx2, also named Cbfa1 or AML3, is the major transcription factor regulating osteoblast commitment and osteogenic differentiation of mesenchymal cells [6–8]. Studies in mice lacking *Runx2* indicated that the expression of Runx2 is critical for mesenchymal cell differentiation toward the osteoblast lineage. Runx2 deficient mice (*Runx2–/–*) completely lack osteoblasts and bone formation, demonstrating a pivotal role for this factor in osteoblastogenesis [6–8]. However, *Runx2* overexpression also impairs bone formation in mice [9], indicating that depending on the stage of osteoblast differentiation, Runx2 could have different effects on the bone formation process. *Runx2* overexpressing mice also show enhanced bone resorption possibly through increased expression of the osteoclast-stimulating factor, RANKL, by osteoprogenitor cells [10]. Human osteoblast differentiation is primarily associated with increased Runx2 activity without changes in mRNA or protein expression [11, 12]. The activation of Runx2/Cbfa1 in human BM stromal and osteoblastic cells induces the expression of the osteoblast markers collagen I, alkaline phosphatase, and osteocalcin during the different stages of the osteoblast maturation [11].

Both the expression and activity of Runx2 are tightly regulated by other transcription factors, as well as protein–DNA or protein–protein interactions. Runx2 itself is regulated by phosphorylation by the ERK/MAP kinase pathway [13]. Hey-1, Hoxa2, Stat1, and Sox9 interact with Runx2 and inhibit its expression and/or transcriptional activity and thus are negative regulators of osteoblast differentiation. Runx2 activity is also positively regulated by transcription factors such as TAZ, Hoxa10, or BAPX-1 [5, 6, 8]. In addition multiple signaling pathways converge to interact with Runx2 to regulate osteoblast differentiation, including binding with AP-1 and ATF4 that with Runx2 regulate osteocalcin and Osterix (Osx) [5, 6, 8]. Osx is a zinc finger transcription factor that is important for osteoblast differentiation. *Osx* deficient mice lack osteoblast formation. Osx acts downstream of Runx2 [5, 6]. In mouse systems osteogenic factors stimulate osteogenesis through the regulation of these transcription factors. BMP-2 promotes *Runx2* and *Osx* expression in murine osteoprogenitor and osteoblastic cells, and TGF-β and FGF-2 may enhance osteoblast differentiation by increasing Runx2 expression and activity [5, 6].

Several studies have demonstrated that Wnt signaling plays a critical role in the regulation of osteoblast formation [14–18]. The canonical Wnt signaling pathway is activated by Wnt 1/3a that triggers the phosphorylation of GSK3/Axin complex, leading to the stabilization and nuclear translocation of the active dephosphorylated (dephospho) β-catenin, which in turn activates the Lef1/TCF transcription system [14–18].

In murine systems activation of canonical Wnt signaling in osteoblast progenitors induces osteogenic differentiation [17, 18]. In particular, bone morphogenic protein (BMP)-2 and other osteogenic molecules induce osteoblastic differentiation of murine mesenchymal stem cells by stimulating Wnt signaling through the modulation of Wnt stimulators and/or inhibitors [18]. Several molecules negatively regulate canonical Wnt signaling by inducing phosphorylation and subsequent degradation of β-catenin. Dickkopfs (DKKs) including DKK-1 [19], the secreted frizzled-related proteins (sFRPs) such as sFRP1-2-3-4 and Wnt inhibitory factor (Wif-1) are the major soluble Wnt inhibitors present in murine osteoblasts, which block early osteoblast formation and induce the death of immature cells [20, 21].

In vivo models support the role of Wnt signaling in the regulation of bone mass [22–24]. Inactivating mutations of the *LRP5* Wnt co-receptor cause osteoporosis [22], indicating that Wnt-mediated signaling via LRP5 affects bone accrual during growth and is important for the establishment of peak bone mass. Constitutive activating *LRP5* mutations impair the action of normal antagonists of the Wnt pathway, such as DKK-1, and increase Wnt signaling, which result in high bone density [23, 24]. These results demonstrate that canonical Wnt signaling plays an important role in human bone formation.

Despite the consistent findings between human genetic studies and mouse studies indicate that activation of canonical Wnt signaling stimulate bone formation, surprisingly, recent in vitro data obtained with human mesenchymal cells indicate that canonical Wnt activation by Wnt3a in human BM cells suppresses osteogenic differentiation [25–28]. These results suggest that Wnt signaling is required to maintain stromal cells in an undifferentiated state.

We can suppose that the effect of canonical Wnt signaling on osteogenesis in human mesenchymal may depend to the level of Wnt activity given that hyperactivation of Wnt signaling by overexpressing LRP5 [23] can enhance osteogenesis whereas exogenous level of Wnt3a inhibits osteoblast differentiation [25, 26]. Alternatively the effect of canonical Wnt signaling may depend on the stage of differentiation of the cells. Accordingly, it has been reported that Wnt signaling antagonizes the terminal steps of osteogenic differentiation as demonstrated by the evidence that mice lacking the Wnt inhibitor DKK-2 are osteopenic [29] and by the increased expression of Wnt antagonists during late osteoblast differentiation [30, 31].

On the other hand it has been reported that activation of the non-canonical Wnt pathway by Wnt5a blunted the inhibitory effect of Wnt3a on osteogenic differentiation of human mesenchymal cells [32, 33]. Similarly, non-canonical Wnt-4 signaling enhances bone regeneration of mesenchymal stem cells in vivo [32]. The pro-osteogenic effect of Wnt5a could be mediated by activation and homodimerization of the Ror2 receptor in mesenchymal cells, whereas Wnt3a has not effect on Ror2 activation and homodimerization [33, 34]. It has been consistently shown that *Ror2* overexpression in human mesenchymal stem cells induces expression of the osteogenic transcription factors Osx and Runx2 and induces osteogenic differentiation [34–36]. These results suggest that the non-canonical Wnt signaling pathway is involved in human mesenchymal cells osteogenic differentiation.

13.3 MM-Induced Suppression of Osteoblast Formation by Inhibiting Runx2 Pathway: Role of Cell-to-Cell Contact and Soluble Factors

The impairment of osteoblasts and bone formation in MM is mainly due to the block of the osteogenic differentiation process of mesenchymal cells induced by MM cells. Co-culture of human MM cells with osteoprogenitor cells inhibited osteoblast differentiation in long-term bone marrow cultures. MM cells reduced both, early osteoblast precursors, fibroblast colony-forming units (CFU-F) and the more differentiated osteoblast precursor, the colony-forming osteoblast units (CFU-OB) as well as the expression of osteoblastic differentiation markers, alkaline phosphatase, osteocalcin, and collagen I [37]. These in vitro observations have been confirmed in vivo in MM patients [38], although this is controversial [39, 40].

The inhibitory effect of MM cells on osteoblast differentiation appears to be mediated by the capacity of MM cells to inhibit Runx2 activity in human mesenchymal stem and osteoprogenitor cells [37]. A significant reduction in the number of osteoblastic cells/mm^2 has been consistently reported in MM patients with osteolysis as compared to patients without bone lesions. Consequently, the number of both stromal and osteoblastic cells positive for Runx2 was reduced as well as the percent of Runx2 positive osteoblastic cells in MM patients with osteolytic lesions in comparison with patients without osteolysis [37]. The suppression of Runx2 activity by MM cells is mediated, at least in part, by the cell-to-cell contact between MM and osteoprogenitor cells. This cell-to-cell contact involves interactions between VLA-4 on MM cells and VCAM-1 on osteoblast progenitors, as demonstrated by the capacity of a neutralizing anti-VLA-4 antibody to reduce the inhibitory effects of MM cells on Runx2/Cbfa1 activity [37]. The role of cell-to-cell contact via VLA-4/VCAM-1 interaction in the development of bone lesions by osteoclast activation and osteoblast inhibition in MM has been recently demonstrated using in vivo mouse models [41]. When the human MM cell line, JJN3, which strongly expresses VLA-4, is implanted in irradiated severe combined immunodeficient (SCID) mice, the mice developed lytic lesions and marked osteoblastopenia with a significant reduction of bone formation [4]. In addition to VLA-4/VCAM-1, other adhesion molecules appear to be involved in the inhibition of osteoblastogenesis by human MM cells. For example, NCAM–NCAM interactions between MM cells and stromal/osteoblastic cells decrease bone matrix production by osteoblastic cells, and may contribute to the development of bone lesions in MM patients [42]. Soluble factors contribute to the inhibitory effects of MM cells on osteoblast differentiation by mesenchymal stem cells and Runx2/Cbfa1 activity [37]. Interleukin-7 (IL-7) decreases Runx2/Cbfa1 promoter activity and the expression of osteoblast markers in osteoblastic cells [43]. Moreover, IL-7 can inhibit bone formation in vivo in mice [43], as well as CFU-F and CFU-OB formation in human bone marrow cultures and reduces Runx2 activity in human osteoprogenitor cells [37]. The potential involvement of IL-7 in MM has been supported by the demonstration of higher IL-7 plasma levels in MM patients compared to normal subjects [44] and by the capacity of blocking antibodies to IL-7 to partially blunt the inhibitory effects of MM cells on osteoblast differentiation [37]. These studies suggest that MM cells block Runx2 activity and osteoblast differentiation either by cell-to-cell contact or by secreting IL-7, which leads to a reduction in the number of more differentiated osteoblastic cells.

Other soluble factors may also be involved in osteoblast suppression by MM cells. The hepatocyte growth factor (HGF) is produced by MM cells and its high levels in BM of MM correlated with those of alkaline phosphatase [45]. HGF inhibits in vitro osteoblastogenesis induced by bone morphogenetic protein (BMP)-2 and BMP-induced expression of alkaline phosphatase in both human and murine mesenchymal cells. Moreover, the expression of transcription factors Runx2 and Osx as well as Smad are reduced by HGF treatment [45].

Transforming growth factor-β (TGF-β) is a multifunctional factor that is released from the bone matrix during osteoclastic bone resorption and acts to inhibit osteoblast differentiation. In addition to inhibiting myeloma growth, inhibition of TGF-β signaling has been shown to block the ability of myeloma cells to inhibit osteoblast differentiation in vitro [46].

TAZ, a Runx2/Cbfa1 transcriptional co-activator, has been recently shown to modulate the osteogenic potential of the human mesenchymal stem cells [8, 47] and to be expressed at lower levels in MM patients as compared to healthy donors [48]. The repressed osteogenesis and TAZ expression were both partially restored by neutralization of TNF-alpha [49].

The inhibition of Runx2 in BM osteoprogenitor cells by MM cells through the above-mentioned mechanisms suggest that Runx2 could be a target to counterbalance the inhibition of osteogenic differentiation in MM. Modulation of Runx2 activity has been shown with anabolic agents such as parathyroid hormone (PTH) amino-terminal peptide 1–34 [49, 50]. Moreover, in vivo mouse models have shown that Runx2 gene transfer enhances osteogenic activity of BM mesenchymal cells [51].

13.4 Role of IL-3 in the Inhibition of Osteoblasts Formation by MM Cells

IL-3 has been reported as a potential osteoblast inhibitor in MM patients [52]. In both murine and human system, IL-3 indirectly inhibited osteoblast formation in a dose-dependent manner, without affecting cell growth at concentrations comparable to those seen in bone marrow plasma from patients with MM. IL-3 levels in bone marrow plasma from patients with MM were increased in approximately 70% of patients compared to normal controls or patients with monoclonal gammopathy of undetermined significance (MGUS) patients [53]. IL-3 is also produced by T lymphocytes in the MM bone microenvironment [54]. Importantly, bone marrow plasma from patients with MM with high levels of IL-3 inhibited osteoblast formation in human cultures, and this inhibition was partially reversed by addition of a neutralizing antibody to human IL-3 [52]. The inhibitory effect of IL-3 was increased in the presence of TNFα, a cytokine-induced in the MM marrow microenvironment. The effect of IL-3 is indirect and mediated by $CD45^+/CD11b^+$ monocyte/macrophages in both human and mouse primary culture systems. IL-3 increased the number of $CD45^+$ hematopoietic cells in stromal cell cultures, and depletion of the $CD45^+$ cells abolished the inhibitory effects of IL-3 on osteoblasts. Importantly, reconstituted $CD45^+$ depleted cultures with $CD45^+$ cells, restored the capacity of IL-3 to inhibit osteoblast differentiation. IL-3 had no direct effect on osteoblast progenitors or on Runx2 expression and activity in both murine and human BM cells [52].

13.5 Role of Wnt Inhibitors in MM-Induced Osteoblast Suppression

The potential involvement of inhibitors of Wnt signaling in the suppression of osteoblast formation and function in MM has been investigated. Primary $CD138^+$ MM cells overexpress the Wnt inhibitors DKK-1 as compared to plasma cells from MGUS patients and normal plasma cells [55]. Further, using gene expression profiling, a tight correlation between *DKK-1* expression by MM cells and the occurrence of focal lytic bone lesions in MM patients has been reported. High DKK-1 levels in bone marrow and peripheral sera in MM patients correlated with the presence of bone lesions [56]. Interestingly, patients with advanced disease, as well as human

MM cell lines did not express DKK-1 [55], suggesting that DKK-1 may mediate bone destruction in the early phases of disease. MM cells also produce other Wnt inhibitors, including SFRP-3/FRZB. FRZB is highly expressed by CD138+ MM cells from patients as compared to MGUS patients, and BM plasma levels are higher in MM patients with bone lesions as compared to those without skeletal involvement [56]. sFRP-2 also has been reported to be produced by some human MM cell lines and by patients with advanced MM bone disease, and can inhibit osteoblast differentiation by murine osteoprogenitor cells [57].

The mechanism by which DKK-1 and the other Wnt inhibitors produced by MM cells is related to bone destruction is not completely understood. Neutralizing anti-DKK-1 antibody can block the inhibitory effect of bone marrow plasma of MM patients on BMP-2-induced alkaline phosphatase expression and osteoblast formation by a murine mesenchymal cell line [55] but failed to block the inhibitory effects of MM cells on human bone marrow osteoblast formation [37]. In addition, only high concentrations of DKK-1 are able to inhibit CFU-F and CFU-OB formation and to block β-catenin signaling in human bone marrow osteoprogenitor cells [37]. Recently it has been reported that MM cells failed to block canonical Wnt signaling in human BM osteoblast progenitors but inhibited this pathway in murine systems suggesting that blockade of the canonical Wnt pathway may not occur in MM patients [56]. Interestingly, it has been shown that human mesenchymal and osteoprogenitor cells express Wnt5a, an activator of the non-canonical Wnt pathway but did not express the main activators of canonical Wnt signaling such as Wnt1, Wnt3a, and Wnt8 as demonstrated in murine osteoprogenitor cells [56]. These results suggest that non-canonical pathway rather than canonical one could be active in human mesenchymal/osteoprogenitor cell. To investigate whether MM cells may affect canonical Wnt signaling, the accumulation and stabilization of β-catenin has been evaluated as a marker for the activation of canonical Wnt signaling in co-cultures of MM cells and osteoprogenitor cells. No significant inhibitory effect on total cytosolic and nuclear dephosphoβ-catenin was observed after co-culture [56]. Moreover, the capacity of Wnt signaling stimulation to block MM-induced suppression of osteoblast formation in vitro has been evaluated. In human BM cultures, Wnt3a did not blunt the inhibitory effect induced by MM cells on bone nodules formation [56]. On the other hand, the activation of Wnt non-canonical pathway in BM mesenchymal and osteoprogenitor cells through Wnt5a overexpression has been recently reported [58].

Other mechanisms could be involved in DDK-1-mediated bone destruction in MM. For example, a link between cell adhesion and the Wnt pathway was recently reported. Wnt inhibitors such as DKK-1 are triggered by cell contact and modulate adhesion of leukemia cells to osteoblasts [59]. Possibly, DKK-1 production by MM cells could be involved in the adhesion of stromal and MM cells, which is critical for osteoclast activation and MM-induced Runx2 inhibition and osteoblast suppression. Further, cross-talk between MM cells and the microenvironment can stimulate both DKK-1 and IL-6 production in human bone marrow cultures [60]. The capacity of DKK-1 to regulate expression of the osteoclast inhibitory factor, osteoprotegerin (OPG), has been reported in murine osteoblasts [61].

Studies in the SCID-human mice model of MM have shown that anti-DKK-1 increases bone mineral density and the number of osteocalcin positive osteoblasts compared to control mice [62]. Interestingly, a reduction of the number of osteoclastic cells was also observed, suggesting that Wnt signaling could be involved in the regulation of bone resorption [62]. Consistently, it has been reported that activation of the Wnt3a signaling pathway in the bone microenvironment is able to block the development of bone lesions and the growth of MM cells in murine MM models [63, 64]. These observations are in line with those showing that canonical Wnt pathway stimulates bone formation in mice. Both anti-DKK-1 antibody and Wnt canonical activation by Wnt3a or by litium [63, 64] are able to blunt the inhibitory effect of MM cells on osteoblast formation independently of the production of DKK-1 by MM cells. These results suggest that the bone microenvironment rather than MM cells is the target of anti-DKK-1 antibody therapy.

13.6 Effect of MM Cells on Osteoblast Proliferation and Survival

In addition to blocking osteoblast formation, several studies suggest that MM cells may directly act on mature osteoblastic cells. MM cells have been reported to inhibit osteoblast proliferation [65] and up-regulate osteoblast apoptosis when co-cultured with osteoblasts [66]. Moreover, osteoblasts obtained from MM patients with extensive bone lesions appear to be highly prone to undergoing apoptosis as compared to osteoblasts from patients without bone lesions [67]. Recently it has been reported that MM cells induce apoptosis of osteoblasts when co-cultured with human osteoblastic cells [68]. Besides killing osteoblasts, human MM cells sensitize osteoblastic cells to cell death mediated by recombinant TRAIL, and in turn osteoblastic cells may also stimulate MM survival by blocking TRAIL-mediated apoptosis of MM cells through the secretion of OPG, a decoy receptor or both RANKL and TRAIL [68, 69]. However, using a triple co-culture system with osteoclasts, osteoblasts, and MM cells, it has been reported that osteoblastic cells may attenuate the stimulatory effect of osteoclastic cells on MM cell survival [70]. Moreover, it has been reported in an MM mouse model that the stimulation of bone formation could inhibit MM cells growth [63, 64, 70].

13.7 Conclusions

Multiple factors are involved in the interactions between MM cells and osteoprogenitor cells in the development of osteolytic bone lesions and the inhibition of osteogenic differentiation in human mesenchymal stem cells. Blockade of Runx2 activity and soluble factors such as IL-3, IL-7, and HGF have recently been identified as osteoblast inhibitors in MM. Many studies have reported that the production of canonical Wnt antagonists such as DKK-1, sFRP-2, and sFRP-3 by MM cells correlates with the presence of osteolytic bone lesions in MM and that stimulating Wnt

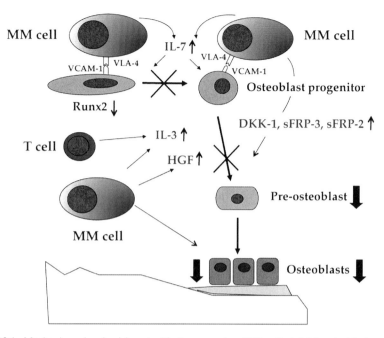

Fig. 13.1 Mechanisms involved in osteoblast suppression MM cells inhibit osteoblastogenesis by blocking Runx2 activity in mesenchymal and osteoprogenitor cells through direct cell-to-cell contact with the involvement of VLA-4/VCAM-1. Soluble factors as IL-7 and HGF may contribute to the suppression of Runx2 activity by MM cells. The direct production of the Wnt inhibitor DKK-1 s-FRP-3 and sFRP-2 by MM cells inhibits osteoblast differentiation. IL-3 overproduction in the MM microenvironment may also be involved in the inhibition of osteoblast formation and differentiation indirectly. A direct inhibitory effect of MM cells on mature osteoblasts has also been reported

signaling in the bone microenvironment could be a potential therapy for MM bone disease (Fig. 13.1). Finally MM cells may directly inhibited osteoblast proliferation and survival and consequently their activity.

References

1. Kyle RA, Rajkumar SV. Multiple myeloma. N Engl J Med. 2004;351:1860–1873.
2. Giuliani N, Rizzoli V, Roodman GD. Multiple myeloma bone disease: pathophysiology of osteoblast inhibition. Blood. 2006;108:3992–3996.
3. Vejlgaard T, Abildgaard N, Jans H, et al. Abnormal bone turnover in monoclonal gammaopathy of undetermined significance: analyses of type I collagen telopeptide, osteocalcin, bone-specific alkaline phosphatase and propeptides of type I and type III procollagens. Eur J Haematol. 1997;58:104–108.
4. Hjorth-Hansen H, Seifert MF, Borset M, et al. Marked osteoblastopenia and reduced bone formation in a model of multiple myeloma bone disease in severe combined imyelomaunodeficiency mice. J Bone Miner Res. 1999;14:256–263.
5. Franceschi RT, Ge C, Xiao G, et al. Transcriptional regulation of osteoblasts. Ann NY Acad Sci. 2007;1116:196–207.

6. Deng ZL, Sharff KA, Tang N, et al. Regulation of osteogenic differentiation during skeletal development. Front Biosci. January 2008;1(13):2001–2021.
7. Ducy P, Zhang R, Geoffroy V, et al. Osf2/Cbfa1: a transcriptional activator of osteoblast differentiation. Cell. 1997;89:747–754.
8. Franceschi RT, Xiao G. Regulation of the osteoblast-specific transcription factor, Runx2: responsiveness to multiple signal transduction pathways. J Cell Biochem. 2003;88:446–454.
9. Liu W, Toyosawa S, Furuichi T, et al. Overexpression of Cbfa1 in osteoblasts inhibits osteoblast maturation and causes osteopenia with multiple fractures. J Cell Biol. 2001;155:157–166.
10. Geoffroy V, Kneissel M, Fournier B, et al. High bone resorption in adult aging transgenic mice overexpressing cbfa1/runx2 in cells of the osteoblastic lineage. Mol Cell Biol. 2002; 22:6222–6233.
11. Shui C, Spelsberg TC, Riggs BL, Khosla S. Changes in Runx2/Cbfa1 expression and activity during osteoblastic differentiation of human bone marrow stromal cells. J Bone Miner Res. 2003;18:213–221.
12. Gronthos S, Zannettino AC, Hay SJ, Shi S, Graves SE, Kortesidis A, Simmons PJ. Molecular and cellular characterisation of highly purified stromal stem cells derived from human bone marrow. J Cell Sci. 2003;116:1827–1835.
13. Xiao G, Jiang D, Thomas P, et al. MAPK pathways activate and phosphorylate the osteoblast-specific transcription factor, Cbfa1. J Biol Chem. 2000;275:4453–4459.
14. Westendorf JJ, Kahler RA, Schroeder TM. Wnt signaling in osteoblasts and bone diseases. Gene. 2004;341:19–39.
15. Krishnan V, Bryant HU, Macdougald OA. Regulation of bone mass by Wnt signaling. J Clin Invest. 2006;116:1202–1209.
16. Gordon MD, Nusse R. Wnt signaling: multiple pathways, multiple receptors, and multiple transcription factors. J Biol Chem. 2006;281:22429–22433.
17. Bennett CN, Longo KA, Wright WS, Suva LJ, Lane TF, Hankenson KD, MacDougald OA. Regulation of osteoblastogenesis and bone mass by Wnt10b. Proc Natl Acad Sci USA. 2005;102:3324–3329.
18. Rawadi G, Vayssiere B, Dunn F, et al. BMP-2 controls alkaline phosphatase expression and osteoblast mineralization by a Wnt autocrine loop. J Bone Miner Res. 2003;18:1842–1853.
19. Niida A, Hiroko T, Kasai M, et al. DKK1, a negative regulator of Wnt signaling, is a target of the beta-catenin/TCF pathway. Oncogene. 2004;23:8520–8526.
20. Galli LM, Barnes T, Cheng T, et al. Differential inhibition of Wnt-3a by Sfrp-1, Sfrp-2, and Sfrp-3. Dev Dyn. 2006;235:681–690.
21. Li J, Sarosi I, Cattley RC, et al. Dkk1-mediated inhibition of Wnt signaling in bone results in osteopenia. Bone. 2006;39:754–766.
22. Boyden LM, Mao J, Belsky J, et al. High bone density due to a mutation in LDL-receptor-related protein 5. N Engl J Med. 2002;346:1513–1521.
23. Gong Y, Slee RB, Fukai N, et al. LDL receptor-related protein 5 (LRP5) affects bone accrual and eye development. Cell. 2001;107:513–523.
24. Ai M, Holmen SL, Van Hul W, et al. Reduced affinity to and inhibition by DKK1 form a common mechanism by which high bone mass-associated missense mutations in LRP5 affect canonical Wnt signaling. Mol Cell Biol. 2005;25:4946–4955.
25. de Boer J, Siddappa R, Gaspar C, et al. Wnt signaling inhibits osteogenic differentiation of human mesenchymal stem cells. Bone. 2004;34:818–826.
26. Boland GM, Perkins G, Hall DJ, et al. Wnt 3a promotes proliferation and suppresses osteogenic differentiation of adult human mesenchymal stem cells. J Cell Biochem. 2004;93:1210–1230.
27. Baksh D, Boland GM, Tuan RS. Cross-talk between Wnt signaling pathways in human mesenchymal stem cells leads to functional antagonism during osteogenic differentiation. J Cell Biochem. 2007;101:1109–1124.
28. Baksh D, Tuan RS. Canonical and non-canonical wnts differentially affect the development potential of primary isolate of human bone marrow mesenchymal stem cells. J Cell Physiol. 2007;212:817–826.

29. Li X, Liu P, Liu W, et al. Dkk2 has a role in terminal osteoblast differentiation and mineralized matrix formation. Nat Genet. 2005;37:945–952.
30. van der Horst G, van der Werf SM, Farih-Sips H, et al. Downregulation of Wnt signaling by increased expression of Dickkopf-1 and -2 is a prerequisite for late-stage osteoblast differentiation of KS483 cells. J Bone Miner Res. 2005;20:1867–1877.
31. Vaes BL, Dechering KJ, van Someren EP, et al. Microarray analysis reveals expression regulation of Wnt antagonists in differentiating osteoblasts. Bone. 2005;36:803–811.
32. Chang J, Sonoyama W, Wang Z, et al. Noncanonical Wnt-4 signaling enhances bone regeneration of mesenchymal stem cells in craniofacial defects through activation of p38 MAPK. J Biol Chem. 2007;282:30938–30948.
33. Liu Y, Rubin B, Bodine PV, et al. Wnt5a induces homodimerization and activation of Ror2 receptor tyrosine kinase. J Cell Biochem. 2008;105:497–502.
34. Liu Y, Ross JF, Bodine PV, et al. Homodimerization of Ror2 tyrosine kinase receptor induces 14-3-3(beta) phosphorylation and promotes osteoblast differentiation and bone formation. Mol Endocrinol. 2007;21:3050–3061.
35. Liu Y, Bhat RA, Seestaller-Wehr LM, et al. The orphan receptor tyrosine kinase Ror2 promotes osteoblast differentiation and enhances ex vivo bone formation. Mol Endocrinol. 2007;21:376–387.
36. Billiard J, Way DS, Seestaller-Wehr LM, et al. The orphan receptor tyrosine kinase Ror2 modulates canonical Wnt signaling in osteoblastic cells. Mol Endocrinol. 2005;19:90–101.
37. Giuliani N, Colla S, Morandi F, et al. myeloma cells block RUNX2/CBFA1 activity in human bone marrow osteoblast progenitors and inhibit osteoblast formation and differentiation. Blood. 2005;106:2472–2483.
38. Corre J, Mahtouk K, Attal M, et al. Bone marrow mesenchymal stem cells are abnormal in multiple myeloma. Leukemia. 2007;21(5):1079–1088.
39. Garderet L, Mazurier C, Chapel A, et al. Mesenchymal stem cell abnormalities in patients with multiple myeloma. Leuk Lymphoma. 2007;48:2032–2041.
40. Arnulf B, Lecourt S, Soulier J, et al. Phenotypic and functional characterization of bone marrow mesenchymal stem cells derived from patients with multiple myeloma. Leukemia. 2007;21:158–163.
41. Mori Y, Shimizu N, Dallas M, et al. Anti-alpha4 integrin antibody suppresses the development of multiple myeloma and associated osteoclastic osteolysis. Blood. 2004;104:2149–2154.
42. Ely SA, Knowles DM. Expression of CD56/neural cell adhesion molecule correlates with the presence of lytic bone lesions in multiple myeloma and distinguishes myeloma from monoclonal gamyelomaopathy of undetermined significance and lymphomas with plasmacytoid differentiation. Am J Pathol. 2002;160:1293–1299.
43. Weitzmann MN, Roggia C, Toraldo G, et al. Increased production of IL-7 uncouples bone formation from bone resorption during estrogen deficiency. J Clin Invest. 2002;110:1643–1650.
44. Giuliani N, Colla S, Sala R, et al. Human myeloma cells stimulate the receptor activator of nuclear factor-kappa B ligand (RANKL) in T lymphocytes: a potential role in multiple myeloma bone disease. Blood. 2002;100:4615–4621.
45. Standal T, Abildgaard N, Fagerli UM, et al. HGF inhibits BMP-induced osteoblastogenesis: possible implications for the bone disease of multiple myeloma. Blood. 2007;109:3024–3030.
46. Edwards CM, Zhuang J, Mundy GR. The pathogenesis of the bone disease of multiple myeloma. Bone. 2008;42:1007–1013.
47. Hong JH, Hwang ES, McManus MT, et al. TAZ, a transcriptional modulator of mesenchymal stem cell differentiation. Science. 2005;309:1074–1078.
48. Li B, Shi M, Li J, et al. Elevated tumor necrosis factor-alpha suppresses TAZ expression and impairs osteogenic potential of Flk-1+ mesenchymal stem cells in patients with multiple myeloma. Stem Cells Dev. 2007;16:921–930.
49. Krishnan V, Moore TL, Ma YL, et al. Parathyroid hormone bone anabolic action requires Cbfa1/Runx2-dependent signaling. Mol Endocrinol. 2003;17:423–435.
50. Jilka RL. Molecular and cellular mechanisms of the anabolic effect of intermittent PTH. Bone. 2007;40:1434–1446.

51. Zhao Z, Zhao M, Xiao G, et al. Gene transfer of the Runx2 transcription factor enhances osteogenic activity of bone marrow stromal cells in vitro and in vivo. Mol Ther. 2005;12: 247–253.
52. Ehrlich LA, Chung HY, Ghobrial I, et al. IL-3 is a potential inhibitor of osteoblast differentiation in multiple myeloma. Blood. 2005;106:1407–1414.
53. Lee JW, Chung HY, Ehrlich LA, et al. IL-3 expression by myeloma cells increases both osteoclast formation and growth of myeloma cells. Blood. 2004;103:2308–2315.
54. Giuliani N, Morandi F, Tagliaferri S, et al. Interleukin-3 (IL-3) is overexpressed by T lymphocytes in multiple myeloma patients. Blood. 2006;107:841–842.
55. Tian E, Zhan F, Walker R, et al. The role of the Wnt-signaling antagonist DKK1 in the development of osteolytic lesions in multiple myeloma. N Engl J Med. 2003;349:2483–2494.
56. Giuliani N, Morandi F, Tagliaferri S, et al. Production of wnt inhibitors by myeloma cells: potential effects on canonical wnt pathway in the bone microenvironment. Cancer Res. 2007;67:7665–7674.
57. Oshima T, Abe M, Asano J, et al. Myeloma cells suppress bone formation by secreting a soluble Wnt inhibitor, sFRP-2. Blood. 2005;106:3160–3165.
58. Giuliani N, Colla S, Storti P, et al. Activation of non-canonical wnt pathway in human mesenchymal cells affects osteogenic differentiation: a potential target in multiple myeloma microenvironment. Blood. 2008;112:2742a.
59. De Toni F, Racaud-Sultan C, Chicanne G, et al. A crosstalk between the Wnt and the adhesion-dependent signaling pathways governs the chemosensitivity of acute myeloid leukemia. Oncogene. 2006;25:3113–3122.
60. Gunn WG, Conley A, Deininger L, et al. A crosstalk between myeloma cells and marrow stromal cells stimulates production of DKK1 and interleukin-6: a potential role in the development of lytic bone disease and tumor progression in multiple myeloma. Stem Cells. 2006;24:986–991.
61. Qiang YW, Chen Y, Stephens O, et al. Myeloma-derived Dickkopf-1 disrupts Wnt-regulated osteoprotegerin and RANKL production by osteoblasts: a potential mechanism underlying osteolytic bone lesions in multiple myeloma. Blood. 2008;112:196–207.
62. Yaccoby S, Ling W, Zhan F, et al. Antibody-based inhibition of DKK1 suppresses tumor-induced bone resorption and multiple myeloma growth in- vivo. Blood. 2007;109:2106–2111.
63. Qiang YW, Shaughnessy JD Jr, Yaccoby S. Wnt3a signaling within bone inhibits multiple myeloma bone disease and tumor growth. Blood. 2008;112:374–382.
64. Edwards CM, Edwards JR, Lwin ST, et al. Increasing Wnt signaling in the bone marrow microenvironment inhibits the development of myeloma bone disease and reduces tumor burden in bone in vivo. Blood. 2008;111:2833–2842.
65. Evans CE, Ward C, Rathour L, Galasko CB. Myeloma affects both the growth and function of human osteoblast-like cells. Clin Exp Metast. 1992;10:33–38.
66. Silvestris F, Cafforio P, Calvani N, Dammacco F. Impaired osteoblastogenesis in myeloma bone disease: role of upregulated apoptosis by cytokines and malignant plasma cells. Br J Haematol. 2004;126:475–486.
67. Silvestris F, Cafforio P, Tucci M, Grinello D, Dammacco F. Upregulation of osteoblast apoptosis by malignant plasma cells: a role in myeloma bone disease. Br J Haematol. 2003;122:39–52.
68. Tinhofer I, Biedermann R, Krismer M, Crazzolara R, Greil R. A role of TRAIL in killing osteoblasts by myeloma cells. FASEB J. 2006;20:759–761.
69. Shipman CM, Croucher PI. Osteoprotegerin is a soluble decoy receptor for tumor necrosis factor-related apoptosis-inducing ligand/Apo2 ligand and can function as a paracrine survival factor for human myeloma cells. Cancer Res. 2003;63:912–916.
70. Yaccoby S, Wezeman MJ, Zangari M, et al. Inhibitory effects of osteoblasts and increased bone formation on myeloma in novel culture systems and a myeloma tous mouse model. Haematologica. 2006;91:192–199.

Index